Anti-Ageing
dietCOOKBOOK

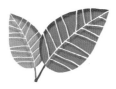

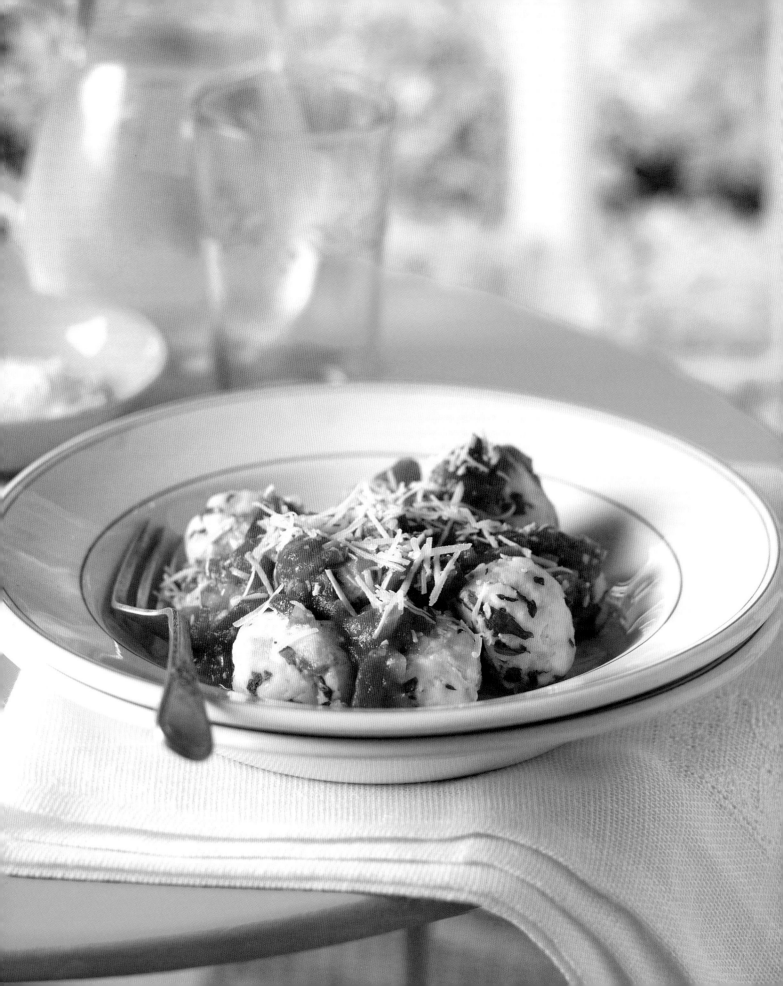

Anti-Ageing diet COOKBOOK

More than 130 recipes for energy and vitality

Reader's Digest

Contents

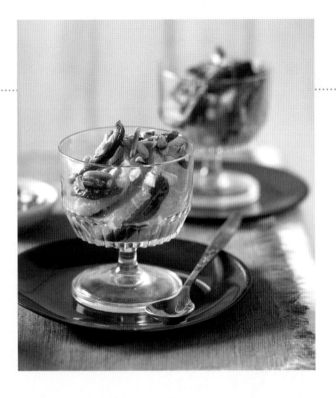

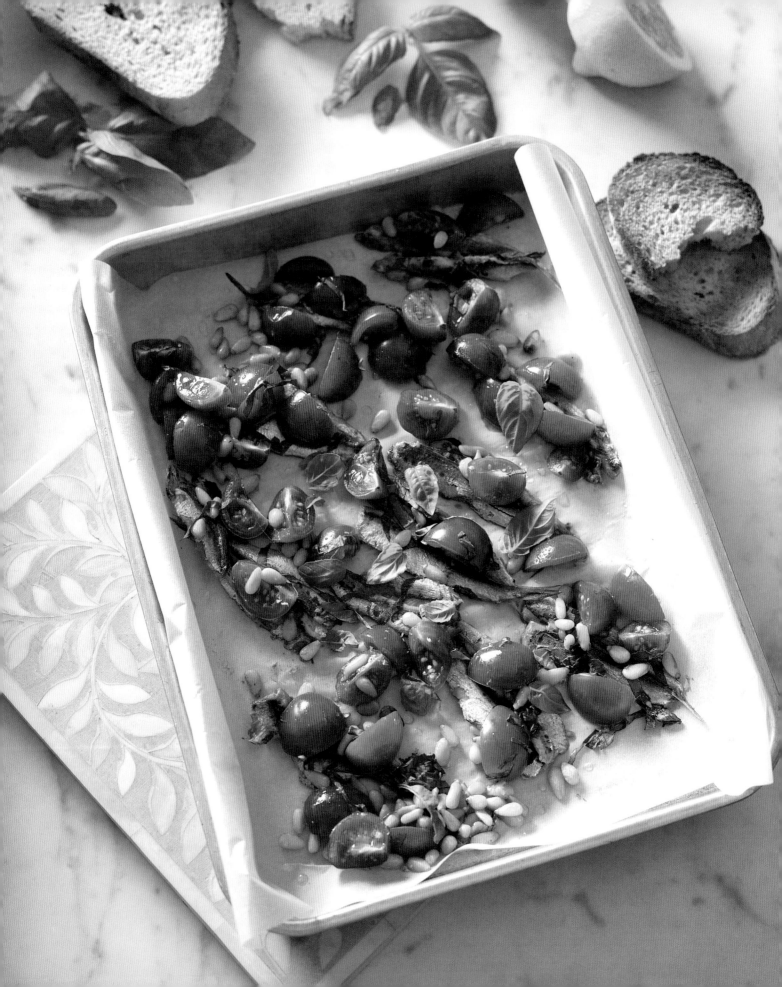

Foreword

For thousands of years, humans have sought easy ways to reverse the signs of ageing and regain youthful health and vitality. While sadly there is no magical fountain of youth, and no way to turn back the clock, there are ways to fight some common degenerative conditions and to slow the processes associated with ageing.

Your lifestyle, and particularly the foods that you eat, will help you take charge. A healthy, well-balanced diet can increase your energy levels, decrease the rate of cellular damage that can cause signs of ageing, and improve your health from within.

The recipes in this book provide you with plenty of fresh ideas on how to go about revitalising your diet and yourself. You won't have to hunt for hard-to-find ingredients, and you'll be able to explore lots of interesting new ways with trusted staples. Salt and saturated fats have been replaced with flavoursome herbs, spices and fresh seasonal produce. And even better, you won't need to spend too long in the kitchen on complicated cooking tasks. Many of the recipes are quick and easy to prepare.

Here you'll find great recipes that are rich in fruit and vegetables, high in fibre and protein, with generous amounts of key anti-ageing nutrients to keep you looking and feeling youthful for longer. Whichever dishes you choose, you are sure to give yourself an age-defying boost of vitality. I hope you enjoy using this cookbook.

Suzie Ferrie
Advanced Accredited Practising Dietitian

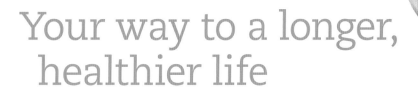

Your way to a longer, healthier life

Minute by minute, *whether we like it or not, we are all getting older. This doesn't automatically mean the quality of our lives dimishes or that we lose enjoyment in it. Far from it, for in many ways, age really is a state of mind. You can choose to look and feel youthful for longer. Here, we show you how!*

WHAT IS AGEING?

Ageing, or 'senescence', is a gradual process that starts after the fertile age 20s to 30s, and continues for the rest of the life span. But it doesn't seem to be the same for everyone. How is it that two people can be the same age, yet one seems much older than the other, both physically and mentally?

Your **chronological age** (the number of years you have lived) and your **physiological age** (how you function in your life) may be two very different numbers. Looking and feeling older can be a result of cellular damage (think wrinkles or declining eyesight and hearing); gradual reduction in muscle mass and bone density; or degenerative conditions such as heart disease, osteoporosis or arthritis.

Some of these changes are genetically influenced, but the good news is that nearly all of these conditions can be improved, or even prevented, with the right lifestyle strategies, especially your food choices.

Living longer, and living better, is possible.

> *If you eat well and make wise lifestyle choices, you can delay the signs of ageing and reduce your risk of developing some of the most common age-related conditions.*

What's food got to do with it?

Food provides the building blocks for your body's tissues, replacing old cells and protecting new cells against damage. Some of the **essential vitamins and minerals** are important in these processes, but these aren't the only substances that count when it comes to enhancing your life span: **anti-oxidants are substances that protect cells against damage,** preventing disease and directly combating the effects of ageing.

ANTI-OXIDANTS have been available in supplement form for many years, but increasingly research indicates that supplements may be ineffective (or even harmful in some cases), and it is far more beneficial to obtain them from food. This is because individual anti-oxidant substances seem to work better as a team, in the combinations that are found naturally in foods.

This means that you can greatly increase the benefits by consuming a wide range of different **anti-oxidant-rich foods** within a diet of **highly nutritious foods**. See pages 10–15.

Why variety really is 'the spice of life'

Apart from providing anti-oxidants, dietary variety is important in other ways. Every single food we eat offers a different profile of essential nutrients, and falling into a repetitive pattern of not eating a variety of foods could increase the chance that you are missing out on some important vitamin or mineral.

As we get older, we need to eat extra amounts of particular nutrients to maintain good health. To solve this problem without simply eating more, the nutrient density of your food needs to increase. **This book features recipes that are rich in the age-defying nutrients** that help to fight disease and increase vitality, so you can look – and feel – youthful for longer.

Follow a diet high in anti-oxidants. It has the potential to slow the appearance of ageing and reduce your risk of chronic diseases that shorten life.

Inflammation and ageing

In a healthy body, inflammation is a process of defending against injury or infection, and preparing for healing. This process should subside when healing is complete. But scientists now think that some people have an ongoing low-level inflammatory process that never switches off. This **chronic inflammation may be a key underlying promoter of ageing processes**, as well as some of the typical age-related conditions such as dementia, diabetes, arthritis, osteoporosis and loss of muscle mass. Inflammation may be worsened by lifestyle factors such as stress and lack of exercise, but some of our food choices can also help to tip the balance towards – or away from – inflammation.

For example, foods with a low glycaemic index (GI) are known to be useful for people with diabetes, as they release their energy slowly without affecting blood glucose levels too much. But low glycaemic index eating may also be an anti-inflammatory (and anti-ageing) strategy, as sudden spikes in blood glucose level may promote chronic inflammation.

THE FOODS TO AVOID

Reducing your intake of foods that have a pro-inflammatory effect may help to keep you younger and healthier. In simple terms, this means eating fewer highly processed foods, but also means cutting down on:

- salt and salty foods (including sauces and soup mixes)
- fried foods, especially deep-fried
- legume- or grain-fed farmed meat, poultry and fish
- food products that have been transported long distances or stored for long periods
- foods high in saturated or trans fats
- processed carbohydrates and sugars with a high glycaemic index
- sugary drinks including soft drinks and undiluted juices
- alcohol, in excess of recommended amounts.

Eating your way to longer life

Target anti-oxidants Always include foods high in anti-oxidants, to protect your cells against damage.

Choose low-GI foods Eat low glycaemic index carbohydrates, for sustained energy without upsetting blood glucose levels.

Cut down on salt and unhealthy fats Minimise your intake of salt and unhealthy fats, to protect your cardiovascular system and reduce inflammation.

Aim for balanced nutrition Make sure that you are meeting your vitamin and mineral needs, to optimise your physical and mental wellbeing.

Eat smaller meals Have smaller portions, more frequently, to give your body time to benefit from the nutrients.

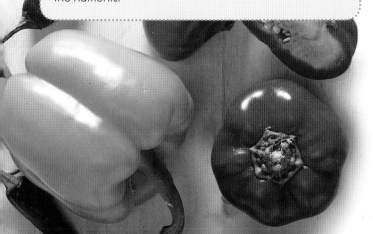

An A–Z of the best anti-ageing foods

*D**id you know** that the most powerful anti-ageing superfoods aren't rare and exotic ingredients, difficult to find and hard to cook? The fact is, mostly they are familiar foods that you can buy in your local greengrocer or supermarket. This is your alphabet of anti-ageing foods: together they spell out all you need for a balanced diet to maximise health and vitality.*

Avocado

Rich in **beneficial oils** and **anti-oxidants**, avocados contain good amounts of **vitamin C** (needed for your immune function as well as to keep your skin looking good), **folate** (essential for good brain function and normal blood) and **vitamin E** (also important for healthy skin).

Berries

One of the best-known sources of **anti-oxidants**, berries appear to be protective against some types of cancer. They also have good amounts of **fibre** (to promote healthy bowel function) and **vitamin C**. Some types, such as cranberry and blueberry, also contain a special substance that protects against urinary tract infections.

Cruciferous vegetables

This family of vegetables includes cabbage, kale, broccoli, cauliflower, bok choy and brussels sprouts. Providing plenty of **fibre**, as well as being rich in **vitamins** and **minerals**, they are also star performers when it comes to **anti-oxidant content**: more than 100 different research studies have shown a link between cruciferous vegetables and cancer prevention.

Dark chocolate

Chocolate tops most people's list of 'naughty' foods, but recent research points to potential health benefits from a small regular intake of cocoa and cocoa products such as dark chocolate. Thanks to its high **anti-oxidant content**, a cup of hot cocoa or a daily square of dark chocolate (check the label – cocoa solids content should be at least 65 per cent for greatest benefit) appears to be protective against cardiovascular disease.

Eggs

One of nature's convenience foods, eggs form the basis of so many quick, easy meals providing balanced, complete **protein** as well as most of the **vitamins** and **minerals** you need every day. They are also a source of **vitamin D**, which is important for healthy bones. Both the white and the yolk are nutritious but most of the vitamins and minerals are concentrated in the yolk. There is no reason to worry unduly about limiting your intake of eggs unless you already have a cholesterol problem.

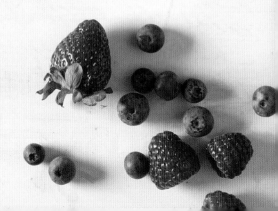

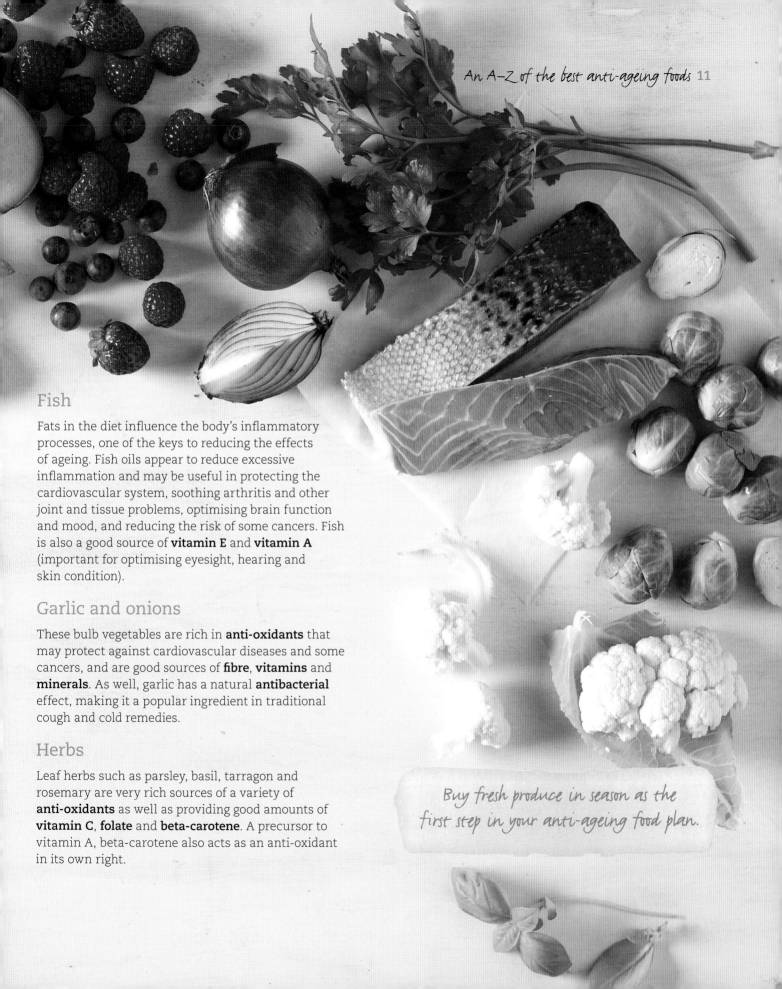

Fish

Fats in the diet influence the body's inflammatory processes, one of the keys to reducing the effects of ageing. Fish oils appear to reduce excessive inflammation and may be useful in protecting the cardiovascular system, soothing arthritis and other joint and tissue problems, optimising brain function and mood, and reducing the risk of some cancers. Fish is also a good source of **vitamin E** and **vitamin A** (important for optimising eyesight, hearing and skin condition).

Garlic and onions

These bulb vegetables are rich in **anti-oxidants** that may protect against cardiovascular diseases and some cancers, and are good sources of **fibre**, **vitamins** and **minerals**. As well, garlic has a natural **antibacterial** effect, making it a popular ingredient in traditional cough and cold remedies.

Herbs

Leaf herbs such as parsley, basil, tarragon and rosemary are very rich sources of a variety of **anti-oxidants** as well as providing good amounts of **vitamin C**, **folate** and **beta-carotene**. A precursor to vitamin A, beta-carotene also acts as an anti-oxidant in its own right.

Buy fresh produce in season as the first step in your anti-ageing food plan.

In-season fresh produce

Buying your fruit and vegetables when they are in season is recommended, not just because they are cheaper: nutritionally, fruit and vegetables contain more of those precious **anti-oxidants** when they are at their peak of ripeness and haven't been stored before sale. The flavour is better, too!

Jerusalem artichoke or 'sunchoke'

This knobbly root vegetable is one of the best known sources of **inulin**, a type of dietary fibre. Inulin directly promotes bowel health and protects against cancers by providing your gut bacteria with the fuel they need to make vitamins and short-chain fatty acids that keep gut cells healthy.

Kidney beans, lentils and other legumes

Dried peas, beans and lentils are a great vegetarian source of **protein** and **iron** (important for carrying oxygen in the blood to fuel the muscles and brain). Unlike meat they also provide good amounts of **fibre**. Legumes have a **low glycaemic index**, that is, they contain a slow-release type of carbohydrate that doesn't cause rapid spikes in blood glucose levels.

Lean, wild or free-range meats and poultry

Lean meat and liver are a **mineral-rich** source of balanced **protein**. Some recent research suggests that, when possible, it is a good idea to choose grass-fed, wild or free-range types when you are buying meat and poultry. Try wild meats such as venison or other game, and look for grass-fed meat. These varieties tend to be lower in fat, with more beneficial types of fat than grain-fed meat raised in more intensive conditions.

To maximise the anti-ageing benefits, aim for a wide variety of foods every day.

Milk

Recommendations to avoid dairy foods are widespread on the internet, but most of these claims are quite exaggerated or just plain wrong. This food group remains the best way for most people to obtain their **calcium** needs, as long as you stick mainly to low-fat milk and yogurt. For heart health and to optimise bone strength, keep your salt and fat intake low by limiting your intake of cheeses and creamy desserts.

Nuts and seeds

The beneficial oils in nuts and seeds have an **anti-inflammatory effect** that may reduce your risk of cardiovascular disease and some cancers, as well as promoting optimal brain function. Nuts also provide **protein**, **fibre** and **minerals**, and a variety of **anti-oxidant substances** including **selenium** (particularly in Brazil nuts) and **vitamin E**.

Olive oil

Olive oil is a central part of the Mediterranean diet which has been claimed to promote longevity and reduce the risk of cancer and cardiovascular disease. This may be due to the monounsaturated fats in the oil. Less-processed oils, such as extra virgin olive oil, are much higher in **anti-oxidants**.

Peppers, chillies and capsicums

Very rich in **vitamin C**, capsicums (bell peppers) and chillies are also an impressive source of a wide variety of **anti-oxidants**. Chilli also has an **antibacterial** and **anti-inflammatory** effect, leading to its traditional use in pain relief remedies for sore joints and muscles.

Quinoa

Unlike most grain foods, quinoa is a good source of complete **protein**, making it valuable in vegetarian diets. It also provides **fibre** as well as **minerals** such as **iron** and **magnesium**.

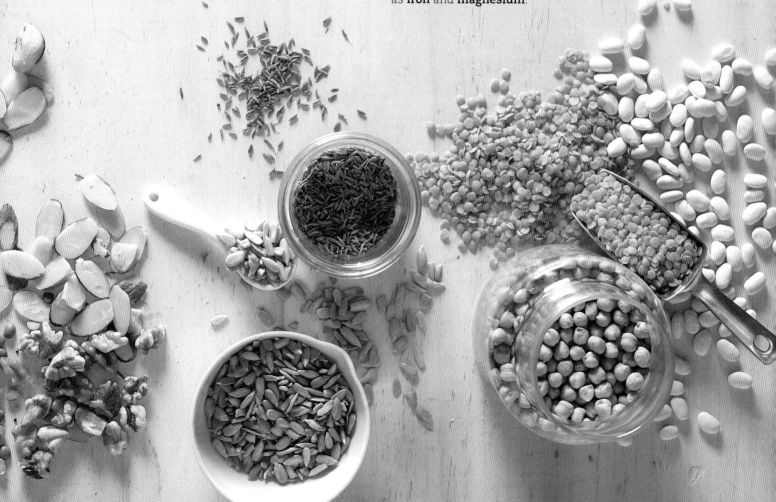

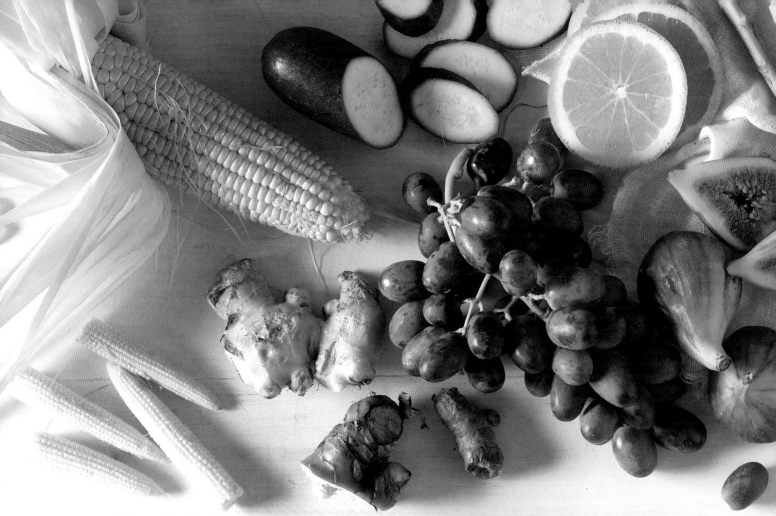

Root ginger and other rhizomes such as galangal and turmeric

Ginger and galangal have traditionally been used to **stimulate appetite** and **soothe the digestive system**, promoting normal gut movement and reducing nausea. Turmeric has potent **anti-inflammatory** benefits, potentially protecting against cardio-vascular disease and dementia.

Spices

Mineral-rich spices such as cumin, cardamom, nutmeg, cinnamon and pepper are very high in **anti-oxidants**. This may explain why spices have been valued for centuries as ingredients in medicinal remedies for indigestion, pain and inflammation.

Tea

There are good amounts of **anti-oxidants** in both black and green tea, although the types differ between the two. Both are associated with reduced risk of cardiovascular disease and some cancers.

Unprocessed foods

Packaged foods tend to contain much larger amounts of salt, harmful fats and refined carbohydrates, and fewer **vitamins** and **minerals**, when compared to unprocessed foods. There are indications that highly processed foods may promote chronic inflammation, accelerating ageing and increasing disease risk.

Vegetables and fruit in general

Apart from the specific ones mentioned here, a high intake of any types of vegetables and fruit is associated with reduced risk of many cancers, cardiovascular disease and dementia. It is highly recommended that you eat **two daily serves of fruit, and five per day of vegetables, for optimal health.**

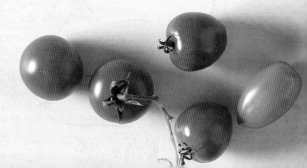

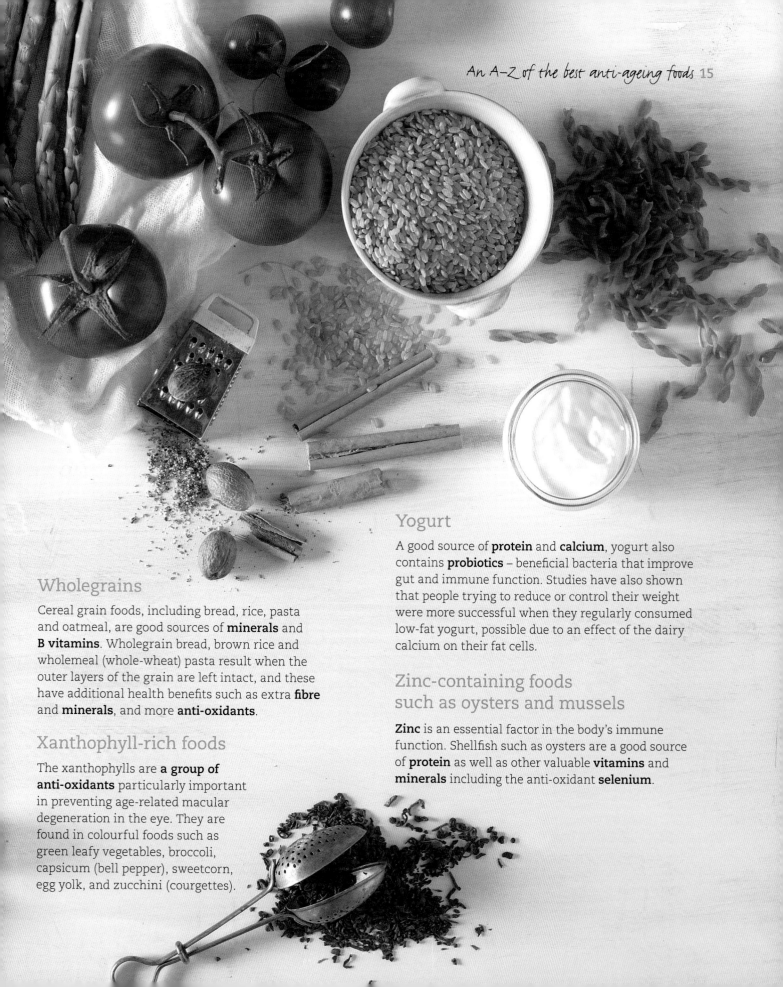

Wholegrains

Cereal grain foods, including bread, rice, pasta and oatmeal, are good sources of **minerals** and **B vitamins**. Wholegrain bread, brown rice and wholemeal (whole-wheat) pasta result when the outer layers of the grain are left intact, and these have additional health benefits such as extra **fibre** and **minerals**, and more **anti-oxidants**.

Xanthophyll-rich foods

The xanthophylls are **a group of anti-oxidants** particularly important in preventing age-related macular degeneration in the eye. They are found in colourful foods such as green leafy vegetables, broccoli, capsicum (bell pepper), sweetcorn, egg yolk, and zucchini (courgettes).

Yogurt

A good source of **protein** and **calcium**, yogurt also contains **probiotics** – beneficial bacteria that improve gut and immune function. Studies have also shown that people trying to reduce or control their weight were more successful when they regularly consumed low-fat yogurt, possible due to an effect of the dairy calcium on their fat cells.

Zinc-containing foods
such as oysters and mussels

Zinc is an essential factor in the body's immune function. Shellfish such as oysters are a good source of **protein** as well as other valuable **vitamins** and **minerals** including the anti-oxidant **selenium**.

Key anti-ageing nutrients

A varied, balanced diet will give you the right nutrition to keep you looking and feeling young for longer. Here are the most important nutrients and their role in your body's wellbeing.

Protein

The structure of your body, its muscles, organs and skin, is made up of protein, so it is important for growth and healing. **A slight increase in protein intake is recommended as you get older, to minimise muscle loss and to help control body weight.** The building blocks of protein, called amino acids, combine in the body to make 'complete' protein when they are eaten together. Some foods are already complete proteins; examples include meat, poultry, fish and seafood, egg, dairy foods, soybeans and quinoa.

Calcium

An adequate calcium intake reduces bone loss, minimising the risk of fractures. For this reason the recommended calcium intake increases with age. Calcium is also required for normal nerve and muscle function. Dairy foods are the main dietary source of calcium, but other good sources include nuts and seeds, green leafy vegetables, canned fish eaten with the bones, and some soy products.

Vitamin D

Most people will need some sun exposure each day in order to obtain vitamin D. **This sun-triggered vitamin is very important for bone strength and for the immune function**. Walking out in the open air with your sleeves rolled up for 30 minutes in winter, or 10 minutes in summer, is enough for most people to get adequate vitamin D. When it comes to sun exposure, little and often is best – once your body has achieved a healthy level of vitamin D, any additional is lost. 'More' does not mean 'better'. If in doubt, take a vitamin D supplement rather than increasing your risk of skin cancer from sun exposure.

Omega-3 oils

Also referred to as omega-3 fats or omega-3 fatty acids, **omega-3 oils are currently being investigated for their inflammation-reducing properties**, which could be used to soothe joint and muscle problems and control blood pressure, as well as reducing the chronic inflammation thought to contribute to premature ageing.

Iodine

Low levels of this important nutrient are common across all community groups. Found in seaweed and seafood, as well as fortified (iodised) salt, **iodine is essential for normal brain function, and is important for regulating the thyroid gland**. An underactive thyroid causes low energy levels and weight gain.

Vitamin B_6

Without vitamin B_6, insomnia and irritability are common. Wholegrains, nuts and fish are good sources of this **mood-enhancing vitamin**.

Folate

Folate deficiency causes weakness and loss of appetite, forgetfulness, insomnia and anaemia, so it is clear how important this vitamin is! Green leafy vegetables are the best source, but avocados, legumes, oranges and broccoli are also rich in folate.

Vitamin B_{12}

This vitamin, needed for healthy blood, is found only in animal foods – meat, poultry, fish and seafood, eggs and dairy foods. Contrary to claims, mushrooms and spirulina are not useable sources of vitamin B_{12}.

Isoflavones (phyto-oestrogens)

Mainly found in legumes (particularly soybean products) and linseeds (flax seeds), **isoflavones are oestrogen-like substances** that are claimed to soothe hot flushes and other menopause complaints.

Vitamin K

Vitamin K is essential for normal blood coagulation and healthy bones. Green leafy vegetables are the richest source.

Anti-oxidants

An enormous number of different anti-oxidant substances have been discovered, each with different benefits. A selection is listed below.

VITAMIN C Vitamin C (ascorbic acid) **participates in detoxification processes and immune function, and helps the body to absorb iron and vitamin E.** When you're stressed, requirements increase and without adequate vitamin C skin and gum condition deteriorates, mood becomes depressed and joints become painful. The best sources of vitamin C are fruit and vegetables.

VITAMIN E **Essential for healthy skin and cells**, vitamin E is in many beauty creams. Its most powerful effect, however, is inside your body – when consumed in your food. Nuts and seeds (and their oils), avocado and green leafy vegetables are all good sources.

VITAMIN A **Beta-carotene is the plant-food precursor of vitamin A (essential for healthy skin, good eyesight and hearing).** It also acts as an anti-oxidant along with other members of the carotenoid family. Carotenoids are found in green vegetables and in orange-coloured foods such as carrots, orange sweet potatoes, mangoes and apricots.

SELENIUM Brazil nuts are particularly high in this **important component of your body's anti-oxidant defence system.** Other good sources are fish and shellfish, offal, wholegrains and seeds.

ZINC **Important in tissue healing, zinc also helps your anti-oxidant system to work.** Shellfish such as oysters and mussels are the best sources, but lean red meat and liver, seeds and legumes are also rich in zinc.

Phytochemicals

While they are not technically nutrients, phytochemicals (beneficial plant substances) still appear to be very important for health, and many are powerful anti-oxidants claimed to have anti-ageing properties. Here are some of the key phytochemical anti-oxidants.

Lycopene Lycopene has been associated with reduced risk of some cancers, particularly prostate cancer. Good sources include tomato products, watermelon, pink or red grapefruit, and red capsicum (bell pepper).

Xanthophylls Lutein and zeaxanthin are xanthophylls, anti-oxidants that appear to reduce the risk of cataracts and age-related macular degeneration. They are found in colourful foods such as green leafy vegetables, corn, citrus fruit and egg yolk.

Catechins Dark chocolate, tea, legumes and berries are rich in catechins, which may help to reduce the risk of heart disease and some cancers.

Resveratrol Resveratrol, found in red grapes and wine, has been shown to extend life span in some animal studies, and to delay the onset of age-related disease and infirmity in others.

Quercetin A variety of plant foods contain quercetin, including apples, onions, broccoli and berries. It has been associated with reduced risk of heart disease and conditions such as asthma, lung cancer and hay fever.

Proanthocyanidins Colourful reddish or purplish foods such as berries, cocoa and red wine are rich in proanthocyanidins, which have been claimed to reduce the risk of some cancers and cardiovascular disease.

CoEnzyme Q10

Also known as ubiquinone, **this enzyme is an essential part of every cell's energy system.** Levels appear to decline with age, and it has been suggested that supplementation could prolong life and reduce chronic disease risk. Until better evidence emerges, it is better to ensure a good intake of CoQ10 by regularly consuming its richest sources: meat, fish and poultry, offal, olive oil, soybeans and seed oils.

Eating for lifelong good health

Every aspect of your wellbeing responds to what you eat. Recent scientific research has given us a nutritional prescription to keep each system of your body working at its best.

Fitness

For sustained energy levels and a healthy cardio-vascular system, a diet rich in **fruit**, **vegetables** and **whole grains** is very important. Carbohydrate foods with a **low glycaemic index (GI)** give long-lasting energy and **anti-oxidants** help to protect the system from damage. Good fats for the heart include **mono-unsaturated fats** and **omega-3 oils**. Saturated and trans fats cause cholesterol levels to increase, promoting blockages, so should be avoided, as should processed carbohydrates including sugary foods, and salty foods, which increase blood pressure.

When asked his secret for an active old age, Clint Eastwood said: 'Enjoy getting older. That's the most important factor.'

Strong muscles, bones and joints, and healthy skin

Adequate amounts of **complete protein** every day are important for maintaining muscle mass as you get older. Spreading protein intake over the day may help the body to use it more effectively. Bones and joints benefit from adequate **calcium**, and it is important to maximise absorption by avoiding salty foods (salt increases calcium losses). Inflammatory conditions such as arthritis may be soothed by **omega-3 oils**, **spices** and **anti-oxidants**. Healthy skin needs plenty of **fluid**, **vitamin C** and **zinc**, as well as **vitamin E** and beneficial fats such as omega-3 oils.

Immune function

Nutrients that are important for your immune system include **vitamin C** and **zinc**, **selenium**, **folate**, **omega-3 oils** and **vitamin E**. It is important to drink adequate **fluid** to keep all these processes working normally. **Garlic**, **tea**, **cruciferous vegetables** and **spices** contain many beneficial immune-supporting substances, as do fruit and vegetables in general.

A healthy gut

Fibre and **fluid** are the essential diet components that keep the gut working normally. The fibre soaks up the fluid to make the stool bulky, stimulating the gut muscles so that everything moves along comfortably. Increasing fibre intake (along with fluid) can be helpful in relieving constipation, as well as encouraging beneficial bacteria, which protect against infection and make vitamins and fuels for gut cells.

Optimal brain and eye function

The eye and the brain both rely on **anti-oxidants** and beneficial fats such as **omega-3 oils** to stay healthy, and both can be damaged by excessive alcohol intake, salty foods and weight gain. Mood can be profoundly affected by what we eat, and a high intake of processed and fatty foods has been shown to promote depression and reduce memory skills. **Tryptophan**, an amino acid found in meat, fish, turkey, dairy foods and bananas, appears to help improve mood and promote restful sleep. Additionally, small, regular amounts of alcohol (taken with meals) appear to be protective against dementia and cognitive impairment.

Women's health

Menstrual problems and menopausal symptoms both seem to respond to a high intake of **isoflavones** (see page 17), which imitate oestrogen and may reduce some of the effects of hormonal changes. Other nutrients that may be important here include **vitamin E**, **vitamin B₆**, **magnesium** and **iron**. **Low-fat dairy foods**, too, may help, perhaps because inadequate **calcium** levels are associated with hormone swings. Avoid salt and salty foods, as they promote fluid retention which can add to symptoms. Caffeine, alcohol and sugary foods may also exacerbate hormonal problems.

Men's health

Zinc is thought to be important in the normal functioning of the prostate. An increased zinc intake appears to help reduce an enlarged prostate, and is recommended along with anti-inflammatory **omega-3 oils** and foods rich in **anti-oxidants** such as cruciferous vegetables and green tea. **Selenium** has been shown to be beneficial in studies of prostate cancer risk, and **lycopene**, found in tomato products, appears to slow its growth. Fatty meat, full-fat dairy foods, excess calcium intake (more than six serves of dairy foods per day) and refined carbohydrates have all been implicated in increasing prostate problems.

Anti-ageing lifestyle changes

Eating well is just one part of healthy living. While many factors will determine your life span, research has identified some other key lifestyle behaviours that can significantly improve your physiological age.

Maintain a healthy weight Carrying too much weight puts a strain on your joints and heart, but being too thin increases the risk of fractures as well as some cancers, so aim for a healthy weight.

Ensure a low alcohol intake Although regularly consuming small amounts of alcohol seems to reduce the risk of heart disease and dementia, any amount of alcohol can increase inflammation and damage the liver. So if you enjoy a drink now and then, remember to have it with a meal and stick to just one or two drinks.

Quit smoking Quitting smoking is difficult, but worth it: someone quitting at age 60 will immediately gain years in life expectancy, because tobacco smoking is the single largest preventable cause of premature death and disease. It is also a promoter of chronic inflammation and physical signs of ageing such as skin wrinkles.

Increase activity level and flexibility Many of the age-related bodily changes result more from disuse than from simple ageing: that is, 'use it or lose it'! Staying active is important if you want to control your weight and maintain your muscle strength, flexibility and bone density. Exercise is also good for the brain.

Improve your sleep There is a good reason why we talk about 'beauty sleep' – sleep is the time when all the cells in your body repair and recover, while your muscles relax. Get plenty of exercise and fresh air earlier in the day, and avoid late-night stress, smoking, heavy meals, caffeine and alcohol, which can all interfere with sleep.

Ensure adequate hydration The thirst response decreases with ageing, so older people are at higher risk of dehydration, particularly when taking medications that increase fluid requirements, or in hot weather. Drink water regularly.

Decrease stress Stress hormones promote weight gain and suppress the immune system, making you vulnerable to infections and accelerating the ageing process. Exercise can help the body to deal with stress; learning to relax is also helpful. Try meditating, yoga, visualisation exercises, deep breathing or relaxation techniques.

Look after your skin Mature skin can become dry very quickly and can benefit from a hydrating moisturiser (make sure it contains sunscreen). Sun damage is the most powerful factor in skin ageing, so keeping out of the sun in the middle of the day is very important for youthful skin.

Take care with food safety The protection of our immune system is reduced as we get older, so it is important to wash hands well before handling food; minimise time that cooked foods are at room temperature; and throw out old food.

Keep your mind active Mental health is as important to wellbeing as physical health: the mind and body are closely linked, so it is essential to look after both. A busy, socially connected life with plenty of close relationships and active interests is important in keeping you young. 'Use it or lose it!'

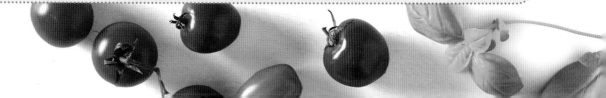

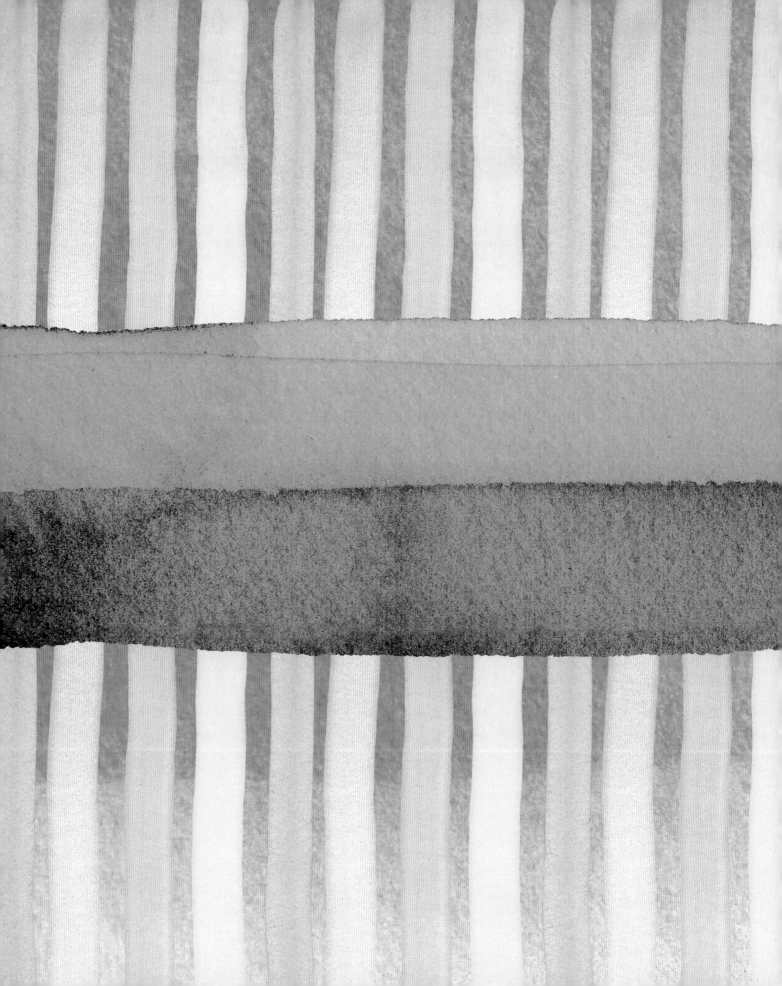

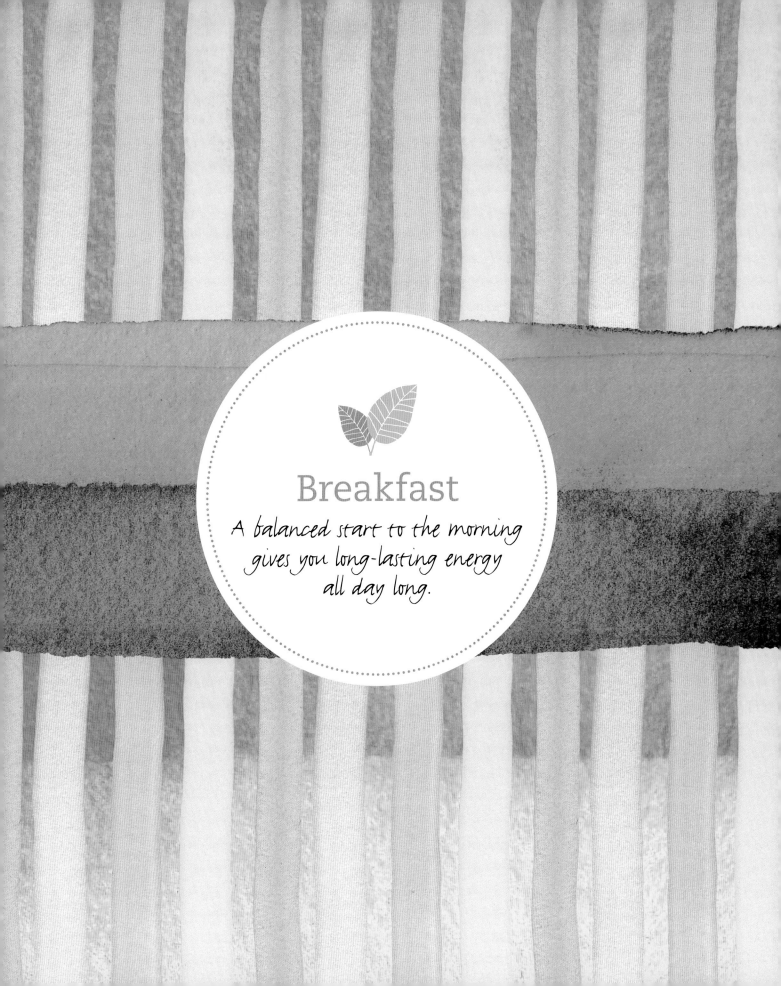

Breakfast

A balanced start to the morning
gives you long-lasting energy
all day long.

Bread and toast

Breakfast is famously the most important meal of the day. What you have will depend on the season, your time frame, your taste and budget. Try incorporating a decent serve of complex carbohydrates, some fresh fruit and protein, which will fuel you through the morning and well into your day. When time is short, you may just want to throw together something 'on toast'.

The simple recipes below should tick all the boxes.

Bread

The base for your breakfast is all-important, and there is an enormous variety of breads to choose from. To maximise nutritional value, choose a **wholemeal** (whole-wheat) or **wholegrain** bread, which will contain many more nutrients than bread made from highly refined flour. There are many 'mixed grain' types available, and **rye** or **pumpernickel** breads are nutritious and taste great. If you can get **sourdough** made using traditional sourdough methods, you will enjoy many favourable digestive benefits. A good-quality **fruit bread** is particularly delicious with the sweet options.

Freezing bread

Bread freezes beautifully, and if you are going to use it for toast you can cook it straight from frozen. If your bread comes pre-sliced in a plastic bag, simply freeze in its original bag. Remember to seal it well (you may want to replace a flimsy clasp with a more sturdy one), and expel excess air each time you open the package. If you buy unsliced bread, you can slice it up yourself, then transfer to a large ziplock bag and expel excess air before sealing.

....

COOK'S TIP These tasty ideas don't have to be strictly for breakfast. They make a great quick lunch or easy supper.

Toppings

Choose the best quality ingredients possible. Look for natural products without large amounts of – or any – added sugar, salt or unnecessary fats. Use fresh produce when it is in season for optimum nutritional value, and buy low-fat or reduced-fat dairy products whenever possible

Divide the quantities given here evenly between 2 average-sized slices of toast to give 1 serve.

- Spread 2 tablespoons natural **peanut butter** over toast slices. Mash or slice 1 large, ripe **banana** and spoon over peanut butter.

- Spread 1 tablespoon **tahini** (sesame paste) over toast slices. Top with ¼ cup (60 g) reduced-fat **ricotta**, and sprinkle with 2 teaspoons **pepitas** (pumpkin seeds) and 2 teaspoons **sunflower seeds**. Drizzle with 2 teaspoons **honey**.

- Slice 6 **strawberries** and put in a small bowl. Drizzle with ½ teaspoon **balsamic vinegar** and sprinkle with a very light grinding of freshly ground **black pepper**. Leave to stand 5 minutes, stirring occasionally. Pile ⅓ cup (60 g) low-fat **cottage cheese** on toast, and top with strawberries. For a quick and easy alternative, you could drizzle the strawberries with 2 teaspoons **orange juice** and 1 teaspoon **honey** and leave to stand for 5 minutes.

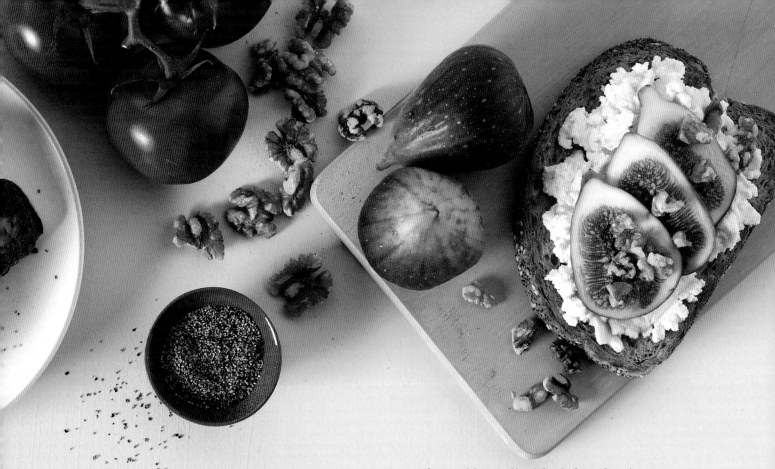

- Mash ½ small ripe **avocado** with 2 teaspoons **lemon juice** and spread over toast. Slice 1 **tomato** and lay slices over avocado. Season with freshly ground **black pepper**.

- Spread toast with ¼ cup (60 g) reduced-fat **ricotta** and top with 1 tablespoon chopped **semi-dried tomatoes** (sun-blushed). Sprinkle with 1 tablespoon finely grated **parmesan** and cook under grill (broiler) preheated to high 1 minute, until lightly golden. Top with 5 finely shredded fresh **basil** leaves if in season.

- Combine ⅓ cup (80 g) reduced-fat **ricotta** with 1 teaspoon **honey**, 1 good pinch ground **cinnamon** and 1 good pinch ground **nutmeg**. Spread on toast and top with ⅓ cup (50 g) fresh or thawed frozen **raspberries** or **blueberries**, or a combination of both. Use a fork to crush berries slightly.

- Combine ⅓ cup (80 g) low-fat **cottage cheese** with the chopped flesh of 1 **orange** or mandarin (discard skin and seeds) and ½ teaspoon **poppyseeds**. Spread the mixture over toast and drizzle with 1 teaspoon **honey**.

- Spread toast with ¼ cup (60 g) reduced-fat **ricotta** and top with 1–2 sliced fresh **figs** when in season. Sprinkle with 1 tablespoon chopped **walnuts**. Drizzle with honey if desired. You can use dried figs, dried apricots or dates, or a combination, if preferred.

- Chop a **hard-boiled egg** (hard-cooked) and mix with 1 teaspoon snipped **chives**. Spread 2 tablespoons low-fat **cottage cheese** on toast and top with egg mixture. Season with freshly ground **black pepper**. If you want this to be more substantial, use 2 eggs. You can cook the egg the night before and keep in the refrigerator, if you prefer.

- Warm 220 g (8 oz) can **baked beans** in a small saucepan. Finely shred ½ cup (25 g) **baby spinach leaves**, add to pan and stir over low heat until spinach wilts. Serve on toast, sprinkled with 2 tablespoons grated low-fat **cheddar**.

- Arrange 1 sliced **tomato** over toast and top with 40 g (1½ oz) chopped lean **ham**. Drain 125 g (4 oz) can **corn kernels** and sprinkle over. Cover with 2 tablespoons grated low-fat **cheddar** and cook under grill (broiler) preheated to high 1 minute, until cheese has melted.

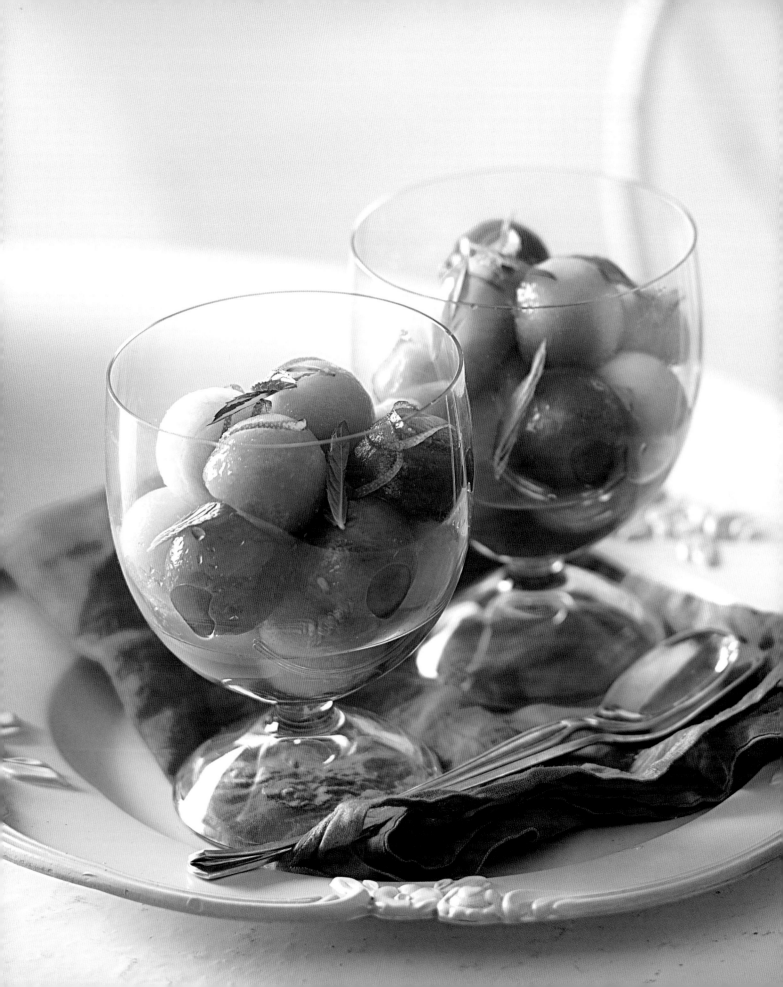

Melon medley

¼ cup (60 ml) water
½ cup (110 g) sugar
2.5 cm (1 inch) piece fresh ginger,
   finely sliced lengthwise
1 lime
1 kg (2 lb) assorted melons, such as
   ¼ rockmelon (cantaloupe), ¼ honeydew
   melon and ¼ small seedless watermelon
low-fat natural (plain) yogurt, to serve
fresh mint leaves, to garnish (optional)

PREPARATION 10 minutes, plus 30 minutes cooling
COOKING 10 minutes SERVES 4

EACH SERVING PROVIDES 837 kJ, 200 kcal, 2 g protein,
1 g fat (<1 g saturated fat), 48 g carbohydrate
(46 g sugars), 3 g fibre, 46 mg sodium

> This recipe features the high anti-oxidant combination of melon and lime, with the stimulating properties of fresh ginger. Ginger has antibacterial and anti-inflammatory properties, as well as settling stomach upsets with its gentle soothing action.

1 Mix water and sugar together in a large heavy-based saucepan. Warm gently over low heat, stirring continuously, until sugar is dissolved.

2 Add ginger slices. Use a zester to remove zest from lime, then add to syrup. (Alternatively, use a sharp knife to remove the surface part of the lime peel, avoiding the bitter white pith, then slice finely before adding to syrup.) Simmer 10 minutes to infuse syrup with fragrance of ginger and lime. Pour syrup into a large bowl and refrigerate 30 minutes, until cool. Remove ginger and discard.

3 Remove seeds from rockmelon and honeydew melon, if using. With a small spoon or melon-baller, scoop balls of flesh from melons. Alternatively, peel melons and cut flesh into bite-sized pieces.

4 Add melon pieces to cooled syrup. Juice lime and sprinkle over melon. Stir gently to combine.

5 Serve with yogurt and a scattering of mint leaves, if desired.

COOK'S TIP Halve the quantities if preparing for two.

To keep the melons after cutting, cover with plastic wrap or place in an airtight container and refrigerate. Avoid eating cut melon that has been left out of the refrigerator for 2 hours or more.

Cinnamon and banana yogurt whip

4 dried apricot halves

4 dried peach halves

4 dried pear halves

¼ cup (30 g) sultanas (small golden raisins)

4 cm (1½ inch) cinnamon stick or
    2 teaspoons ground cinnamon

2 tablespoons wheat germ

2 large bananas (about 300–350 g/10–12 oz
    in total before peeling)

2 tablespoons honey, or to taste

200 g (7 oz) low-fat natural (plain) yogurt
    (about ¾ cup)

1 teaspoon powdered gelatin

PREPARATION 10 minutes, plus overnight soaking
SERVES 4

EACH SERVING PROVIDES 982 kJ, 235 kcal, 7 g protein,
<1 g fat (<1 g saturated fat), 52 g carbohydrate
(45 g sugars), 6 g fibre, 48 mg sodium

1 Place dried apricots, peaches, pears and sultanas in a small bowl and pour over cold water to cover. Cover and leave to soak in refrigerator overnight.

2 Meanwhile, put cinnamon and wheat germ in a food processor or blender and process until ground. Add bananas and honey and blend until smooth. Stir yogurt through banana mixture to combine well.

3 Pour 3½ tablespoons (50 ml) water into a large heatproof bowl and sprinkle gelatin over. Warm gelatin in a microwave, or over a saucepan of boiling water, until it dissolves completely. Slowly pour banana yogurt mixture over gelatin, stirring rapidly.

4 Divide yogurt mixture between four glasses or small bowls. Put in refrigerator to set overnight.

5 To serve, remove dried fruits from soaking liquid and divide between four yogurt whips.

COOK'S TIP The gelatin in the yogurt whips sets overnight, at the same time that the dried fruits are soaking. For a quicker version that you can serve immediately after making, omit the gelatin and dried fruits and serve the yogurt whips topped with slices of fresh fruit.

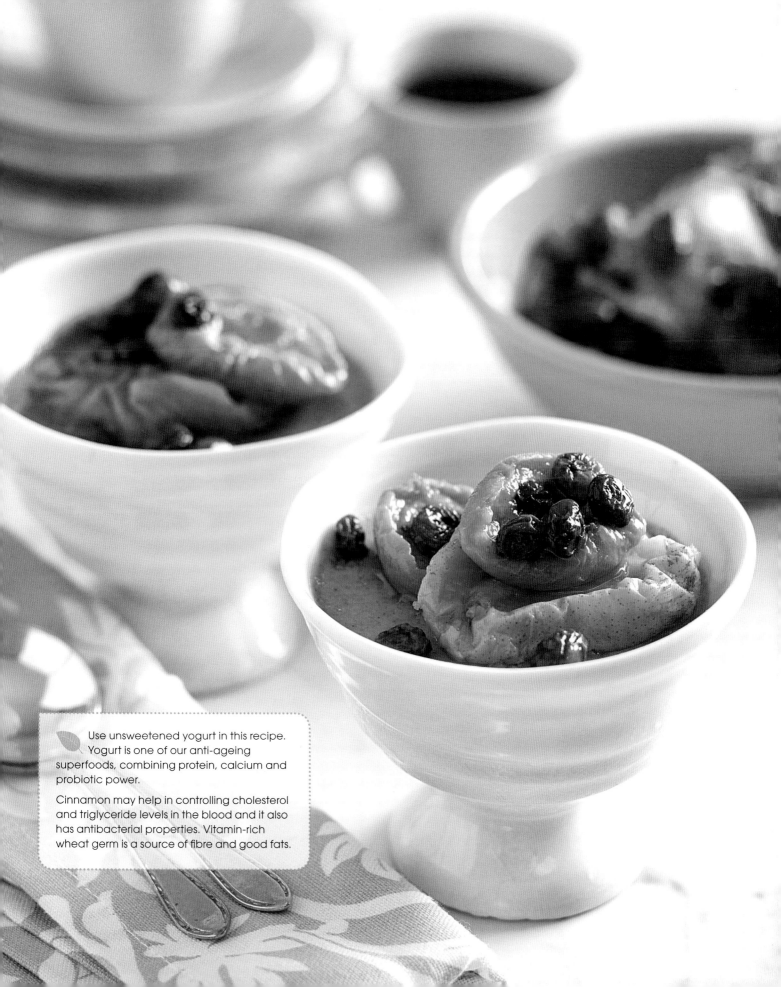

Use unsweetened yogurt in this recipe. Yogurt is one of our anti-ageing superfoods, combining protein, calcium and probiotic power.

Cinnamon may help in controlling cholesterol and triglyceride levels in the blood and it also has antibacterial properties. Vitamin-rich wheat germ is a source of fibre and good fats.

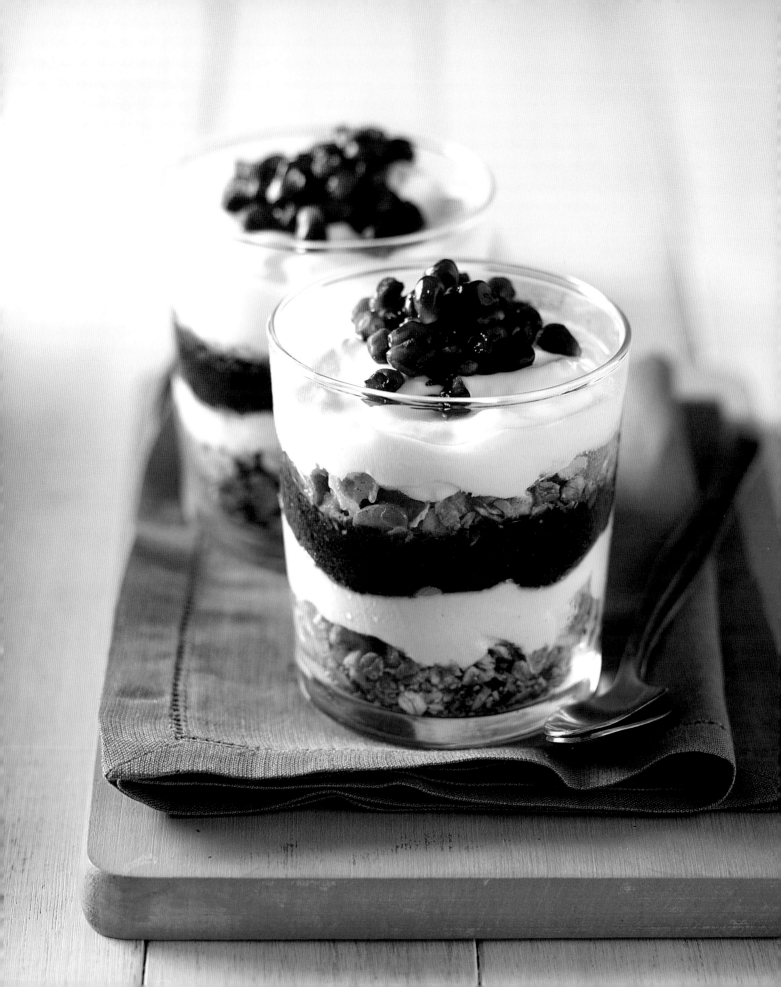

Yogurt berry parfait

250 g (8 oz) fresh or frozen mixed berries,
   such as strawberries, raspberries and
   blackberries
1 tablespoon lemon juice
2 tablespoons caster (superfine) sugar
1 cup (125 g) toasted muesli
½ cup (50 g) walnut halves, roughly
   chopped
1 pomegranate (optional)
2⅓ cups (600 g) low-fat Greek-style yogurt

PREPARATION 10 minutes SERVES 4

EACH SERVING PROVIDES 1840 kJ, 439 kcal, 17 g protein,
16 g fat (5 g saturated fat), 54 g carbohydrate
(32 g sugars), 6 g fibre, 356 mg sodium

> Berries are among the best food
> sources of anti-oxidants. This breakfast
> is a great source of fibre too, thanks to the
> berries and nutrient-rich whole grains.
>
> Pomegranate has recently been discovered
> to have inflammation-reducing properties.

1 Chill four tall glasses in the refrigerator.

2 Combine berries, lemon juice and caster sugar
in a food processor or blender and process to make
a smooth coulis.

3 Stir toasted muesli and walnuts in a bowl so that
the walnuts are evenly distributed.

4 If using pomegranate, fill a large bowl with water.
Use a small sharp knife to make a shallow cut in the
pomegranate skin (not penetrating the flesh) in a
circle around the top of the pomegranate, then peel
off this top section of skin to reveal the pomegranate
seeds and white membranes separating the sections.
Make shallow cuts in the skin down the sides of the
pomegranate, in line with each white membrane.
Hold the pomegranate under the water in the bowl
and gently tear the sections apart and separate the
seeds. (This prevents the juice squirting.)

5 Put a spoonful of muesli mixture in the bottom of
each glass. Top with a spoonful of yogurt. Add a layer
of berry coulis and top with another spoonful of
yogurt. Repeat until each glass is filled. Top with
pomegranate seeds, if using, or a spoonful of coulis
to serve.

COOK'S TIP Use the toasted Nut and cranberry
muesli, see page 33, or a good-quality shop-bought
toasted muesli.

The berry coulis can be prepared ahead of time and
stored in the refrigerator for 2 days or, alternatively,
it can be frozen.

Grilled spiced grapefruit

2 tablespoons soft brown sugar
1 teaspoon ground cardamom
1 teaspoon ground cinnamon
1/2 teaspoon ground ginger
2 ruby red or pink grapefruits or large
oranges
low-fat thick Greek-style yogurt, to serve

PREPARATION 5 minutes
COOKING 5 minutes SERVES 4

EACH SERVING PROVIDES 185 kJ, 44 kcal, 1 g protein,
<1 g fat (<1 g saturated fat), 10 g carbohydrate
(9 g sugars), 1 g fibre, 5 mg sodium

COOK'S TIP For a dessert, remove grapefruit
skin and slice flesh 1 cm (1/2 inch) thick. Put
overlapping slices in a heatproof dish, sprinkle
with the spiced sugar and grill 5 minutes.

1 Preheat grill (broiler) to hot.

2 Put brown sugar, cardamom, cinnamon and ginger
in a bowl and stir to combine well.

3 With a sharp knife, cut grapefruits in half. Trim a
thin slice off the base if needed, so that each half sits
flat. Run knife between skin and grapefruit segments
to loosen them. Make several cuts from the centre to
the outside of the flesh (but do not cut the skin) to
divide into bite-sized chunks. With a large spoon,
scoop under segments to free them from the skin,
then pat them back in so that they are flat.

4 Heap sugar mixture evenly onto flesh of grapefruit
halves. (Do not press down as this makes the sugar
too wet.)

5 Grill grapefruits 5 minutes, or until sugar is
bubbling all over and edges of skin are beginning
to char.

6 Serve each grapefruit half with a dollop of yogurt.

Citrus fruits are a great source of fibre
and vitamin C. Pink or red grapefruits
also contain lycopene, the cancer-protective
pigment found in tomatoes. Grapefruit and
oranges are both rich in substances called
polyamines, which are thought to be related
to the ageing process. Researchers have found
reduced polyamine levels in experimental
animals as they grow older, and adding
polyamines to the diet increases their life span.

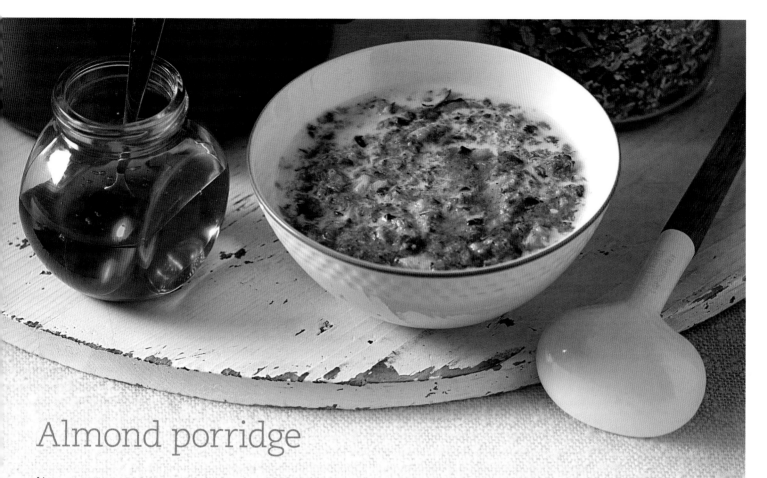

Almond porridge

½ cup (80 g) whole raw almonds or ½ cup
   (55 g) almond meal (ground almonds)
1½ cups (150 g) rolled (porridge) grains,
   such as oats, barley and rye
4 cups (1 litre) water
1 teaspoon ground cinnamon
1 teaspoon ground nutmeg
low-fat milk or soy milk, to serve
honey, to serve

PREPARATION 5 minutes
COOKING 15 minutes SERVES 4

EACH SERVING PROVIDES 1098 kJ, 262 kcal, 8 g protein,
14 g fat (2 g saturated fat), 23 g carbohydrate (1 g sugars),
5 g fibre, 4 mg sodium

> The almonds put a new twist (as well as extra anti-oxidants and vitamins) into the traditional high-protein, high-fibre porridge breakfast.

1 If using whole almonds, put in a food processor or blender and process to your preferred coarseness. (Leave quite chunky for a textured porridge.)

2 Combine processed almonds or almond meal, rolled grains, water, cinnamon and nutmeg in a large heavy-based saucepan and bring to a boil. Reduce heat and simmer until soft and creamy, about 15 minutes.

3 Serve with milk or soy milk, and a little honey, if desired.

COOK'S TIP You can replace the water with low-fat milk for a creamier result. Stir frequently during cooking to prevent burning.

If you use whole almonds, grind enough for 2–3 days and store in an airtight container in the refrigerator.

The cooked porridge will store for 2 days in the refrigerator and can be reheated in the microwave.

Anti-ageing cereals

The Muesli recipe is the basis for two great recipes that make the most of anti-ageing cereals. To simplify the preparation process, make a batch of this Muesli at the beginning of the week.

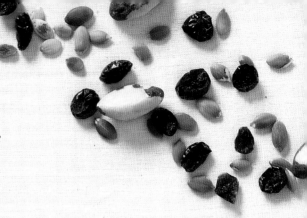

Muesli

2 cups (250 g) rolled (porridge) oats
1 cup (100 g) rolled triticale or rye
1/2 cup (60 g) rolled barley or spelt
1/2 cup (60 g) rolled quinoa or rice
1/4 cup (30 g) pepitas (pumpkin seeds)
1/4 cup (30 g) sunflower seeds
1/4 cup (40 g) linseeds (flax seeds)
1/4 cup (45 g) unhulled sesame seeds
   or chia seeds

Combine all ingredients and store in an airtight container in the cupboard, ready for use.

....

COOK'S TIP For this recipe, you can adjust the balance of ingredients according to your taste and the choices at your local store. Supermarkets now sell a variety of different grains, or check the stock at your local health food store; you may find some new grains that you haven't seen before. Quinoa is a small round grain, high in protein, that originates in the mountainous areas of South America. Spelt is an ancient grain, related to wheat; triticale is the result of breeding wheat with rye.

The combination of grains you use will determine the Muesli's final texture. Triticale and rye provide a firm, chewy texture. Spelt and barley are softer and produce a moist result when milk or yogurt is added. Quinoa and rice stay quite dry and crunchy even when wet. Double or triple the quantities and store in an airtight container; it will keep for several weeks.

PREPARATION 5 minutes MAKES 5 cups (10 serves)

EACH SERVING PROVIDES 1005 kJ, 240 kcal, 9 g protein, 9 g fat (2 g saturated fat), 32 g carbohydrate (1 g sugars), 9 g fibre, 9 mg sodium

Bircher muesli

1 cup (120 g) Muesli, see left
1/3 cup (40 g) sultanas (small golden raisins)
8 prunes, pitted and chopped
juice of 2 large oranges
2 large green or red apples, unpeeled,
   cored and grated
1/2 cup (80 g) raw almonds, roughly chopped
1 teaspoon ground cinnamon
1 teaspoon ground nutmeg
200 g (7 oz) low-fat natural (plain) yogurt
   (about 3/4 cup)

1 Stir together Muesli, sultanas and prunes in a glass dish with a lid. Spread the ingredients out evenly. Pour orange juice over. Add a little water, if needed, so mixture is completely covered with liquid. Leave to soak overnight in the refrigerator.

2 In the morning, stir apples, almonds, cinnamon and nutmeg into mixture to evenly distribute.

3 Stir through yogurt, divide among four bowls and serve.

....

COOK'S TIP You can prepare this muesli and store it in the refrigerator for a few days. However, don't stir in the grated apple until just before eating. Vary the muesli by using different nuts, spices or a different fruit juice to soak the grains.

PREPARATION 10 minutes, plus overnight soaking
MAKES 4 cups (8 serves)

EACH SERVING PROVIDES 808 kJ, 193 kcal, 6 g protein, 8 g fat (1 g saturated fat), 25 g carbohydrate (15 g sugars), 5 g fibre, 24 mg sodium

Nut and cranberry muesli

1½ cups (180 g) Muesli, see left
1 tablespoon ground cinnamon
1 teaspoon ground mixed spice (allspice)
¼ cup (40 g) Brazil nuts, sliced
¼ cup (35 g) hazelnuts, roughly chopped
1 tablespoon maple syrup, honey or
   agave syrup
1 tablespoon canola or light olive oil
½ cup (35 g) dried apple, chopped
1 cup (120 g) dried cranberries
½ cup (60 g) sultanas (small golden raisins)
low-fat milk or low-fat plain (natural) yogurt,
   to serve

PREPARATION 5 minutes, plus 20 minutes cooling
COOKING 10 minutes SERVES 4

EACH SERVING PROVIDES 2174 kJ, 519 kcal, 11 g protein,
23 g fat (3 g saturated fat), 71 g carbohydrate
(29 g sugars), 20 g fibre, 18 mg sodium

1 Preheat oven to 200°C (400°F/Gas 6).

2 In a large bowl combine Muesli, cinnamon, mixed spice, Brazil nuts and hazelnuts and toss together to mix well. Drizzle maple syrup, honey or agave syrup over and mix thoroughly. Add oil and mix again.

3 Spread mixture on a baking tray (sheet) and bake until it starts to turn light golden brown, about 10 minutes. Stir every 3–4 minutes with a spatula or spoon so mixture toasts evenly. Remove from oven and allow to cool on the tray, about 20 minutes.

4 Tip toasted mixture into a large bowl. Add apple, cranberries and sultanas and mix well. Divide among four bowls and serve with milk or yogurt.

COOK'S TIP After cooling in step 3, you can store the toasted mixture in an airtight container and use it as the base for alternative muesli recipes by altering the dried fruit in step 4. It is also delicious in recipes such as Yogurt berry parfait, see pages 28–29.

Bircher muesli This traditional high-fibre breakfast is also high in protein and anti-oxidants, and a single serve will provide you with the recommended daily intake of fruit and nuts.

Nut and cranberry muesli This muesli provides a good amount of complete protein thanks to its combination of grains, seeds and nuts, and is particularly high in fibre as well as selenium from the Brazil nuts. Seeds that are high in omega-3 oils, such as linseeds (flax seeds) and chia seeds, are a good addition. The cranberries are high in anti-oxidants and protect the urinary system with a special antibacterial action.

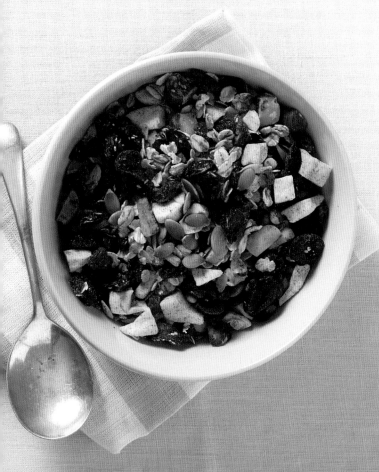

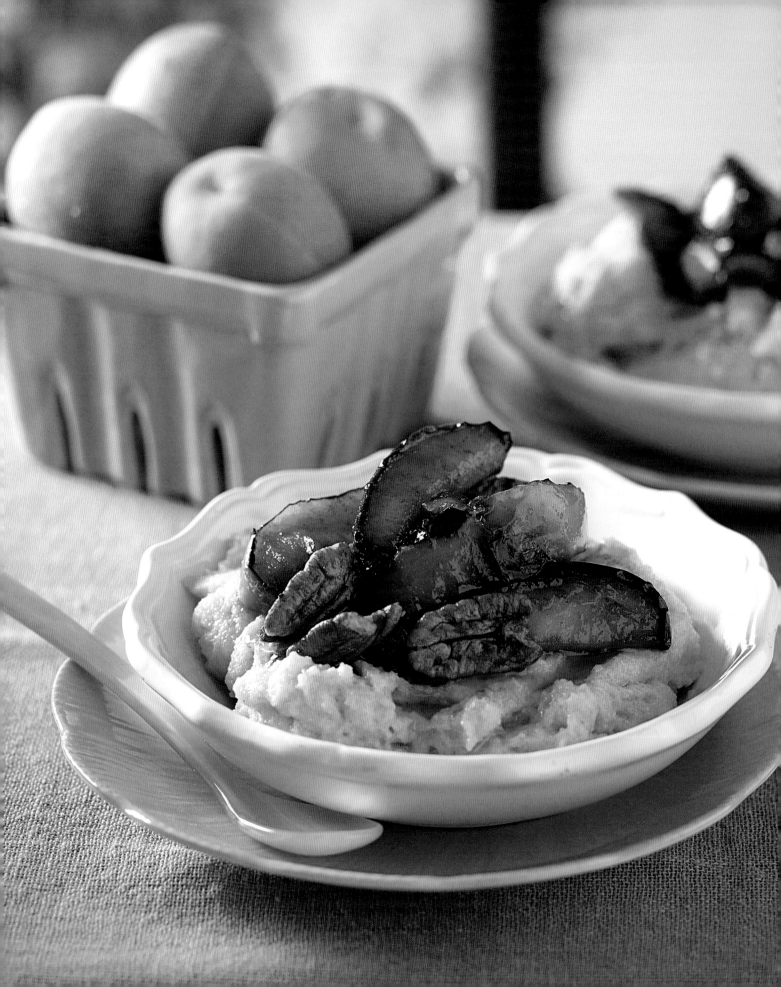

Homestyle polenta cereal

½ cup (60 g) pecan halves
1 tablespoon canola or light olive oil
2 apples, unpeeled, cored and cut
    into wedges
2 tablespoons maple syrup or honey
1 teaspoon cinnamon
4 cups (1 litre) low-fat milk or soy milk
1 cup (150 g) polenta or cornmeal

PREPARATION 5 minutes
COOKING 25 minutes SERVES 4

EACH SERVING PROVIDES 1931 kJ, 461 kcal, 17 g protein,
17 g fat (1 g saturated fat), 62 g carbohydrate
(34 g sugars), 4 g fibre, 153 mg sodium

> Polenta is a high-protein whole grain that provides good amounts of fibre and B-group vitamins. The combination of polenta, low-fat milk and nuts in this recipe means that it provides high-quality protein, healthy fats and calcium.

1 Spread out pecans in a large heavy-based saucepan and stir over medium heat about 3 minutes, until fragrant. Remove and leave to cool.

2 Heat oil in the pan. Add apples and cook, stirring and turning frequently, 5 minutes, or until wedges are golden brown on both sides. Drizzle maple syrup or honey over, add half the cinnamon and cook, stirring continuously, a further 3 minutes, or until apple is soft. Add apple mixture to the pecans and toss together well.

3 Put milk and remaining cinnamon in the pan over high heat. Sprinkle in polenta or cornmeal, stirring continuously to avoid lumps forming. Bring to a boil, then reduce heat and simmer, stirring frequently, 10–15 minutes, until the polenta is thickened and cooked through.

4 Serve polenta in individual bowls, topped with the apple and pecan mixture.

COOK'S TIP Coarse semolina can be used like the polenta in this recipe for a breakfast that is warming and nutritious.

Try with a combination of pistachios with pears or quinces and a little rosewater for a Middle East–inspired breakfast, or use almonds with apricots or peaches.

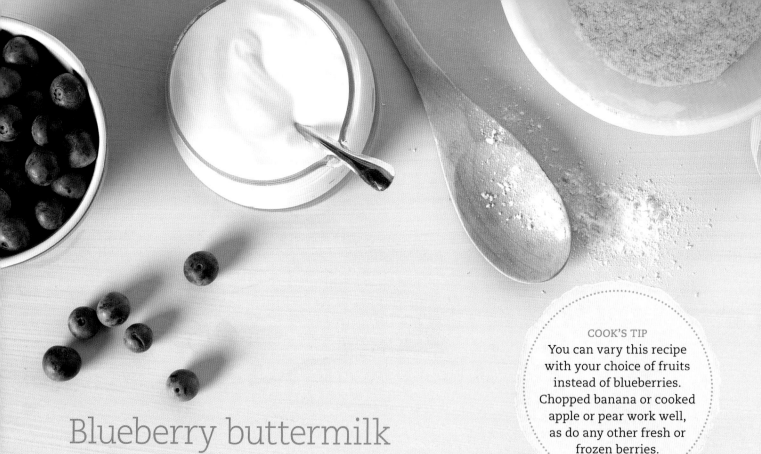

Blueberry buttermilk pancakes

½ cup (80 g) self-raising wholemeal
    (whole-wheat) flour
½ cup (75 g) self-raising flour
1 teaspoon baking powder
1 tablespoon caster (superfine) sugar
1 egg
1 eggwhite
¾ cup (180 ml) buttermilk
1 cup (155 g) fresh or frozen blueberries
light olive oil or canola oil, for frying
½ cup (125 g) low-fat natural (plain) yogurt,
    to serve
2 tablespoons maple syrup, to serve

PREPARATION 10 minutes, plus 15 minutes standing
COOKING 20 minutes SERVES 4 (makes 8 pancakes)

EACH SERVING PROVIDES 1124 kJ, 269 kcal, 11 g protein,
7 g fat (1 g saturated fat), 38 g carbohydrate
(13 g sugars), 3 g fibre, 228 mg sodium

COOK'S TIP
You can vary this recipe
with your choice of fruits
instead of blueberries.
Chopped banana or cooked
apple or pear work well,
as do any other fresh or
frozen berries.

1 Sift together wholemeal flour, flour, baking powder
and sugar into a medium bowl. Tip husks left in sieve
into to the bowl. Put egg, eggwhite and buttermilk
in a jug and whisk until combined. Make a well in
centre of flour mixture and pour in egg mixture.
Whisk until smooth. Gently stir in blueberries. Leave
batter to stand 15 minutes.

2 Heat a little oil in a large non-stick frying pan over
medium heat. Spoon ¼ cup (60 ml) of batter into
pan and spread out with a spoon to 1 cm (½ inch)
thickness. Cook 1–2 minutes, or until bubbles appear
in surface. Turn and cook a further 1–2 minutes, or
until pancake is golden brown. Transfer to a plate
and cover to keep warm. Repeat with remaining
batter to make 8 pancakes.

3 Serve pancakes warm, topped with yogurt and
a drizzle of maple syrup.

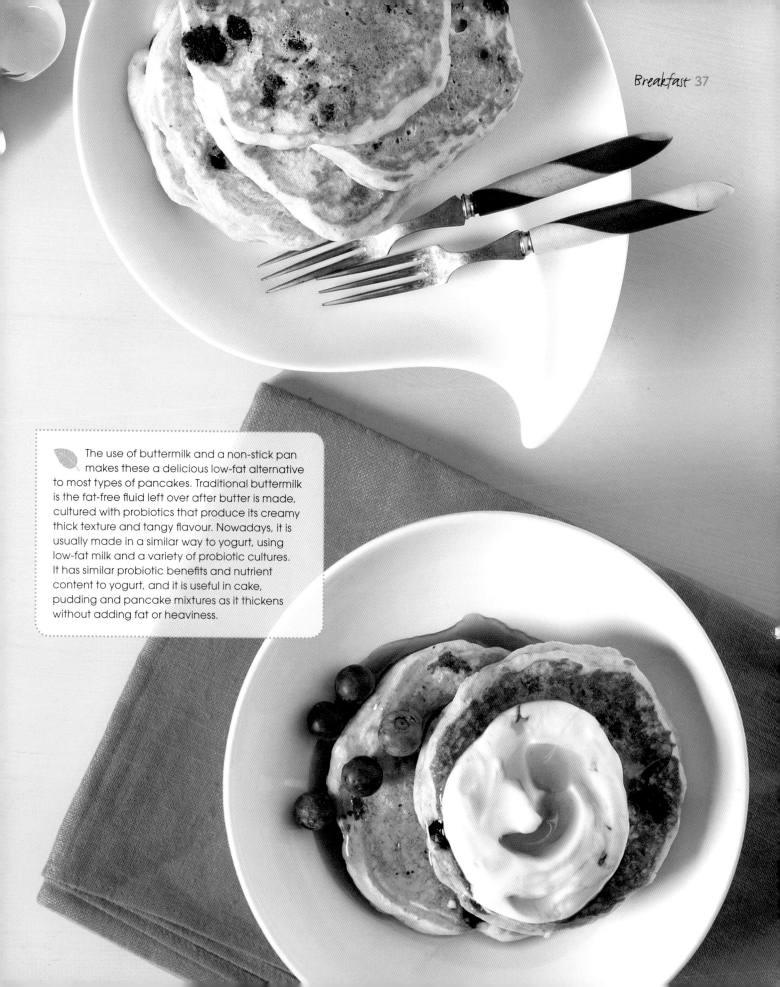

The use of buttermilk and a non-stick pan makes these a delicious low-fat alternative to most types of pancakes. Traditional buttermilk is the fat-free fluid left over after butter is made, cultured with probiotics that produce its creamy thick texture and tangy flavour. Nowadays, it is usually made in a similar way to yogurt, using low-fat milk and a variety of probiotic cultures. It has similar probiotic benefits and nutrient content to yogurt, and it is useful in cake, pudding and pancake mixtures as it thickens without adding fat or heaviness.

Oat crepes

¾ cup (110 g) plain (all-purpose) flour
⅓ cup (40 g) rolled (porridge) oats
3 eggs
1 tablespoon olive oil, plus extra, for frying
¾ cup (180 ml) low-fat milk

Filling

2 tablespoons olive oil
1 small brown (yellow) onion, finely chopped
1 clove garlic, crushed
250 g (8 oz) button mushrooms, thinly sliced
2 tablespoons plain (all-purpose) flour
1 cup (250 ml) low-fat milk
2 tablespoons finely snipped fresh chives

PREPARATION 20 minutes, plus 15 minutes standing
COOKING 25 minutes SERVES 4 (makes 8 crepes)

EACH SERVING PROVIDES 1651 kJ, 394 kcal, 17 g protein,
19 g fat (4 g saturated fat), 38 g carbohydrate
(8 g sugars), 4 g fibre, 121 mg sodium

Like the oatcakes of northern England, these fine-textured crepes are made with a blend of flour and ground rolled oats for extra fibre and a nutty flavour. In this recipe, nutrient-rich mushrooms are cooked in a low-fat white sauce for the filling.

1 Put flour and rolled oats in a food processor or blender and process at high speed until finely ground. Tip into a large bowl.

2 Put eggs, 1 tablespoon oil and milk in a jug and whisk until combined. Make a well in centre of flour mixture and pour in egg mixture. Whisk until smooth. Leave batter to stand 15 minutes.

3 Meanwhile, for the filling, heat oil in a large saucepan over medium–high heat. Add onion and cook, stirring, 2–3 minutes, or until soft. Add garlic and mushrooms and cook, stirring, 3–4 minutes, or until mushrooms are tender.

4 Reduce heat to medium. Sprinkle flour evenly over mushrooms and cook, stirring quickly, 1 minute. Gradually whisk in milk until smooth. Cook, stirring, 3–4 minutes, or until mixture boils and thickens. Stir in chives. Remove from heat and cover to keep warm.

5 Heat a little oil in a medium crepe pan or frying pan over medium heat. Spoon ¼ cup (60 ml) of batter into pan and swirl around to coat base. Cook 1 minute, then turn and cook a further 1 minute, or until golden brown. Transfer to a plate and cover to keep warm. Repeat with remaining batter to make 8 crepes.

6 Divide mushroom mixture among crepes. Fold crepes to enclose filling, then serve.

COOK'S TIP These oat crepes can be served spread with jam, or with a range of fillings, such as fresh berries and low-fat vanilla yogurt, or sliced banana and low-fat ricotta flavoured with honey and ground cinnamon.

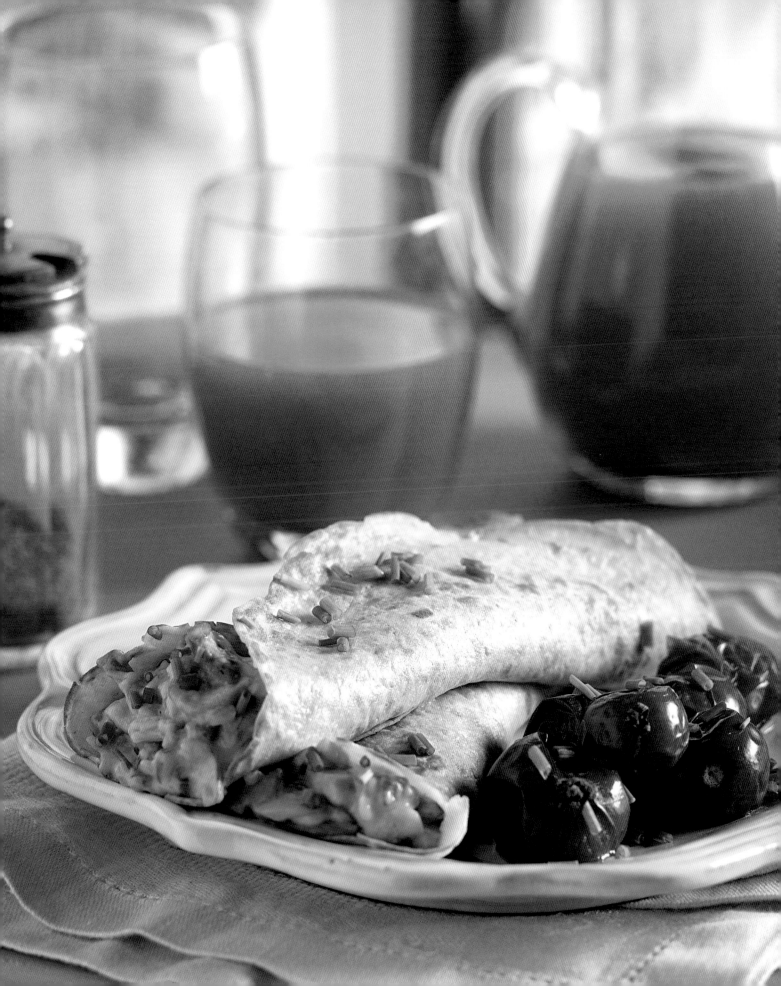

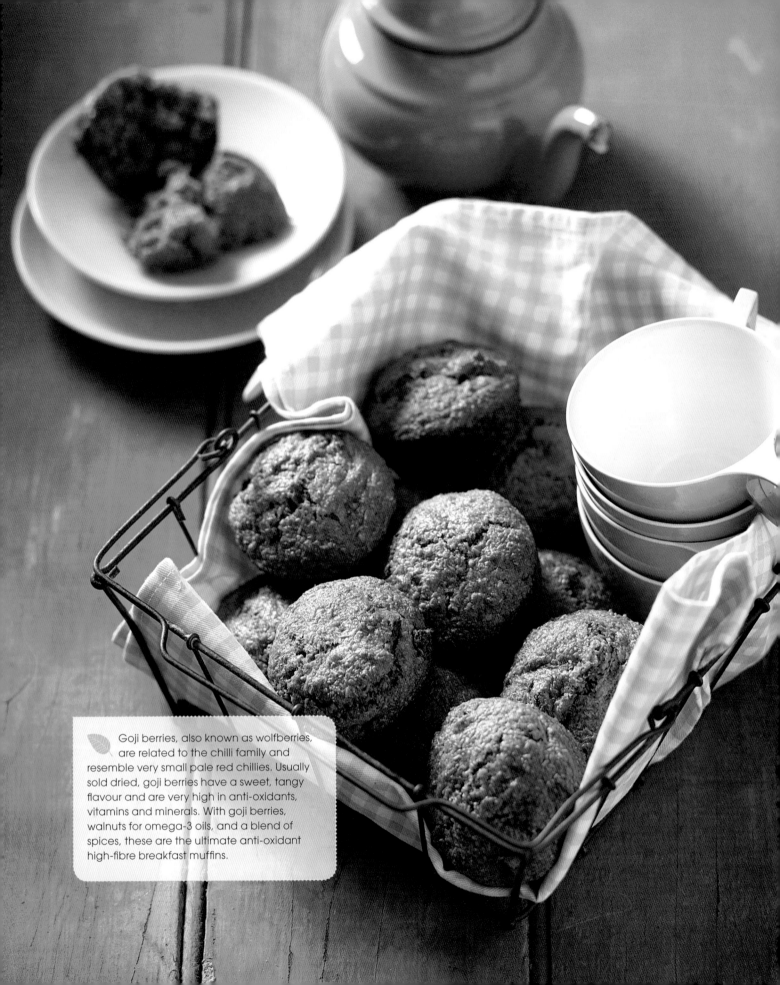

Goji berries, also known as wolfberries, are related to the chilli family and resemble very small pale red chillies. Usually sold dried, goji berries have a sweet, tangy flavour and are very high in anti-oxidants, vitamins and minerals. With goji berries, walnuts for omega-3 oils, and a blend of spices, these are the ultimate anti-oxidant high-fibre breakfast muffins.

Spicy bran muffins

1 cup (150 g) self-raising flour
1 teaspoon ground mixed
    (pumpkin pie) spice
1 teaspoon bicarbonate of soda
    (baking soda)
½ cup (115 g) firmly packed soft brown sugar
1¾ cups (75 g) unprocessed bran
½ cup (60 g) goji berries or currants
½ cup (60 g) chopped walnuts
1 egg
1¼ cups (310 ml) buttermilk
⅓ cup (80 ml) canola oil
reduced-fat canola spread, for greasing

PREPARATION 15 minutes, plus overnight standing
COOKING 25 minutes MAKES 12 muffins

EACH SERVING PROVIDES 930 kJ, 222 kcal, 5 g protein,
11 g fat (1 g saturated fat), 26 g carbohydrate
(12 g sugars), 3 g fibre, 163 mg sodium

1 Sift flour, mixed spice and bicarbonate of soda into a medium bowl. Stir in sugar, bran, goji berries or currants and walnuts. Put egg, buttermilk and oil in a separate bowl and whisk until combined. Stir egg mixture into dry ingredients, but do not overmix; it should remain lumpy. Cover and stand in the refrigerator overnight.

2 Preheat oven to 180°C (350°F/Gas 4). Grease a 12-hole standard muffin tin.

3 Spoon mixture into muffin tin. Bake 20–25 minutes, or until a skewer inserted in the centre of a muffin comes out clean. Stand muffins in tin 5 minutes before turning them onto a wire rack to cool.

COOK'S TIP Refrigerating the mixture overnight allows the bran to soften and the flavours to develop. It also saves time in the morning – you just have to bake them!

The muffins can be stored in an airtight container for 2 days, or in the freezer for up to 2 months.

Yogurt cheese on toast

1 pide (Turkish flat bread), halved crosswise
   and cut into pieces, toasted
2 large ripe tomatoes, sliced
1 tablespoon extra virgin olive oil
1 teaspoon sumac (optional)

Labna

2 cups (500 g) low-fat thick Greek-style yogurt
1½ teaspoons fine table salt
½ teaspoon freshly ground black pepper
1 clove garlic, crushed

PREPARATION 15 minutes, plus 24 hours draining
SERVES 8

EACH SERVING PROVIDES 862 kJ, 206 kcal, 9 g protein,
5 g fat (2 g saturated fat), 30 g carbohydrate
(6 g sugars), 2 g fibre, 792 mg sodium

1 To make the labna, combine yogurt, salt, pepper and garlic in a medium bowl. Put a medium mesh strainer over a bowl. Rinse a 25 cm (10 inch) piece of muslin (cheesecloth) in hot water. Wring out, then line strainer with muslin. Put yogurt mixture in strainer and cover with plastic wrap. Refrigerate at least 24 hours to drain.

2 Turn labna onto a plate and remove muslin.

3 Spread toasted pide with labna. Top each piece with a slice of tomato, drizzle over oil and sprinkle with sumac, if using, then serve.

COOK'S TIP Labna, also spelt labne, labneh or labnah, is a drained yogurt-based cheese popular on mezze platters in Middle Eastern cuisine. It can be drained for longer than 24 hours; the longer it is drained, the firmer it will become. Labna will keep for up to 1 week in the refrigerator.

Fine muslin or cheesecloth is available from fabric stores and some kitchenware stores.

Sumac is a dried berry that is ground and used in Middle Eastern dishes to add a lemony flavour.

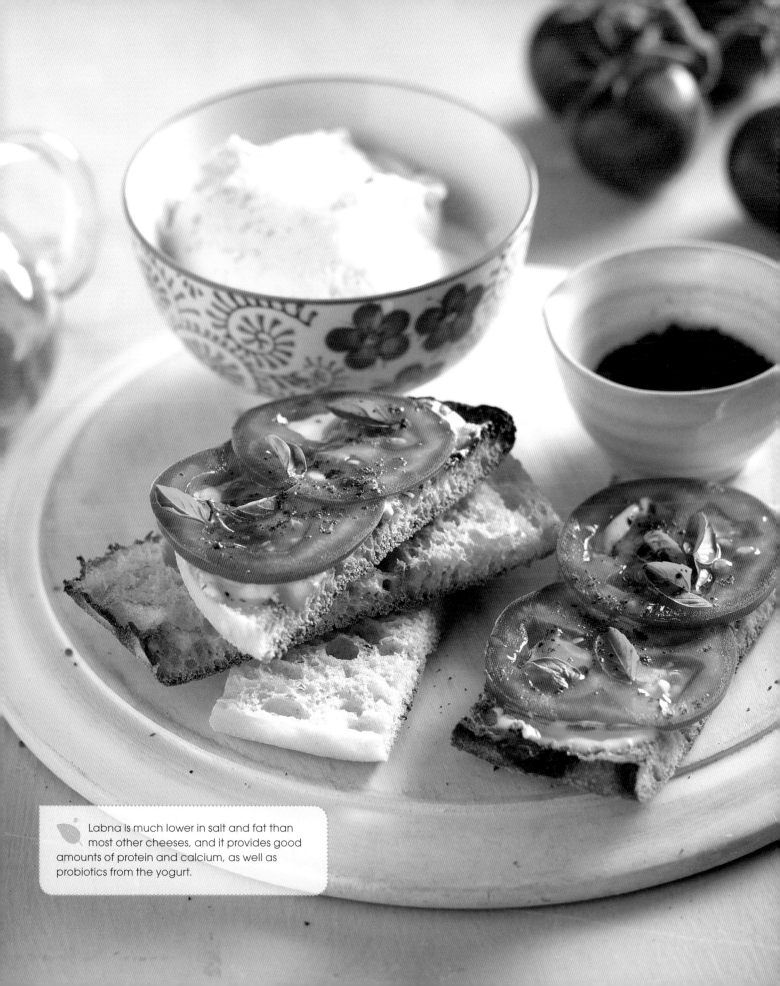

Labna is much lower in salt and fat than most other cheeses, and it provides good amounts of protein and calcium, as well as probiotics from the yogurt.

French toast

2 eggs
½ cup (125 ml) light evaporated milk
2 teaspoons caster (superfine) sugar
½ teaspoon ground cinnamon
1 tablespoon olive oil spread
4 thick slices wholemeal (whole-wheat)
   sourdough
200 g (7 oz) fresh mixed berries
½ cup (125 g) low-fat vanilla yogurt

PREPARATION 15 minutes
COOKING 10 minutes SERVES 4

EACH SERVING PROVIDES 961 kJ, 230 kcal, 109 g protein,
8 g fat (2 g saturated fat), 30 g carbohydrate
(11 g sugars), 5 g fibre, 286 mg sodium

This is a reduced-fat, high-protein
version of French toast, made with light
evaporated milk, which has a creamy taste while
being low in fat and high in protein. It is served
with berries, which are rich in anti-oxidants.

1 In a medium bowl, lightly whisk eggs and add milk until combined. Mix together sugar and cinnamon in a separate small bowl.

2 Heat the olive oil spread in a large non-stick frying pan over medium heat.

3 Dip two slices of sourdough into egg mixture until evenly coated, allow excess to drip off, then place the sourdough in the pan. Cook 1–2 minutes on each side, or until golden brown. Transfer to a plate. Sprinkle with a little cinnamon sugar and cover to keep warm. Repeat with remaining slices of sourdough.

4 Cut French toast slices in half. Top with berries and a dollop of yogurt, and serve warm.

COOK'S TIP Light evaporated milk is a reduced-fat option that gives a rich, creamy taste. It is a good substitute for cream, and it works well in cooking as it does not curdle when heated.

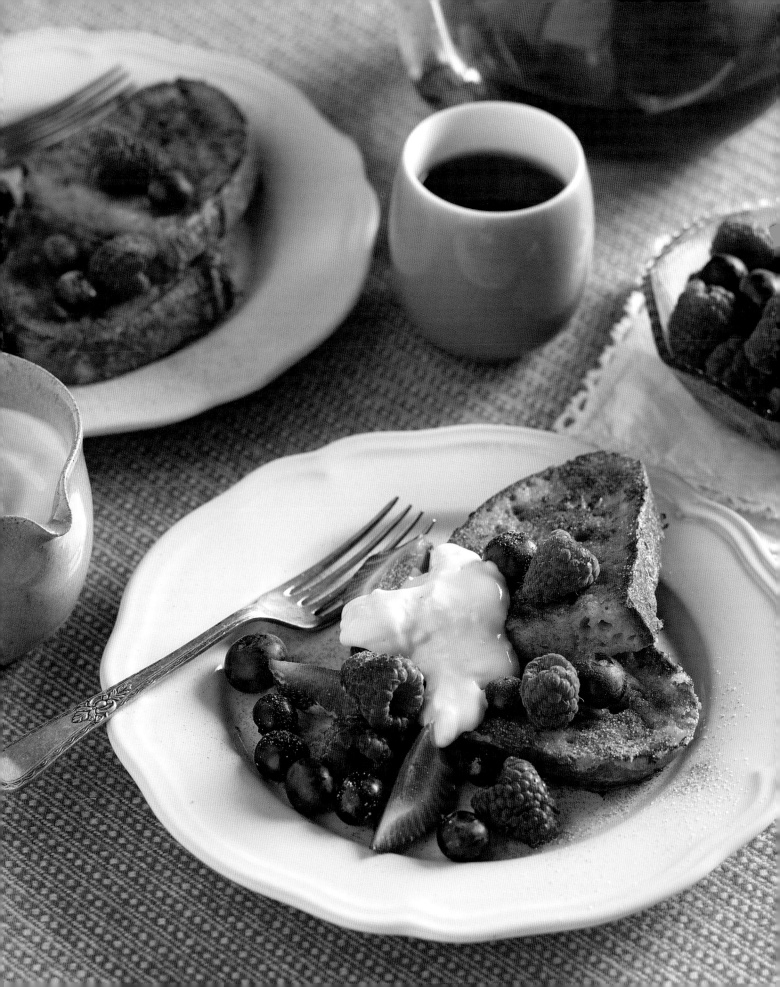

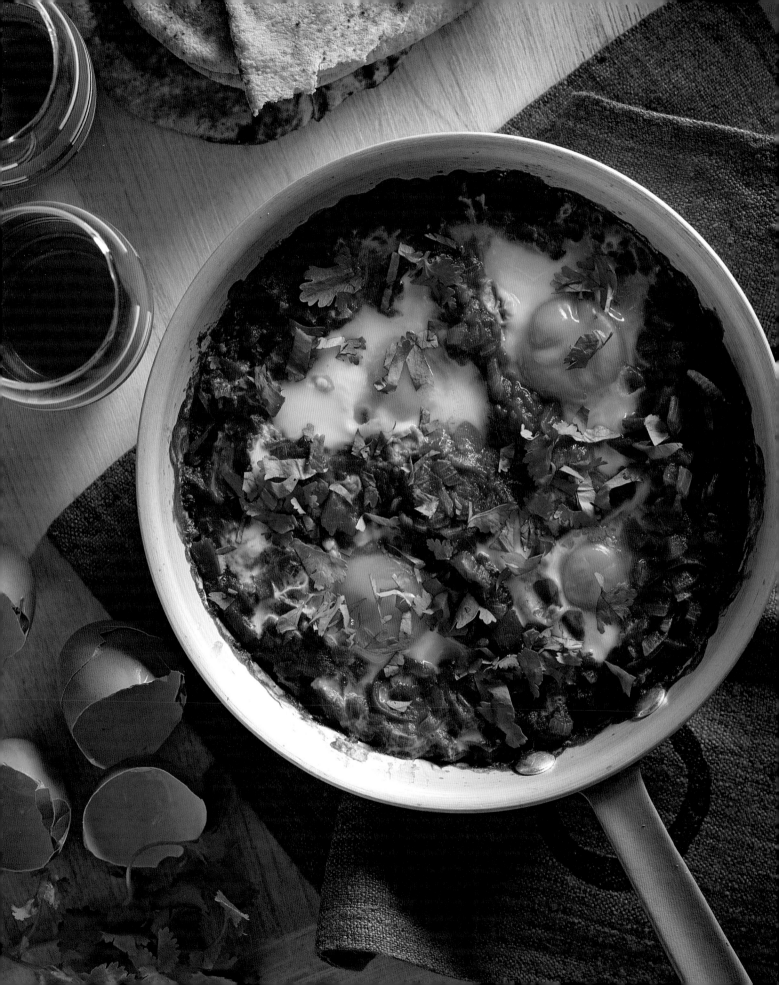

Spicy vegetables with eggs

1 tablespoon olive oil
1 small brown (yellow) onion, finely chopped
1 red capsicum (bell pepper), chopped
1 long red chilli, thinly sliced
1 clove garlic, crushed
1 teaspoon cumin seeds
½ teaspoon ground coriander
410 g (15 oz) can chopped tomatoes
4 eggs
2 tablespoons roughly chopped fresh
    coriander (cilantro) leaves
wholemeal (whole-wheat) pitas, warmed,
    to serve (optional)

PREPARATION 15 minutes
COOKING 15 minutes SERVES 4

EACH SERVING PROVIDES 615 kJ, 147 kcal, 8 g protein,
10 g fat (2 g saturated fat), 8 g carbohydrate
(5 g sugars), 2 g fibre, 135 mg sodium

1 Heat oil in a large frying pan over medium–high heat. Add onion and capsicum and cook, stirring, 3–4 minutes, or until soft. Add chilli, garlic, cumin and ground coriander and cook, stirring, 1 minute, or until fragrant.

2 Add tomatoes and bring to a boil. Reduce heat to low and simmer, uncovered, 5 minutes, or until thickened slightly. With a large spoon, make four indentations in tomato mixture. Gently break 1 egg into each indentation. Cover and cook 5–6 minutes, or until eggwhites are set and yolks are still soft.

3 Sprinkle with fresh coriander and serve with warmed pitas, if desired.

....

COOK'S TIP This popular breakfast dish from North Africa is known as *chakchouka*. To make a heartier version for lunch or supper, brown 400 g (14 oz) minced (ground) lean beef with the onion in step 1.

This is a delicious high-protein breakfast with bonus health benefits. Cooked tomato appears to protect against prostate cancer. Capsicum, tomato, garlic and spices such as cumin and coriander are all excellent sources of anti-oxidants.

Coddled eggs with herbs and yogurt

olive oil, for greasing
1 tablespoon finely snipped fresh chives
1 tablespoon finely chopped fresh flat-leaf
    (Italian) parsley
2 spring onions (scallions), thinly sliced
200 g (7 oz) low-fat thick Greek-style yogurt
    (about ¾ cup)
8 eggs, at room temperature
freshly ground black pepper
4 slices wholegrain bread, toasted

PREPARATION 10 minutes, plus 5 minutes standing
COOKING 15 minutes SERVES 4

EACH SERVING PROVIDES 1274 kJ, 304 kcal, 22 g protein,
15 g fat (5 g saturated fat), 17 g carbohydrate
(5 g sugars), 5 g fibre, 314 mg sodium

1 Preheat oven to 180°C (350°F/Gas 4). Grease four 1 cup (250 ml) ovenproof dishes with a little oil. Put dishes on a baking tray (sheet). Combine chives, parsley and spring onions in a small bowl.

2 Dollop half the yogurt into the base of the prepared dishes. Sprinkle with half the herb mixture. Crack 2 eggs into each dish. Dot with remaining yogurt and sprinkle over remaining herb mixture. Season with plenty of pepper.

3 Bake 12–15 minutes, or until eggwhites are just starting to set. Remove from oven and leave to stand 5 minutes before serving with toast.

COOK'S TIP The eggs should be at room temperature before you start cooking this recipe, as this ensures they cook evenly.

For a variation, use different herbs, such as fresh basil and mint, or sprinkle chopped tomato or red capsicum (bell pepper) or a little crumbled feta over the eggs before baking.

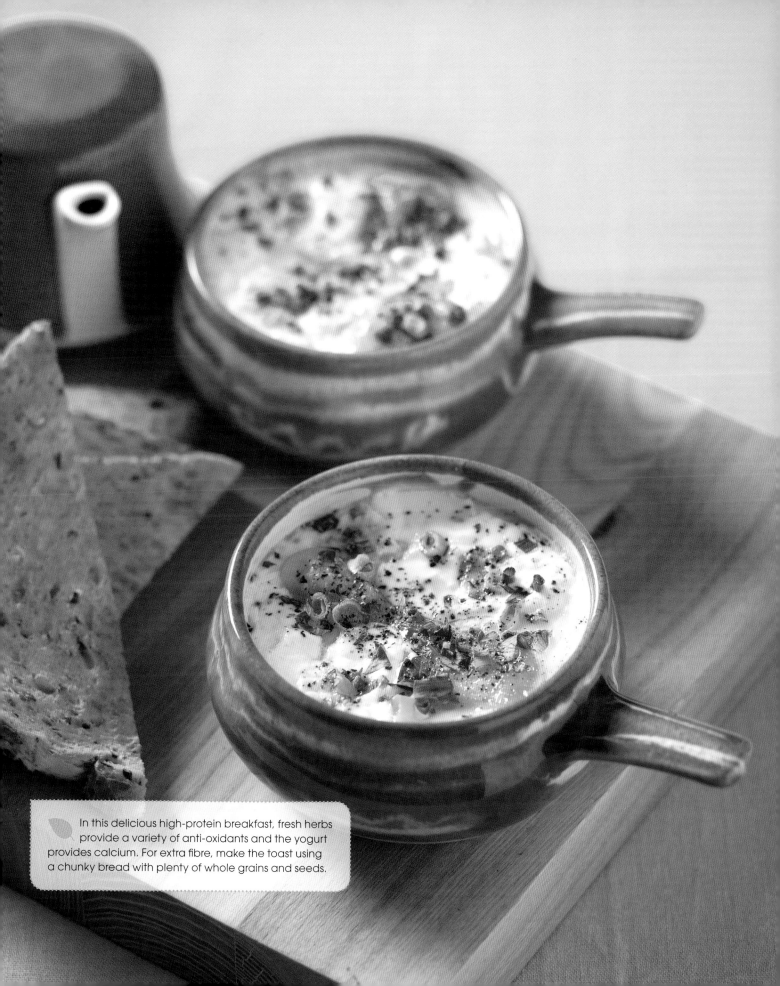

In this delicious high-protein breakfast, fresh herbs provide a variety of anti-oxidants and the yogurt provides calcium. For extra fibre, make the toast using a chunky bread with plenty of whole grains and seeds.

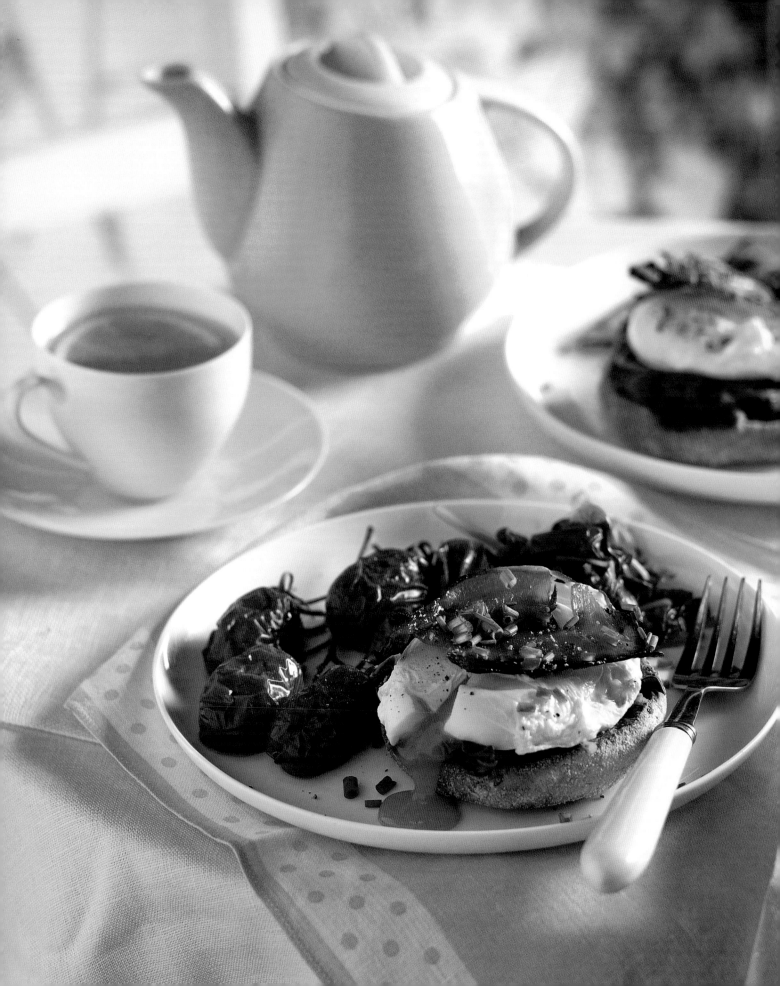

Poached eggs with bacon wafer

1 tablespoon olive oil, plus extra, for greasing
4 slices rindless bacon (bacon strips)
   (about 150 g/5 oz)
2 teaspoons maple syrup
250 g (8 oz) ripe red cocktail tomatoes, small
   truss tomatoes or cherry tomatoes
4 eggs
2 wholegrain English muffins, halved
   crosswise, toasted

PREPARATION 10 minutes
COOKING 10 minutes **SERVES** 4

EACH SERVING PROVIDES 1106 kJ, 264 kcal, 18 g protein,
15 g fat (4 g saturated fat), 15 g carbohydrate
(4 g sugars), 3 g fibre, 755 mg sodium

> Bacon is usually on lists of 'foods to avoid' when people try to improve their diets, but they also tend to be among the 'foods most missed'. This recipe shows how to incorporate a small but delicious taste of bacon in the form of delicate crispy bacon 'wafers'.

1 Preheat oven to 200°C (400°F/Gas 6). Lightly grease a baking tray (sheet) with a little oil. Put bacon on tray and drizzle with maple syrup. Press another baking tray on top to sandwich bacon. Put tomatoes on a separate baking tray and drizzle with oil. Put trays with bacon and tomatoes in oven and bake 8–10 minutes, or until bacon is crisp and tomatoes are just soft. Drain bacon on paper towel.

2 Meanwhile, half-fill a large frying pan with water and bring to a simmer. Carefully crack 1 egg into a cup, then slide egg out of cup into water. Repeat with remaining eggs. Gently poach eggs 2–3 minutes, or until eggwhites are set and yolks are soft.

3 Serve each toasted muffin half topped with a poached egg and a bacon wafer, with tomatoes on the side.

··

COOK'S TIP A variety of vegetable side dishes can be served with this dish. Try blanched English spinach or baby spinach leaves, steamed asparagus, grilled tomatoes or mushrooms sautéed in a little olive oil.

Garlic and spinach omelette

3 teaspoons extra virgin olive oil

2 garlic cloves, finely chopped

1 bunch (350 g/12 oz) English spinach,
    washed and drained, stems discarded,
    leaves cut into thirds

4 small or 2 large spring onions (scallions),
    thinly sliced

freshly ground black pepper

4 eggs

1 teaspoon chopped fresh oregano,
    marjoram or basil

2 tablespoons shredded parmesan

PREPARATION 10 minutes

COOKING 10 minutes SERVES 2

EACH SERVING PROVIDES 1135 kJ, 271 kcal, 20 g protein,
20 g fat (5 g saturated fat), 3 g carbohydrate
(3 g sugars), 6 g fibre, 272 mg sodium

This delicious omelette is high in protein as well as the anti-oxidants and minerals found in spinach and garlic. Green leafy vegetables are an important anti-ageing superfood, with benefits for your skin, heart and bone strength, and this dish provides a complete recommended daily serving of them.

1 Heat 1 teaspoon oil in a medium saucepan over medium–high heat. Add garlic and cook 1 minute. Add spinach and spring onions. Cover and cook, tossing frequently, 3 minutes, or until spinach is wilted and tender. Season well with pepper. Cover and set aside.

2 Put eggs, oregano, marjoram or basil and pepper in a medium bowl and whisk to combine. Heat remaining oil in an omelette pan or small frying pan over medium heat. Pour in eggs and cook, using a spatula to stir gently until egg is beginning to set. Sprinkle with parmesan and cook 3–5 minutes, or until set underneath and almost set on top.

3 Spoon the warm spinach onto one side of the omelette, then use a spatula to carefully fold the other side over the top. Cut in half and lift onto serving plates.

COOK'S TIP Be careful not to overcook the omelette or it will taste dry. If you leave it a little uncooked on the surface, it will continue to set while it is being folded and served, and it will be delicious and moist.

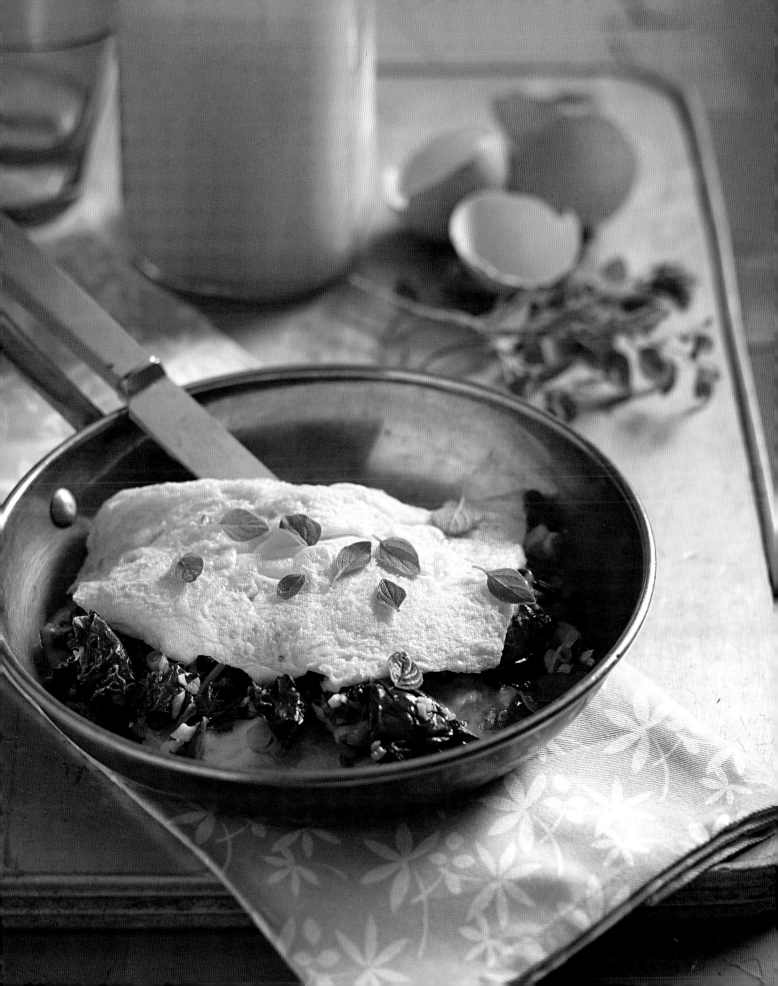

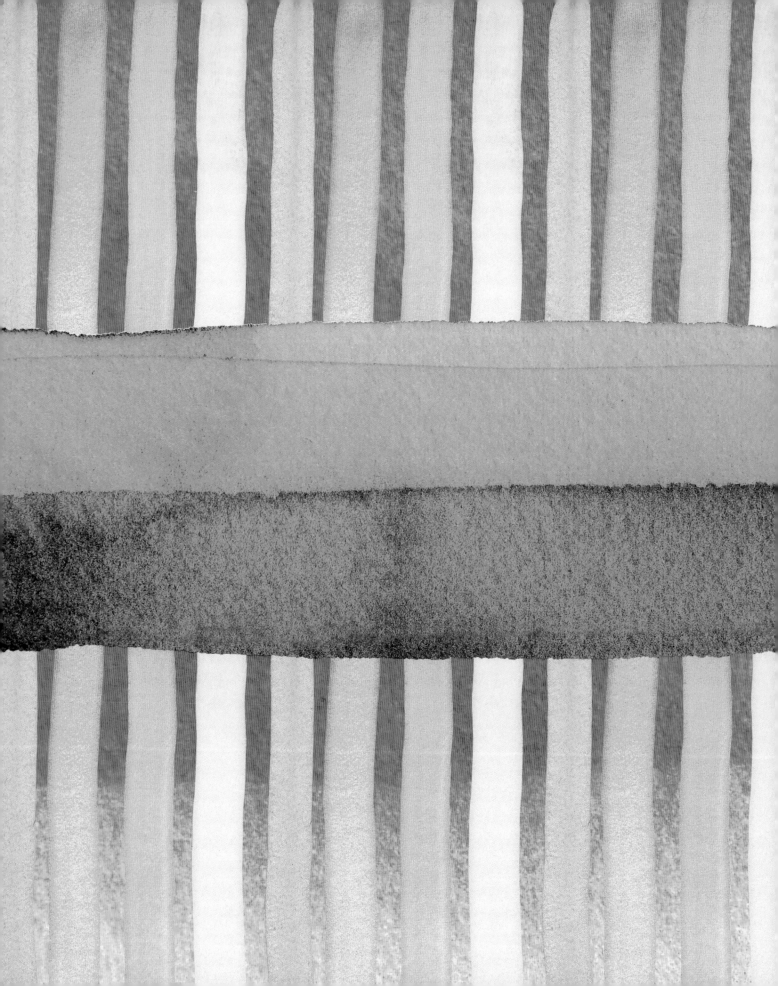

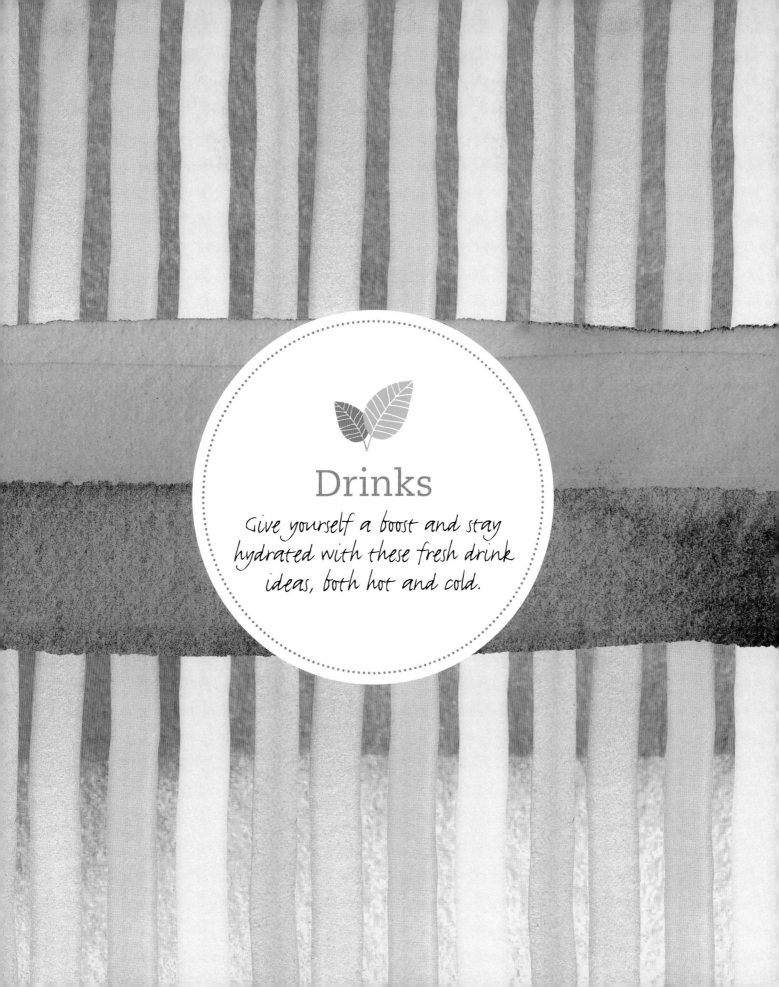

Drinks

Give yourself a boost and stay hydrated with these fresh drink ideas, both hot and cold.

Berry drink

½ cup (70 g) frozen or fresh berries, such as
    raspberries, strawberries or blueberries
½ cup (125 ml) apple juice
1 cup (250 ml) sparkling mineral water

Put berries and apple juice in a blender and blend
until smooth. Pour into two serving glasses. Slowly
add mineral water, taking care not to create too
much froth as it may overflow. Serve immediately.

COOK'S TIP Use any type of berry, or better still,
use a mixture. Don't thaw the frozen berries, as
the iciness adds a nice texture to the drink.

PREPARATION 5 minutes
SERVES 2 (makes about 2 cups/500 ml)

EACH SERVING PROVIDES 199 kJ, 48 kcal, <1 g protein,
<1 g fat (<1 g saturated fat), 10 g carbohydrate
(9 g sugars), 2 g fibre, 18 mg sodium

Grape juice drink

1 cup (250 ml) purple grape juice
1 tablespoon lime juice
6 fresh basil leaves, roughly chopped
4 ice cubes
1 cup (250 ml) sparkling mineral water

Put grape juice, lime juice, basil and ice cubes in a
blender and blend until well combined. Pour through
a mesh strainer into two serving glasses. Slowly pour
in mineral water, taking care not to let it overflow.
Serve immediately.

PREPARATION 5 minutes
SERVES 2 (makes about 2 cups/500 ml)

EACH SERVING PROVIDES 304 kJ, 72 kcal, <1 g protein,
<1 g fat (0 g saturated fat), 18 g carbohydrate
(18 g sugars), <1 g fibre, 27 mg sodium

Melon refresher

¼ honeydew melon (about 400 g/14 oz)
1 tablespoon firmly packed roughly chopped
    fresh mint
2 teaspoons elderflower or lime cordial
1 cup (250 ml) sparkling mineral water

Remove skin and seeds from honeydew melon.
Roughly chop melon flesh. Put melon, mint, cordial
and 2 tablespoons water in a blender and process until
smooth and evenly blended. Pour into two serving
glasses. Slowly add mineral water, taking care not to
create too much froth as it may overflow. Stir gently
to combine, then serve immediately.

PREPARATION 10 minutes
SERVES 2 (makes about 2 cups/500 ml)

EACH SERVING PROVIDES 276 kJ, 66 kcal, 1 g protein,
<1 g fat (<1 g saturated fat), 14 g carbohydrate
(13 g sugars), 2 g fibre, 97 mg sodium

Pink grapefruit yogurt shake

1 ruby red or pink grapefruit
1 lime
½ cup (125 g) low-fat natural (plain) yogurt
2 teaspoons honey

Remove skin and all white pith from grapefruit. Chop
flesh and discard any seeds. Repeat with lime. Put
grapefruit, lime, yogurt and honey in a blender, and
blend until smooth. Pour into two serving glasses
and serve.

PREPARATION 10 minutes
SERVES 2 (makes 1½ cups/375 ml)

EACH SERVING PROVIDES 443 kJ, 106 kcal, 4 g protein,
2 g fat (1 g saturated fat), 17 g carbohydrate
(14 g sugars), 1 g fibre, 41 mg sodium

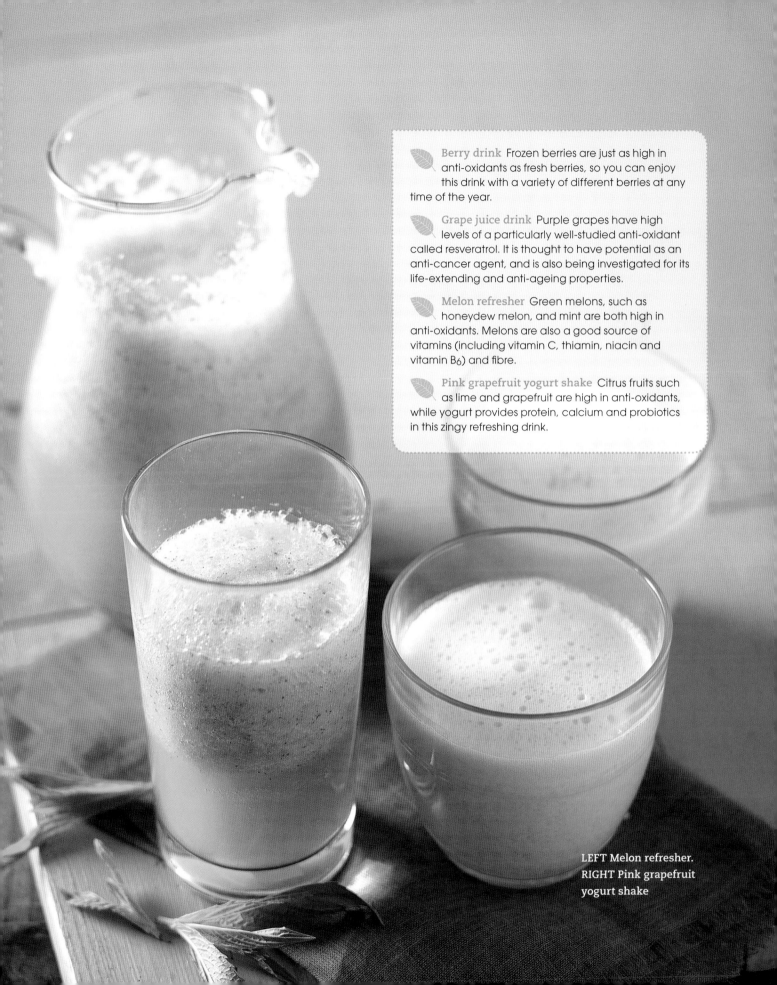

Berry drink Frozen berries are just as high in anti-oxidants as fresh berries, so you can enjoy this drink with a variety of different berries at any time of the year.

Grape juice drink Purple grapes have high levels of a particularly well-studied anti-oxidant called resveratrol. It is thought to have potential as an anti-cancer agent, and is also being investigated for its life-extending and anti-ageing properties.

Melon refresher Green melons, such as honeydew melon, and mint are both high in anti-oxidants. Melons are also a good source of vitamins (including vitamin C, thiamin, niacin and vitamin B6) and fibre.

Pink grapefruit yogurt shake Citrus fruits such as lime and grapefruit are high in anti-oxidants, while yogurt provides protein, calcium and probiotics in this zingy refreshing drink.

LEFT Melon refresher.
RIGHT Pink grapefruit yogurt shake

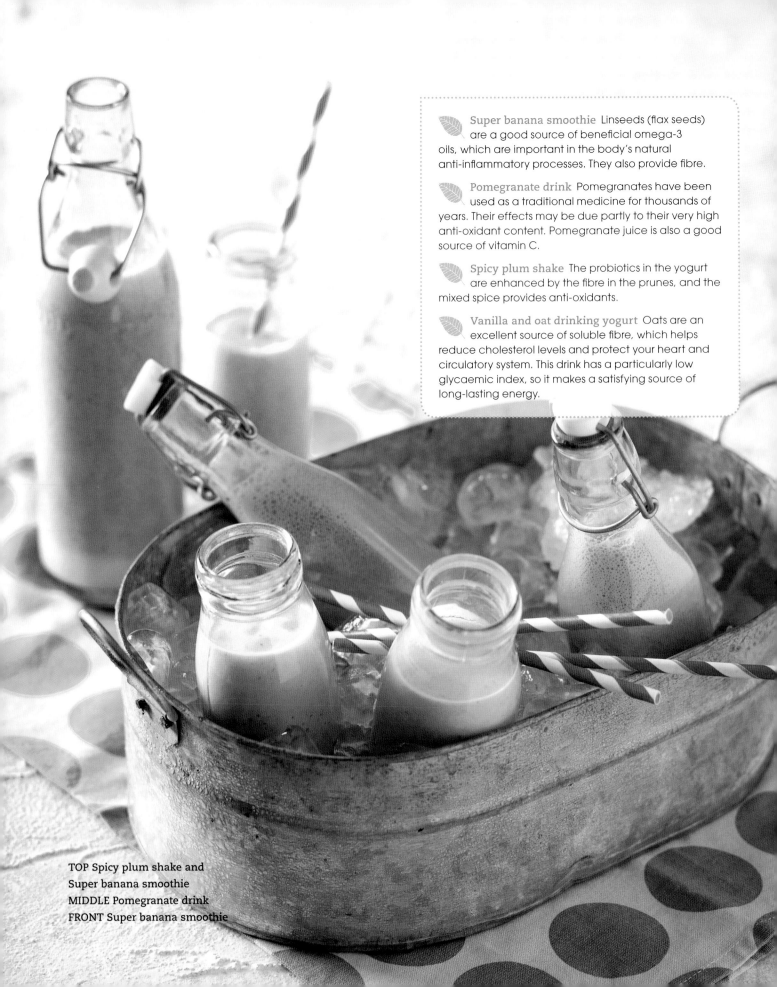

Super banana smoothie Linseeds (flax seeds) are a good source of beneficial omega-3 oils, which are important in the body's natural anti-inflammatory processes. They also provide fibre.

Pomegranate drink Pomegranates have been used as a traditional medicine for thousands of years. Their effects may be due partly to their very high anti-oxidant content. Pomegranate juice is also a good source of vitamin C.

Spicy plum shake The probiotics in the yogurt are enhanced by the fibre in the prunes, and the mixed spice provides anti-oxidants.

Vanilla and oat drinking yogurt Oats are an excellent source of soluble fibre, which helps reduce cholesterol levels and protect your heart and circulatory system. This drink has a particularly low glycaemic index, so it makes a satisfying source of long-lasting energy.

TOP Spicy plum shake and
Super banana smoothie
MIDDLE Pomegranate drink
FRONT Super banana smoothie

Super banana smoothie

1/3 cup (60 g) dried apricots, chopped
1 ripe banana
1 cup (250 g) low-fat natural (plain) yogurt
1 tablespoon linseeds (flax seeds)

Combine apricots with 1/2 cup (125 ml) water in a small saucepan. Bring to a boil, then reduce heat to low and simmer 5 minutes, until apricots are soft and liquid has reduced. Do not allow to boil dry. Transfer to a bowl to cool 10 minutes. Put apricots, banana, yogurt and linseeds in a blender, and blend until smooth and frothy. Pour into two serving glasses and serve immediately.

PREPARATION 5 minutes, plus 10 minutes cooling
COOKING 5 minutes **SERVES** 2 (makes 2 cups/500 ml)

EACH SERVING PROVIDES 430 kJ, 103 kcal, 4 g protein,
3 g fat (1 g saturated fat), 13 g carbohydrate
(11 g sugars), 2 g fibre, 39 mg sodium

Pomegranate drink

1 orange
1 cup (250 ml) pomegranate juice
1 cup (250 g) low-fat berry yogurt

Peel orange and chop flesh, discarding any seeds. Put orange, pomegranate juice and berry yogurt in a blender and blend until smooth. Pour into two serving glasses and serve immediately.

PREPARATION 5 minutes
SERVES 2 (makes 2 cups/500 ml)

EACH SERVING PROVIDES 981 kJ, 234 kcal, 8 g protein,
4 g fat (2 g saturated fat), 42 g carbohydrate
(40 g sugars), 1 g fibre, 85 mg sodium

Spicy plum shake

1/4 cup (55 g) pitted prunes, chopped
1 cup (250 ml) low-fat milk
1/2 cup (125 g) low-fat natural (plain) yogurt
1 teaspoon soft brown sugar
1/4 teaspoon mixed (pumpkin pie) spice

Combine prunes with 1/2 cup (125 ml) water in a small saucepan over high heat. Bring to a boil, then reduce heat to low and simmer 5 minutes, until prunes are soft and liquid has reduced. Do not allow to boil dry. Transfer to a bowl to cool, 10 minutes. Put prunes, milk, yogurt, sugar and mixed spice in a blender, and blend until smooth. Pour into two serving glasses and serve immediately.

PREPARATION 5 minutes, plus 10 minutes cooling
COOKING 5 minutes **SERVES** 2 (makes 2 cups/500 ml)

EACH SERVING PROVIDES 698 kJ, 167 kcal, 9 g protein,
4 g fat (3 g saturated fat), 23 g carbohydrate
(19 g sugars), 2 g fibre, 100 mg sodium

Vanilla and oat drinking yogurt

1/4 cup (30 g) rolled (porridge) oats
1 cup (250 g) low-fat natural (plain) yogurt
1/2 cup (125 ml) freshly squeezed orange juice
1/2 teaspoon vanilla extract

Put oats in a small bowl and add 1/4 cup (60 ml) hot water. Leave to soak 10 minutes, or until soft. Put oats and any soaking water in a blender with yogurt, orange juice and vanilla extract. Blend until smooth. Pour into two serving glasses and serve immediately.

PREPARATION 5 minutes, plus 10 minutes soaking
SERVES 2 (makes 2 cups/500 ml)

EACH SERVING PROVIDES 435 kJ, 104 kcal, 4 g protein,
2 g fat (1 g saturated fat), 16 g carbohydrate
(12 g sugars), 2 g fibre, 37 mg sodium

Warm mulled apple drink

2 cups (500 ml) apple juice
2 allspice berries
4 cloves
2 star anise
1 cinnamon stick
2 teaspoons maple syrup

Combine apple juice, allspice berries, cloves, star anise and cinnamon in a small saucepan. Heat slowly over medium–low heat, until very hot but not boiling. Turn off heat and leave to stand 10 minutes. Stir in maple syrup. Strain through a mesh strainer into a warmed jug, then pour into serving cups and serve.

PREPARATION 5 minutes, plus 10 minutes standing
COOKING 5 minutes SERVES 2 (makes 2 cups/500 ml)

EACH SERVING PROVIDES 530 kJ, 127 kcal, <1 g protein, <1 g fat (<1 g saturated fat), 32 g carbohydrate (30 g sugars), <1 g fibre, 26 mg sodium

Cinnamon drink

2 cups (500 ml) milk
1 cinnamon stick
1 vanilla bean, split lengthwise
1 large pinch ground nutmeg
2 teaspoons honey

Combine milk, cinnamon, vanilla bean, nutmeg and honey in a small saucepan. Heat slowly over medium–low heat until mixture just begins to come to a boil. Turn off heat and leave to stand 10 minutes, until the flavours have infused. Strain through a mesh strainer into a warm jug, then pour into two serving cups.

PREPARATION 5 minutes, plus 10 minutes standing
COOKING 5 minutes SERVES 2 (makes 2 cups/500 ml)

EACH SERVING PROVIDES 832 kJ, 199 kcal, 8 g protein, 10 g fat (6 g saturated fat), 19 g carbohydrate (18 g sugars), <1 g fibre, 107 mg sodium

Creamy chai

1 cup (250 ml) milk
3 cardamom pods, bruised
1 cinnamon stick
½ teaspoon ground ginger
4 cloves
4 peppercorns
2 tablespoons tea leaves
2 teaspoons honey

Combine milk with 1 cup (250 ml) water, cardamom, cinnamon, ginger, cloves and peppercorns in a small saucepan. Bring slowly to a boil over medium–low heat. As soon as it boils, turn off heat and add tea leaves. Leave to stand 10 minutes. Stir in honey, then pour through a mesh strainer into a warmed serving jug. Pour into two serving glasses.

PREPARATION 5 minutes, plus 10 minutes standing
COOKING 5 minutes SERVES 2 (makes 2 cups/500 ml)

EACH SERVING PROVIDES 494 kJ, 118 kcal, 4 g protein, 5 g fat (3 g saturated fat), 14 g carbohydrate (12 g sugars), 1 g fibre, 56 mg sodium

Ginger soother

4 cm (1½ inch) piece fresh ginger, thinly
    sliced
grated zest and juice of ½ lemon
1 tablespoon agave syrup or honey
1½ cups (375 ml) boiling water

Put ginger, lemon zest and juice, and agave syrup or honey in a heatproof jug. Pour over boiling water and leave to stand 5 minutes, until the flavours have infused. Pour through a mesh strainer into two serving cups.

PREPARATION 5 minutes, plus 5 minutes standing
SERVES 2 (makes 1½ cups/375 ml)

EACH SERVING PROVIDES 245 kJ, 59 kcal, <1 g protein, 1 g fat (<1 g saturated fat), 14 g carbohydrate (11 g sugars), 1 g fibre, 2 mg sodium

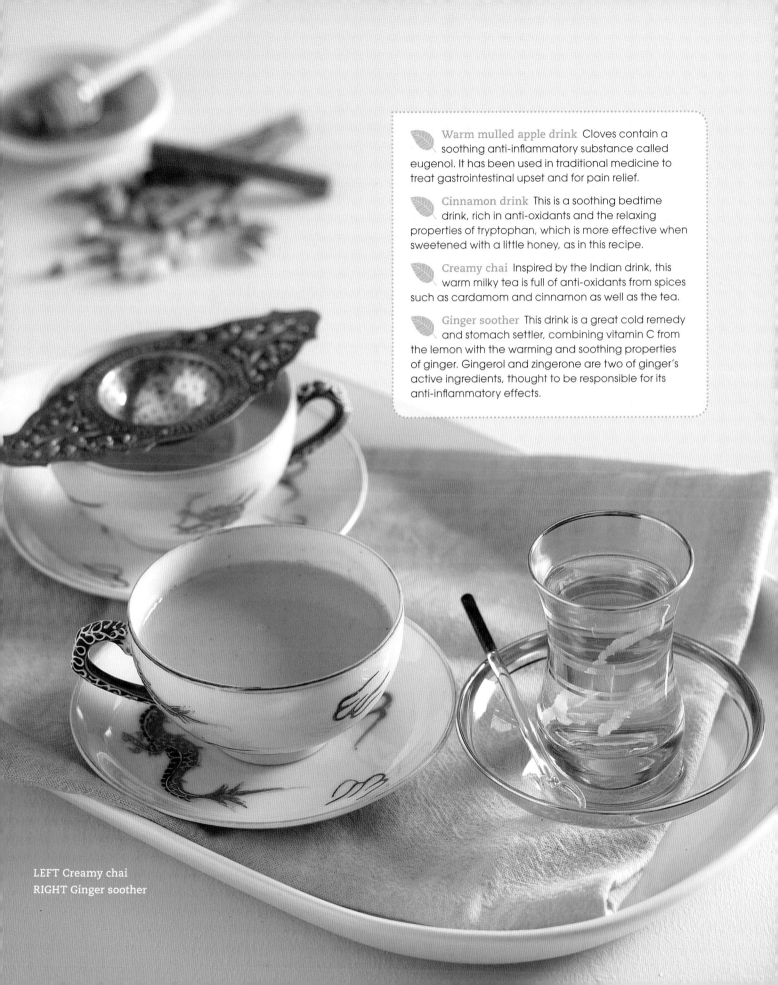

Warm mulled apple drink Cloves contain a soothing anti-inflammatory substance called eugenol. It has been used in traditional medicine to treat gastrointestinal upset and for pain relief.

Cinnamon drink This is a soothing bedtime drink, rich in anti-oxidants and the relaxing properties of tryptophan, which is more effective when sweetened with a little honey, as in this recipe.

Creamy chai Inspired by the Indian drink, this warm milky tea is full of anti-oxidants from spices such as cardamom and cinnamon as well as the tea.

Ginger soother This drink is a great cold remedy and stomach settler, combining vitamin C from the lemon with the warming and soothing properties of ginger. Gingerol and zingerone are two of ginger's active ingredients, thought to be responsible for its anti-inflammatory effects.

LEFT Creamy chai
RIGHT Ginger soother

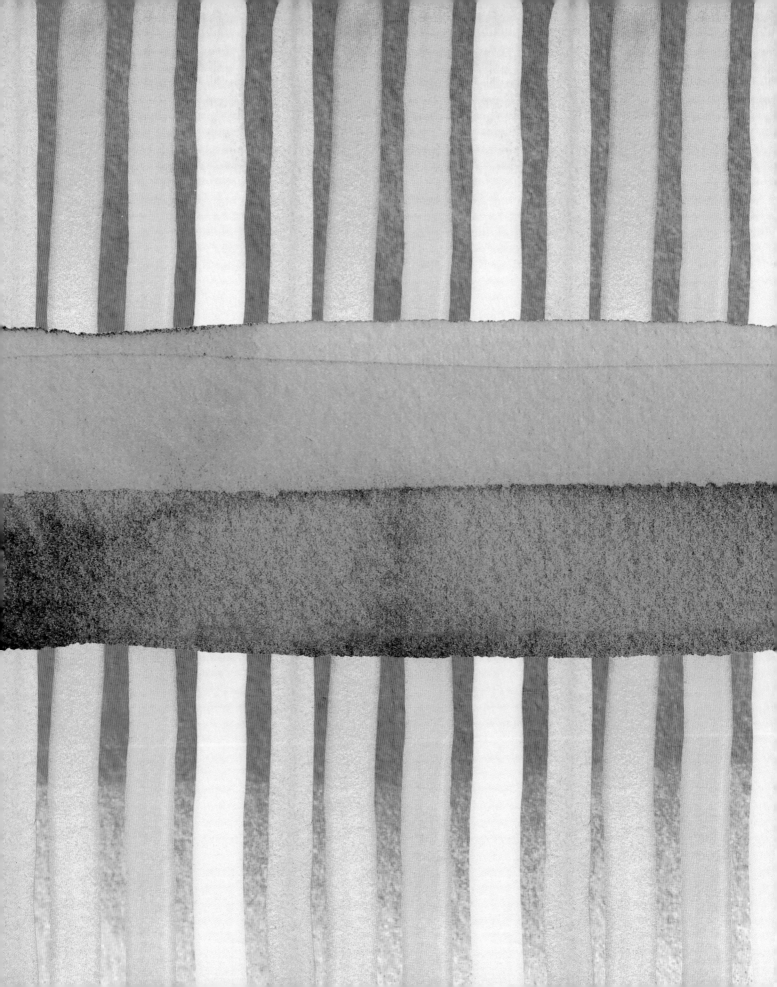

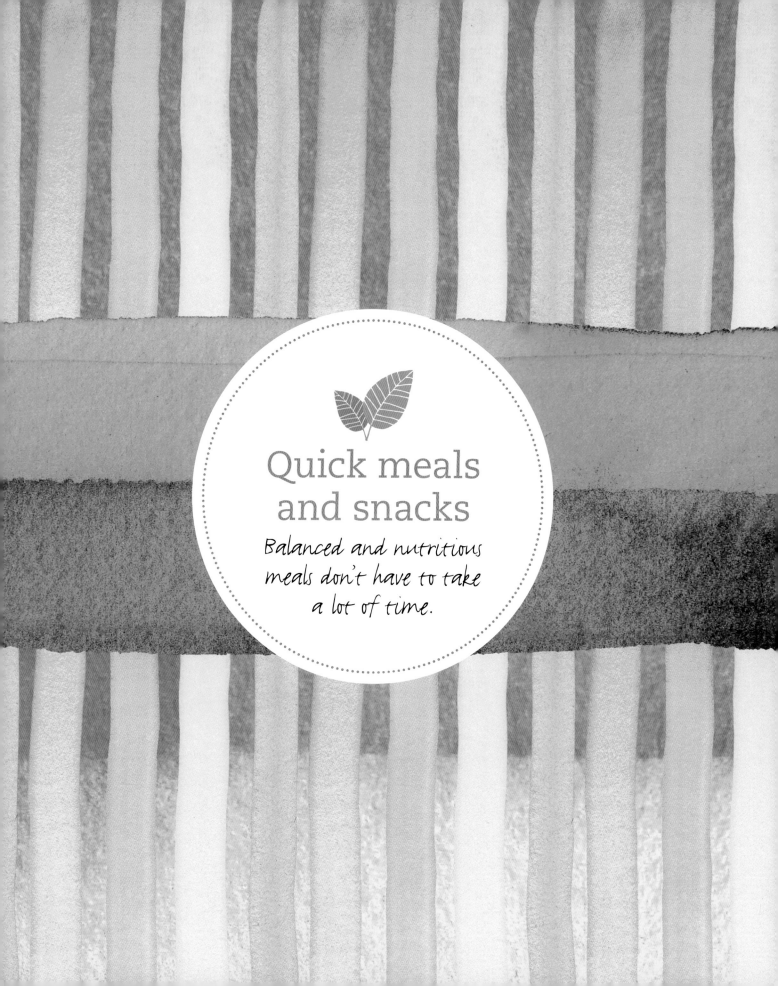

Quick meals
and snacks

Balanced and nutritious
meals don't have to take
a lot of time.

Canned white bean soup

2 tablespoons olive oil
1 large onion
3 cloves garlic
400 g (14 oz) can butterbeans (lima beans)
   or cannellini beans, rinsed and drained
2 large sprigs fresh rosemary
½ cup (125 ml) salt-reduced stock,
   milk or water
grated parmesan or cheddar, to serve
freshly ground black pepper

PREPARATION 5 minutes
COOKING 15 minutes SERVES 2

EACH SERVING PROVIDES 1181 kJ, 282 kcal, 9 g protein,
19 g fat (3 g saturated fat), 18 g carbohydrate
(6 g sugars), 10 g fibre, 335 mg sodium

1 Heat oil in a medium saucepan or soup pot. Add onion and garlic and cook gently over a low heat about 10 minutes, until softened.

2 Put onion, garlic and half the beans in a food processor or blender and process until very smooth.

3 Return mixture to saucepan. Add remaining beans, rosemary and stock, milk or water, and simmer a further 5 minutes to infuse with aroma of rosemary. Add extra water if soup becomes thick or too dry.

4 Ladle soup into bowls and serve topped with a sprinkling of parmesan or cheddar and a little pepper.

Legumes are an anti-ageing superfood because of their protein content and blend of fibres that help promote heart and gut health. Rosemary has powerful anti-oxidant and anti-inflammatory properties that enhance the beneficial substances in the onion and garlic.

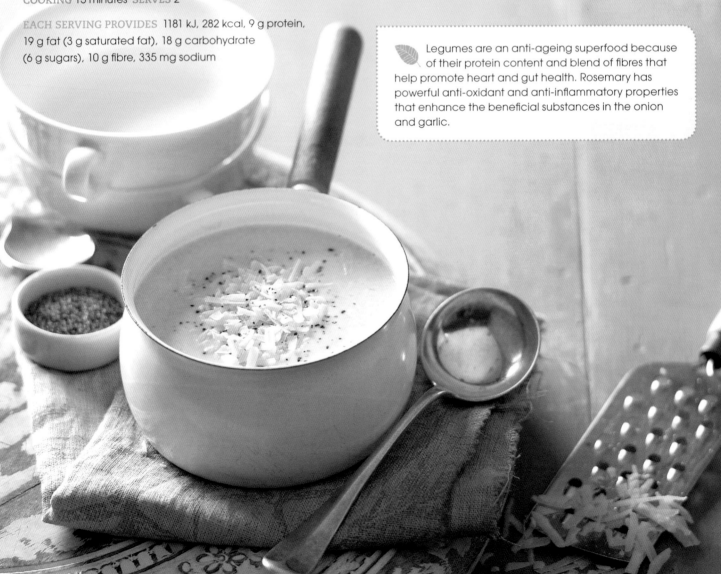

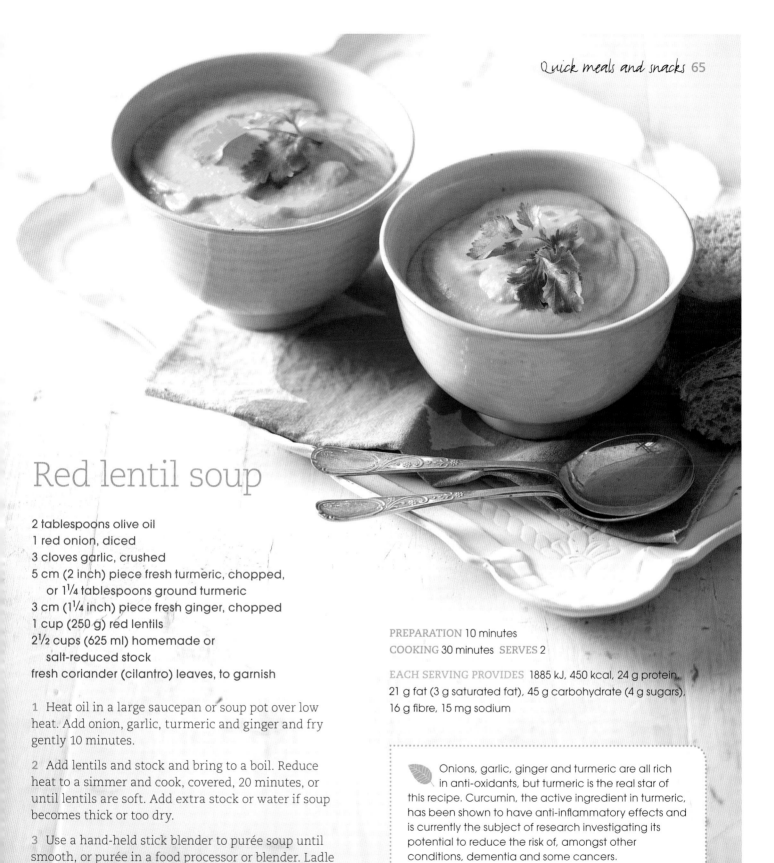

Red lentil soup

2 tablespoons olive oil
1 red onion, diced
3 cloves garlic, crushed
5 cm (2 inch) piece fresh turmeric, chopped,
    or 1¼ tablespoons ground turmeric
3 cm (1¼ inch) piece fresh ginger, chopped
1 cup (250 g) red lentils
2½ cups (625 ml) homemade or
    salt-reduced stock
fresh coriander (cilantro) leaves, to garnish

1 Heat oil in a large saucepan or soup pot over low heat. Add onion, garlic, turmeric and ginger and fry gently 10 minutes.

2 Add lentils and stock and bring to a boil. Reduce heat to a simmer and cook, covered, 20 minutes, or until lentils are soft. Add extra stock or water if soup becomes thick or too dry.

3 Use a hand-held stick blender to purée soup until smooth, or purée in a food processor or blender. Ladle into bowls, scatter with coriander and serve.

PREPARATION 10 minutes
COOKING 30 minutes SERVES 2

EACH SERVING PROVIDES 1885 kJ, 450 kcal, 24 g protein, 21 g fat (3 g saturated fat), 45 g carbohydrate (4 g sugars), 16 g fibre, 15 mg sodium

Onions, garlic, ginger and turmeric are all rich in anti-oxidants, but turmeric is the real star of this recipe. Curcumin, the active ingredient in turmeric, has been shown to have anti-inflammatory effects and is currently the subject of research investigating its potential to reduce the risk of, amongst other conditions, dementia and some cancers.

Frozen pea soup

1 tablespoon olive oil

1 large or 2 small leeks, white part only, chopped

2 cloves garlic, finely chopped

3½ cups (875 ml) homemade or salt-reduced chicken or vegetable stock

4 cups (600 g) frozen peas

1 cup (20 g) fresh mint, chopped

½ cup (125 g) low-fat natural (plain) yogurt, plus 4 tablespoons extra, to serve

freshly ground black pepper

sumac or paprika, to serve

PREPARATION 10 minutes, plus 10 minutes cooling

COOKING 20 minutes SERVES 4

EACH SERVING PROVIDES 775 kJ, 185 kcal, 16 g protein, 6 g fat (1 g saturated fat), 16 g carbohydrate (10 g sugars), 2 g fibre, 606 mg sodium

> Like all of the alliums (onion family), leeks contain flavonoids with powerful anti-oxidant effects. Here, they are combined with nutrient-rich green peas and the anti-oxidants in mint.

1 Heat oil in a large saucepan over medium heat. Add leek and cook, stirring occasionally, 8 minutes, until softened. Stir in garlic and cook 1 minute.

2 Add stock and bring to a boil. Reduce heat to a simmer and cook, covered, 5 minutes. Add peas and return to a boil, then reduce heat and cook, covered, 5 minutes. Remove from heat and allow to cool slightly, about 10 minutes.

3 Add mint and ½ cup yogurt and use a hand-held stick blender to purée, or purée in batches in a food processor or blender. Return soup to pan if using a food processor. Season well with pepper and heat gently until hot but not boiling.

4 Ladle soup into serving bowls, top each with 1 tablespoon yogurt and a light sprinkling of sumac or paprika, and serve.

....

COOK'S TIP If using bought salt-reduced stock, use half stock and half water to keep the salt content at a healthy level.

Frozen vegetables are convenient yet just as nutritious as fresh.

Sumac is a dried berry that is ground and used in Middle Eastern dishes to add a lemony flavour.

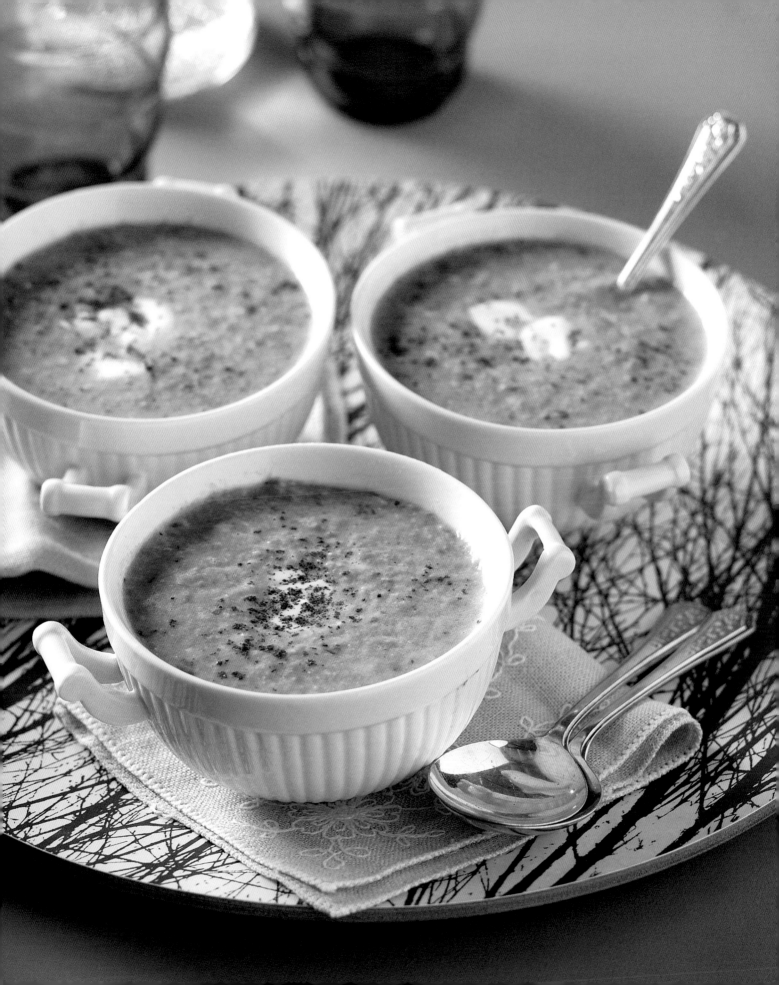

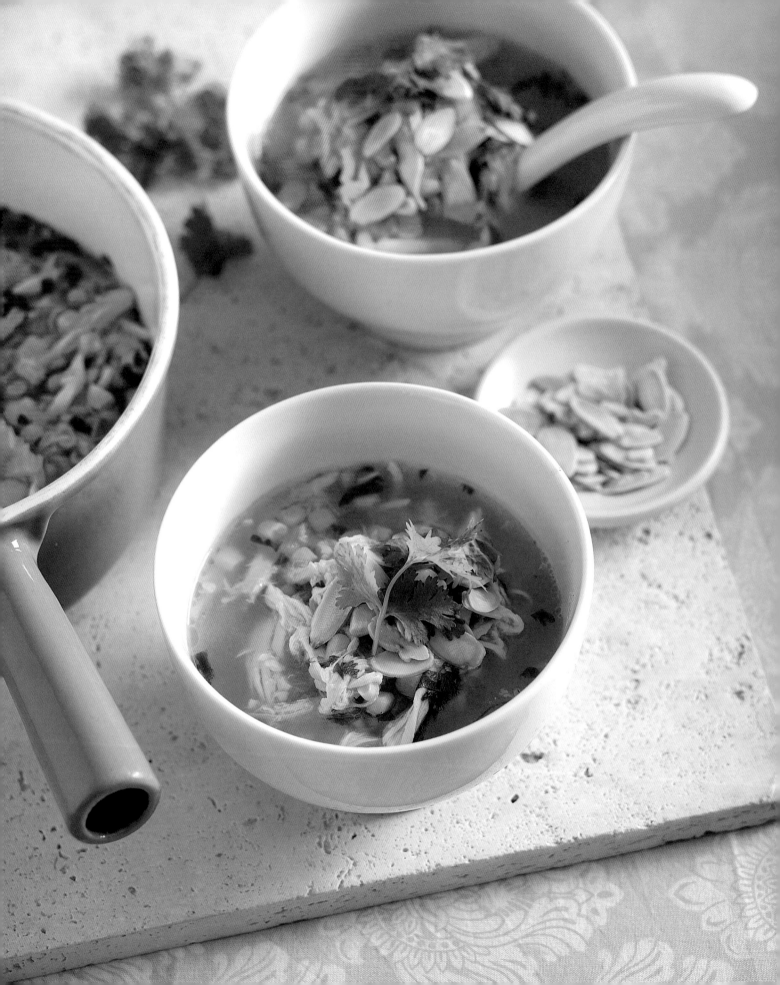

Quick corn and chicken soup

3 teaspoons canola oil
1 onion, finely diced
1 teaspoon finely grated fresh ginger
1 garlic clove, crushed
½ teaspoon ground turmeric
4 cups (1 litre) boiling water
½ roasted or barbecued chicken,
    bones removed and reserved
3 corn cobs, kernels removed
1 teaspoon sesame oil
2 tablespoons chopped fresh coriander
    (cilantro) leaves; extra leaves, to garnish
freshly ground black pepper
2 tablespoons flaked almonds, to garnish

PREPARATION 15 minutes
COOKING 20 minutes SERVES 4

EACH SERVING PROVIDES 1686 kJ, 403 kcal, 29 g protein,
20 g fat (6 g saturated fat), 27 g carbohydrate (3 g sugars),
6 g fibre, 469 mg sodium

Chicken soup has long been used as a comfort food for the sick, and it appears that science now supports its effects, with research discovering a sulfur substance in chicken, released into soup during long cooking, that appears to have anti-bacterial properties. In this recipe corn adds fibre and anti-oxidants.

1 Heat canola oil in a large saucepan over medium heat. Add onion and cook, stirring frequently, 4 minutes. Add ginger, garlic and turmeric and stir until fragrant.

2 Stir in water, chicken bones and corn kernels and bring to a boil. Reduce heat and simmer, covered, 15 minutes.

3 Meanwhile, discard skin and any visible fat from chicken. Shred chicken meat.

4 Use tongs to remove and discard all chicken bones from the soup. Stir chicken meat, sesame oil and 2 tablespoons coriander into the soup. Season well with pepper and cook 1 minute to heat through.

5 Ladle soup into serving bowls and sprinkle with remaining coriander and almonds.

COOK'S TIP This recipe is good for using leftover chicken and chicken bones.

You can use frozen or canned corn kernels if you want to reduce preparation time. You will need 2 cups (300 g) kernels.

Lamb cutlets with herb and lemon crust

1 egg
50 g (1¾ oz) wholemeal (whole-wheat)
    bread crusts or slices
2 sprigs fresh parsley
10 fresh mint leaves
grated zest of ½ lemon
1 small clove garlic
30 g (1 oz) parmesan, grated
freshly ground black pepper
8 lamb cutlets or lean lamb chops,
    bone ends trimmed and cleaned

PREPARATION 5 minutes
COOKING 10 minutes SERVES 4

EACH SERVING PROVIDES 883 kJ, 211 kcal, 23 g protein,
12 g fat (5 g saturated fat), 5 g carbohydrate
(<1 g sugars), 1 g fibre, 241 mg sodium

A lemony crust makes ordinary grilled
cutlets or chops more exciting as well as
boosting the anti-oxidant content of the dish.

1 Preheat grill (broiler) to medium. Line grill tray with foil.

2 Beat egg in a shallow bowl.

3 Put bread, parsley, mint, lemon zest, garlic, parmesan and pepper to taste in a food processor or blender and blend to a fine crumb mixture. Tip out onto a large plate.

4 Dip cutlets or chops in beaten egg and turn to coat well on all sides. Then firmly press each into crumb mixture so that both sides are well coated. Put on grill tray.

5 Grill cutlets about 5 minutes each side, or until crumbs are dark golden. Serve hot.

COOK'S TIP Serve the lamb with a green salad.

Vary the recipe by using different herbs in the crumb mixture. Lime zest instead of lemon zest works well.

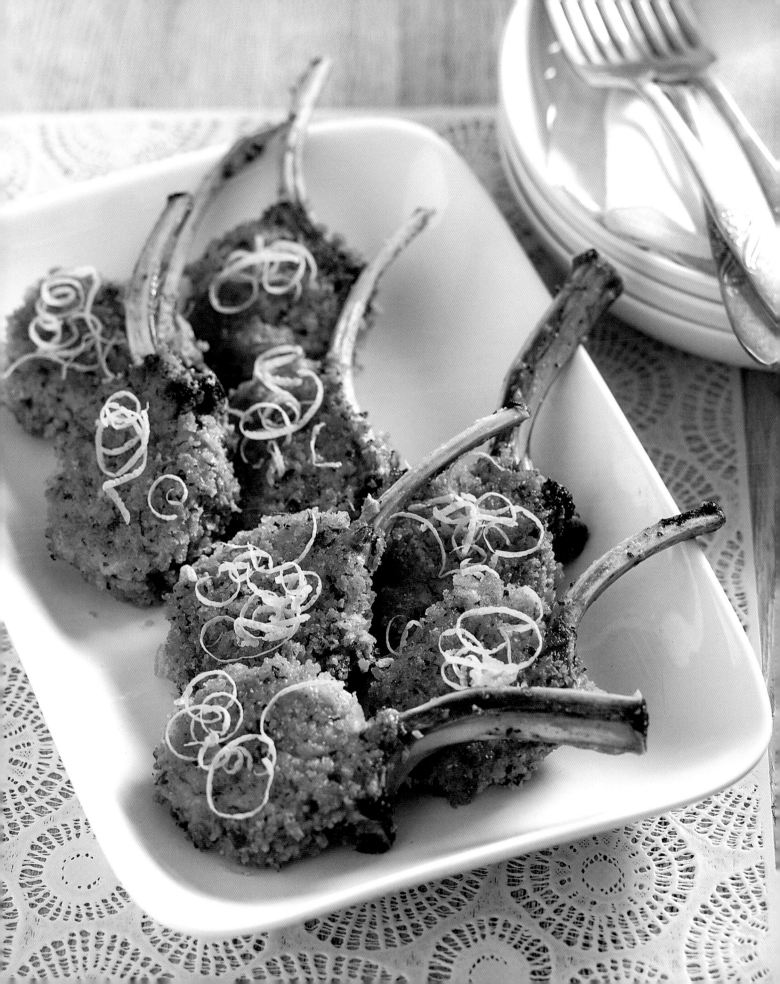

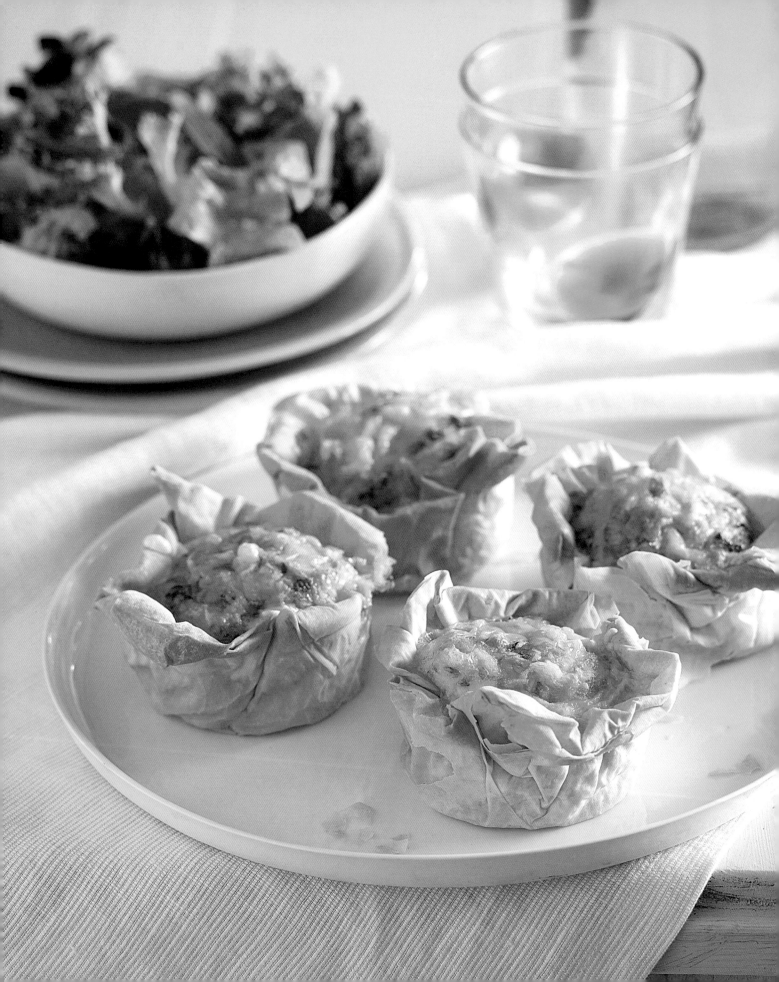

Tuna and egg filo tartlets

olive oil cooking spray
4 sheets filo pastry
2 teaspoons olive oil
1 small onion, finely chopped
½ teaspoon smoked paprika
5 eggs
180 g (6 oz) can tuna in olive oil,
    well drained and flaked
⅓ cup (10 g) chopped fresh flat-leaf
    (Italian) parsley
freshly ground black pepper
2 tablespoons grated reduced-fat cheddar

PREPARATION 10 minutes, plus 10 minutes cooling
COOKING 30 minutes MAKES 4

EACH SERVING PROVIDES 1028 kJ, 246 kcal, 21 g protein,
14 g fat (4 g saturated fat), 8 g carbohydrate
(<1 g sugars), 1 g fibre, 268 mg sodium

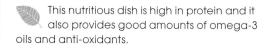 This nutritious dish is high in protein and it also provides good amounts of omega-3 oils and anti-oxidants.

1 Preheat oven to 180°C (350°F/Gas 4). Lightly spray 4 holes of a 6-hole giant muffin tin with cooking spray.

2 Lightly spray 1 sheet filo pastry with cooking spray. Fold in half crosswise, then spray lightly. Fold in half crosswise again, then use to line a muffin hole, overlapping the pastry edges and pressing together to completely line the hole. Fold pointed edges of pastry back and tuck into the muffin hole. Repeat with remaining sheets of pastry.

3 Heat oil in a small saucepan over medium heat. Add onion and cook, stirring occasionally, 5 minutes, until soft. Add paprika and stir 30 seconds. Set aside to cool 10 minutes.

4 Whisk eggs in a bowl. Stir in onion mixture, tuna and parsley. Season with pepper and spoon into pastry in muffin holes. Sprinkle with cheese and bake 25 minutes, or until puffed and set in the centre.

5 Carefully lift tartlets out of muffin tin, transfer to individual plates and serve immediately.

COOK'S TIP You can use canned salmon instead of tuna if you prefer.

The pastry is lovely and crisp after cooking but will soften if the tartlets are left to stand.

Lentil, ricotta and herb muffins

¼ cup (60 g) red lentils
olive oil, for greasing
1⅓ cups (330 ml) low-fat milk
150 g (5 oz) low-fat ricotta
2 eggs
¼ cup (60 g) salt-reduced tomato paste
    (concentrated purée)
½ cup (60 g) finely chopped spring onions
    (scallions)
⅓ cup (35 g) grated parmesan
3 tablespoons chopped fresh parsley
2 tablespoons snipped fresh chives
1½ cups (225 g) wholemeal (whole-wheat)
    self-raising flour
½ cup (75 g) white self-raising flour

PREPARATION 20 minutes, plus 10 minutes cooling
COOKING 30 minutes MAKES 12 muffins

EACH SERVING PROVIDES 649 kJ, 155 kcal, 9 g protein,
4 g fat (2 g saturated fat), 21 g carbohydrate
(3 g sugars), 4 g fibre, 265 mg sodium

1 Put lentils in a small saucepan of boiling water and cook 4–5 minutes, or until just cooked. Drain and leave to cool, about 10 minutes.

2 Meanwhile, preheat oven to 180°C (350°F/Gas 4). Lightly grease a 12-hole standard muffin tin with oil.

3 Whisk together milk, ricotta, eggs and tomato paste in a large bowl. Stir in lentils, spring onions, parmesan, parsley and chives. Sift wholemeal and white flour over mixture, adding the husks from the sifter. Stir until combined.

4 Spoon mixture into prepared muffin tin and bake 25 minutes, or until golden and cooked through. Serve warm.

COOK'S TIP Don't overcook the lentils. They should still hold their shape when cooked.

You'll need about 4 spring onions to obtain ½ cup finely chopped spring onions.

While all forms of tomato are very nutritious and rich in anti-oxidants, the process of concentrating tomato into paste (concentrated purée) releases more of the substances that are believed to be protective against prostate cancer. The lentils and ricotta make these muffins a high-protein snack.

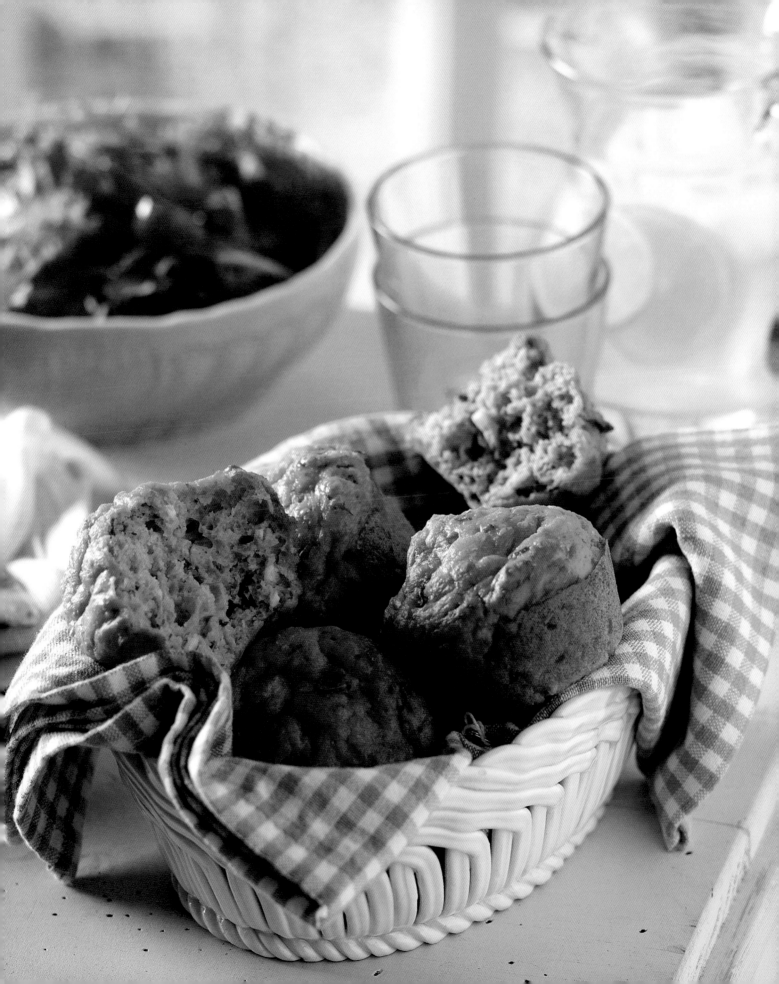

Vegetable lentil spread on toast

1 tablespoon olive oil
1 onion, finely chopped
1 carrot, finely diced
2 cloves garlic, finely chopped
125 g (4 oz) button mushrooms, finely diced
1 small zucchini (courgette), finely diced
½ cup (125 ml) homemade or salt-reduced
   chicken stock or water
2 tablespoons salt-reduced tomato paste
   (concentrated tomato purée)
400 g (14 oz) can brown lentils,
   rinsed and drained
2 tablespoons chopped fresh flat-leaf
   (Italian) parsley
2 tablespoons chopped fresh coriander
   (cilantro) leaves
1 tablespoon lemon juice
freshly ground black pepper
4 slices wholemeal (whole-wheat)
   sourdough, toasted, to serve

PREPARATION 15 minutes
COOKING 15 minutes SERVES 4

EACH SERVING PROVIDES 222 kJ, 105 kcal, 6 g protein,
5 g fat (<1 g saturated fat), 9 g carbohydrate
(4 g sugars), 4 g fibre, 270 mg sodium

1 Heat oil in medium saucepan over medium heat. Add onion and carrot and cook, stirring occasionally, 5 minutes, or until soft. Add garlic and cook, stirring, 1 minute.

2 Add mushrooms, zucchini, stock or water and tomato paste and simmer, covered, 6 minutes, or until mushrooms are tender.

3 Put lentils in a bowl and mash roughly with a fork. Add to pan with parsley, coriander and lemon juice. Mix well and heat through, then season with pepper.

4 Spread lentil mixture thickly on toast and serve.

COOK'S TIP You can mash the lentils in a small food processor or blender if you prefer. Use short bursts to process coarsely.

If using homemade stock, don't add salt. If using bought salt-reduced stock, use half stock and half water to keep the salt at a healthy level.

Adding canned brown lentils to a mixture of finely diced onion, carrot, mushroom and zucchini makes for a quick high-protein and high-fibre snack.

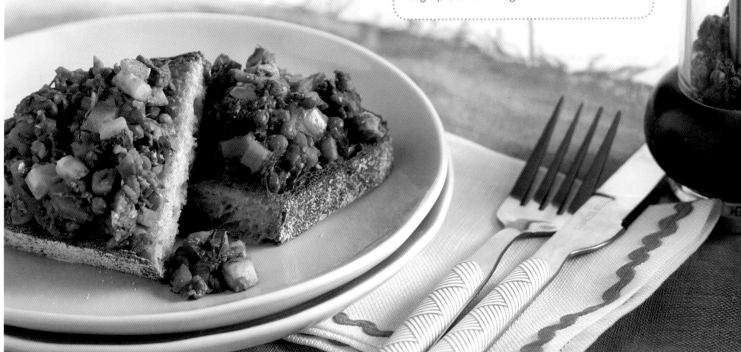

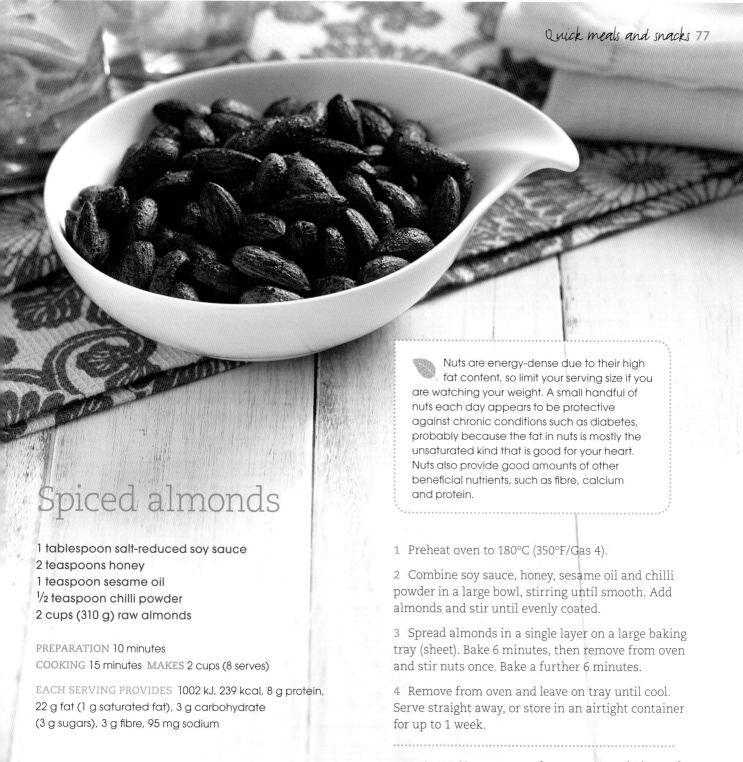

Spiced almonds

1 tablespoon salt-reduced soy sauce
2 teaspoons honey
1 teaspoon sesame oil
½ teaspoon chilli powder
2 cups (310 g) raw almonds

PREPARATION 10 minutes
COOKING 15 minutes MAKES 2 cups (8 serves)

EACH SERVING PROVIDES 1002 kJ, 239 kcal, 8 g protein,
22 g fat (1 g saturated fat), 3 g carbohydrate
(3 g sugars), 3 g fibre, 95 mg sodium

> Nuts are energy-dense due to their high fat content, so limit your serving size if you are watching your weight. A small handful of nuts each day appears to be protective against chronic conditions such as diabetes, probably because the fat in nuts is mostly the unsaturated kind that is good for your heart. Nuts also provide good amounts of other beneficial nutrients, such as fibre, calcium and protein.

1 Preheat oven to 180°C (350°F/Gas 4).

2 Combine soy sauce, honey, sesame oil and chilli powder in a large bowl, stirring until smooth. Add almonds and stir until evenly coated.

3 Spread almonds in a single layer on a large baking tray (sheet). Bake 6 minutes, then remove from oven and stir nuts once. Bake a further 6 minutes.

4 Remove from oven and leave on tray until cool. Serve straight away, or store in an airtight container for up to 1 week.

COOK'S TIP You can use other raw nut varieties such as cashew nuts, macadamia nuts or pecans. Maple syrup or agave syrup can replace the honey. Try other spices instead of chilli – ground paprika, ground cumin, curry powder or Chinese five-spice are all delicious.

Scrambled tofu

2 teaspoons light olive oil

1 teaspoon sesame oil

½ green capsicum (bell pepper), finely
   diced

1 teaspoon grated fresh ginger

½ large green chilli, seeds removed,
   finely chopped

⅓ cup (40 g) finely chopped spring onions
   (scallions)

300 g (10 oz) silken tofu, drained

2 teaspoons salt-reduced soy sauce

1 tablespoon snipped fresh chives

2 slices wholegrain bread, toasted

PREPARATION 15 minutes
COOKING 10 minutes SERVES 2

EACH SERVING PROVIDES 1052 kJ, 251 kcal, 14 g protein,
13 g fat (2 g saturated fat), 17 g carbohydrate
(4 g sugars), 6 g fibre, 299 mg sodium

Soy foods may help to reduce the risk of
dementia, osteoporosis and heart disease,
and may also ameliorate the symptoms of
menopause. Served with wholegrain toast, this
dish makes a delicious alternative to scrambled
eggs, with a similar protein content but extra
health benefits.

1 Heat olive oil and sesame oil in a small frying pan over medium–high heat. Add capsicum, ginger and chilli, and cook, stirring frequently, 3 minutes, or until softened. Add spring onions and cook, stirring, 2 minutes, until softened.

2 Reduce heat to medium. Add tofu and soy sauce. With a wooden spoon, break up tofu into small pieces while gently mixing it into capsicum mixture and cooking, 2 minutes, or until heated through and combined. Add chives and stir carefully to combine.

3 Spoon scrambled tofu on top of toasted wholegrain bread and serve hot.

COOK'S TIP Cook the tofu gently. If it is overcooked it will weep liquid.

You could add 1 diced small tomato with the spring onions if you like. You'll need about 3 spring onions to obtain ⅓ cup finely chopped spring onions.

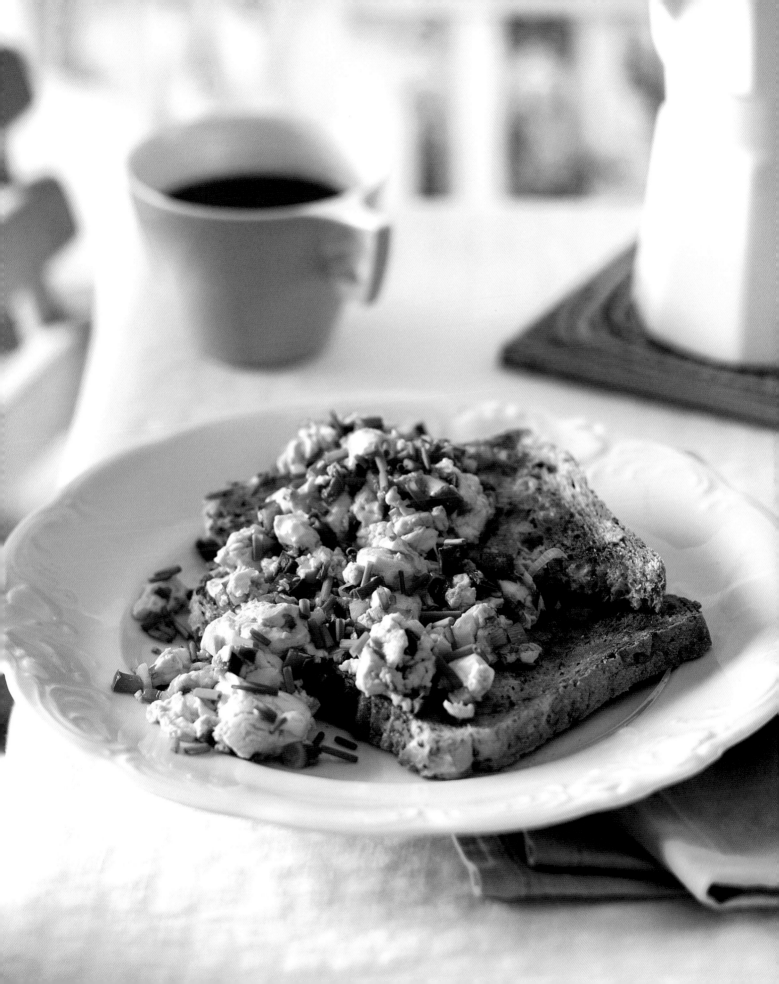

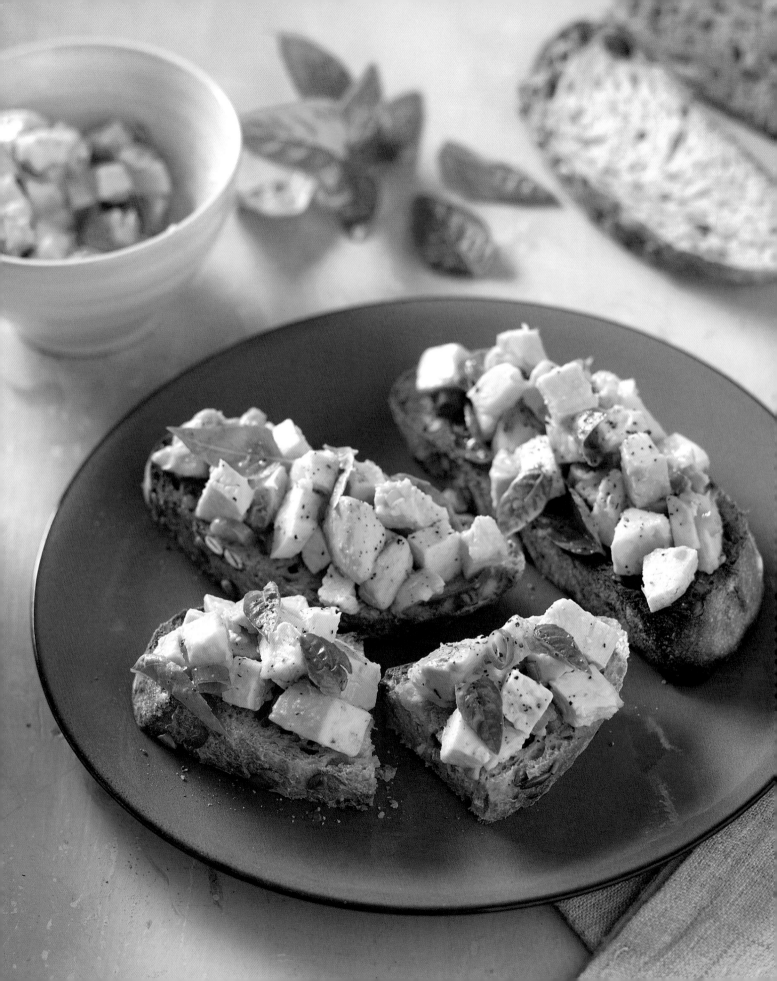

Chicken and avocado bruschetta

1 bay leaf

6 black peppercorns

1 large boneless, skinless chicken breast
(about 350 g/12 oz)

1½ tablespoons extra virgin olive oil

grated zest of 1 lemon

1½ tablespoons lemon juice

freshly ground black pepper

1 ripe avocado, diced

1 spring onion (scallion), finely chopped

2 tablespoons small basil leaves

4 thick slices wholegrain or wholemeal
(whole-wheat) sourdough

1 large garlic clove, halved

PREPARATION 15 minutes, plus 10 minutes cooling
COOKING 20 minutes SERVES 4

EACH SERVING PROVIDES 1718 kJ, 410 kcal, 26 g protein,
28 g fat (6 g saturated fat), 12 g carbohydrate
(1 g sugars), 7 g fibre, 158 mg sodium

Avocado is one of the anti-ageing
superfoods due to its good fats and
anti-oxidant substances. Here it is combined with
other ingredients rich in anti-oxidants, such as
citrus, olive oil and garlic, in a satisfying high-
protein snack.

1 Half-fill a medium saucepan with water and add the bay leaf and peppercorns. Cover and simmer 5 minutes. Add chicken, cover and simmer 10 minutes, or until just cooked. Remove chicken from water and transfer to a plate, cover loosely with plastic wrap and set aside in refrigerator to cool 10 minutes.

2 Whisk 1 tablespoon oil, lemon zest, lemon juice and pepper to taste in a large bowl. Finely dice chicken and add to bowl with avocado, spring onion and basil leaves. Combine gently with a spoon.

3 Preheat grill (broiler) to high. Rub both sides of bread thoroughly with garlic. Drizzle over remaining oil. Toast bread under grill 1–2 minutes each side, until lightly browned.

4 Spoon chicken mixture over toast and serve.

COOK'S TIP You can use bought roasted or barbecued chicken if you prefer. You can make the chicken mixture up to 6 hours before you need it and store in the refrigerator.

Pumpkin and ricotta fritters with capsicum and red onion relish

500 g (1 lb) pumpkin (winter squash),
 peeled, seeds removed, cut into
 1 cm (½ inch) chunks
2 teaspoons light olive oil, plus extra, for
 frying
¼ cup (60 ml) buttermilk
2 eggs
½ cup (125 g) low-fat ricotta
2 tablespoons chopped fresh sage
½ teaspoon ground cumin
½ cup (75 g) plain (all-purpose) flour
freshly ground black pepper

Capsicum and red onion relish

2 tablespoons currants
1¼ tablespoons aged balsamic vinegar
2 red capsicums (bell peppers), quartered,
 seeds removed
1½ tablespoons extra virgin olive oil
1 large red onion, halved, thinly sliced
½ teaspoon soft brown sugar
freshly ground black pepper

PREPARATION 25 minutes, plus 10 minutes cooling
COOKING 40 minutes SERVES 4 (makes 16 fritters)

EACH SERVING PROVIDES 1307 kJ, 312 kcal, 13 g protein,
15 g fat (4 g saturated fat), 30 g carbohydrate
(12 g sugars), 4 g fibre, 108 mg sodium

> This dish is very colourful, reflecting the great range of different anti-oxidants that it provides. Buttermilk and ricotta are both low in fat and good sources of calcium and protein.

1 To make the relish, preheat grill (broiler) or chargrill pan to high. Put currants and vinegar in a small bowl and leave to soak. Put capsicum quarters on grill tray or chargrill and grill, turning occasionally, 5–10 minutes, or until skin is blackened and blistered. When capsicums are cool enough to handle, peel off skin and cut flesh into thin strips.

2 While capsicum is cooling, heat 1 tablespoon oil in a medium frying pan over medium heat. Add onion and cook, stirring often, 10 minutes, or until soft and lightly browned. Add sugar, currants and half the soaking vinegar. Cook, stirring, 2 minutes, then transfer to a bowl. Add remaining soaking vinegar, remaining oil, capsicum strips and pepper to taste and mix well. Set aside.

3 Meanwhile, preheat oven to 180°C (350°F/Gas 4) and line a baking tray with baking paper (baking sheet with parchment paper). Toss pumpkin in 2 teaspoons oil and spread on tray in a single layer. Bake 15 minutes, then leave to cool 10 minutes.

4 Put buttermilk, eggs, ricotta, sage and cumin in a medium bowl and whisk until combined. Whisk in flour and pepper to taste until combined. Add pumpkin and gently fold through.

5 Heat a large non-stick frying pan over medium heat. Lightly grease with oil. Add 4 individual heaped tablespoons of batter to pan and spread out to form 4 fritters; make sure the pumpkin pieces are not heaped up. Cook 2 minutes, or until browned. Turn and cook a further 2 minutes until the other side is browned. Transfer to a plate and keep warm. Repeat to use up remaining mixture.

6 Serve warm fritters with the relish.

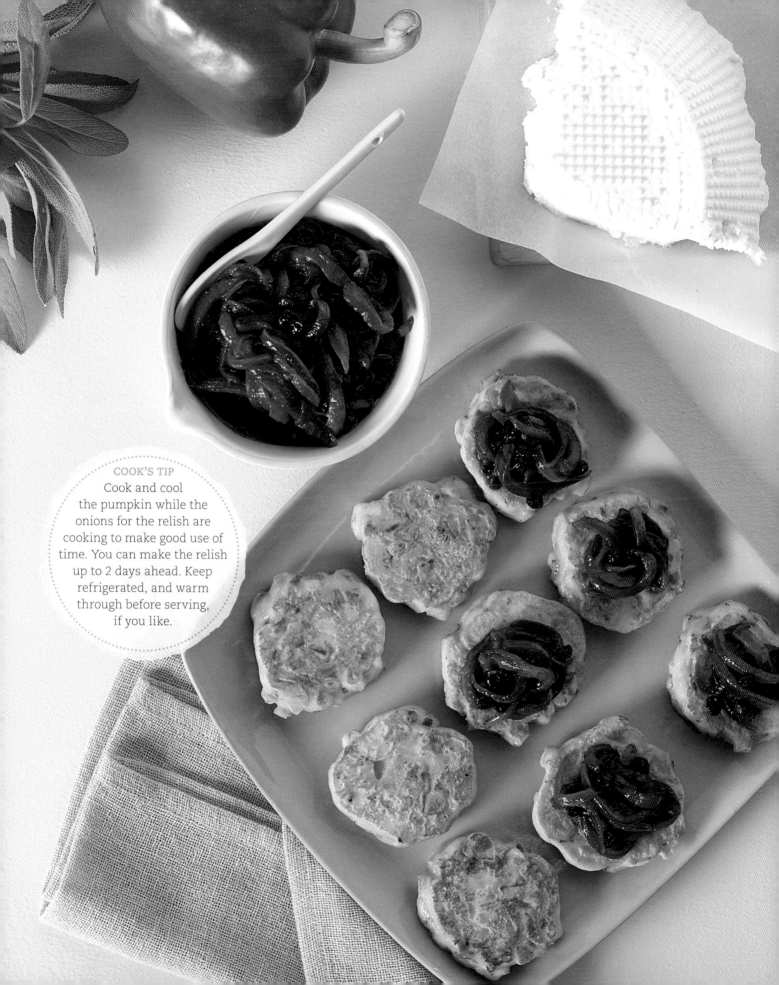

COOK'S TIP
Cook and cool
the pumpkin while the
onions for the relish are
cooking to make good use of
time. You can make the relish
up to 2 days ahead. Keep
refrigerated, and warm
through before serving,
if you like.

Grilled vegetables with romesco sauce

1 red, 1 yellow and 1 green capsicum
    (bell pepper), quartered, seeds removed
1 medium eggplant (aubergine), cut into
    5 mm (¼ inch) slices
1 large zucchini (courgette), cut lengthwise
    into 3 mm (⅛ inch) slices
olive oil, for brushing

Romesco sauce

½ cup (80 g) blanched almonds, toasted
½ cup (70 g) hazelnuts, toasted,
    skins removed
½ large red chilli
3 cloves garlic, crushed
2 large ripe tomatoes (about 375 g/¾ lb in
    total), skins removed, roughly chopped
¼ teaspoon smoked paprika
2 tablespoons extra virgin olive oil
1 tablespoon red wine vinegar
freshly ground black pepper

PREPARATION 20 minutes
COOKING 20 minutes SERVES 4

EACH SERVING PROVIDES 1543 kJ, 368 kcal, 10 g protein,
33 g fat (3 g saturated fat), 9 g carbohydrate
(9 g sugars), 8 g fibre, 12 mg sodium

1 Preheat chargrill pan or grill (broiler) to high. Put capsicum quarters on chargrill or under grill, skin side towards the heat source, and cook, turning occasionally, 5–10 minutes, or until skin is blackened and blistered. When cool enough to handle, peel off skin and cut flesh into thin strips.

2 While capsicums are cooling, brush eggplant slices and zucchini slices with a little oil and grill in batches 2–3 minutes on each side, or until lightly browned and tender.

3 To make the romesco sauce, put almonds and hazelnuts in a food processor or blender and process until finely ground. Add the chilli and garlic and process until finely chopped. Add tomatoes, paprika, oil, vinegar and pepper to taste and process to a paste. Transfer to a serving bowl.

4 Cut eggplant slices in half. Put eggplant, zucchini and capsicums in a serving bowl. Toss gently to combine, then serve with the bowl of romesco sauce.

COOK'S TIP The romesco sauce and grilled vegetables can be made the day before and stored in the refrigerator. Serve at room temperature.

The variety of grilled vegetables of different colours in this recipe, served Italian-style with a romesco sauce, blends anti-oxidant-rich ingredients such as garlic, tomato, hazelnuts and almonds with olive oil.

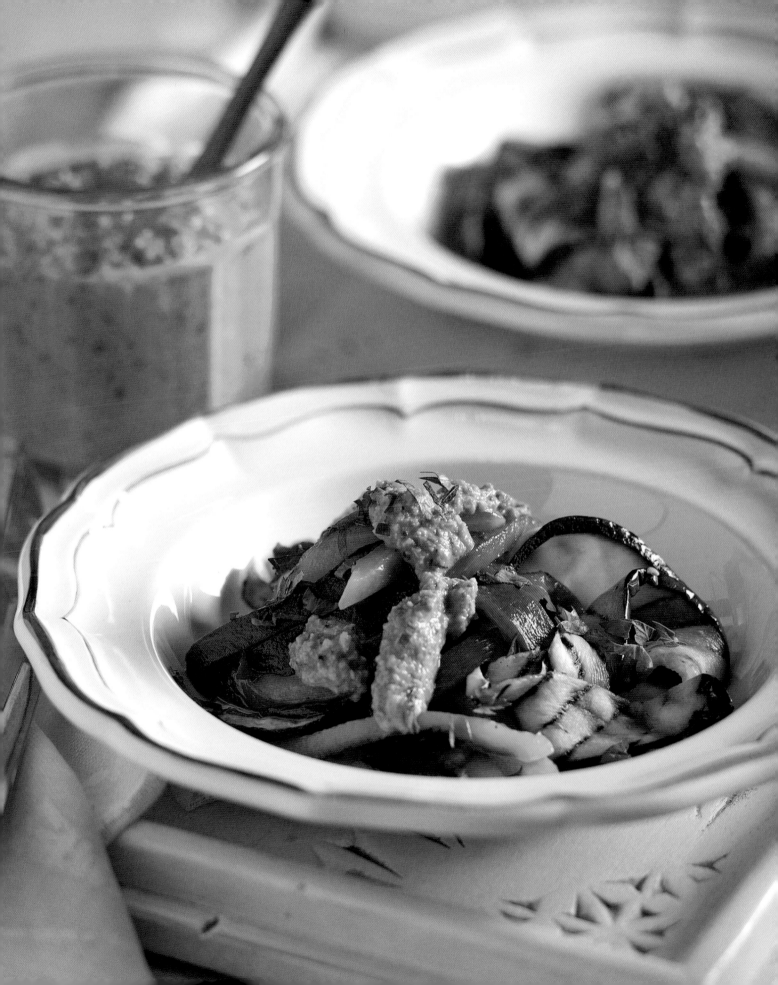

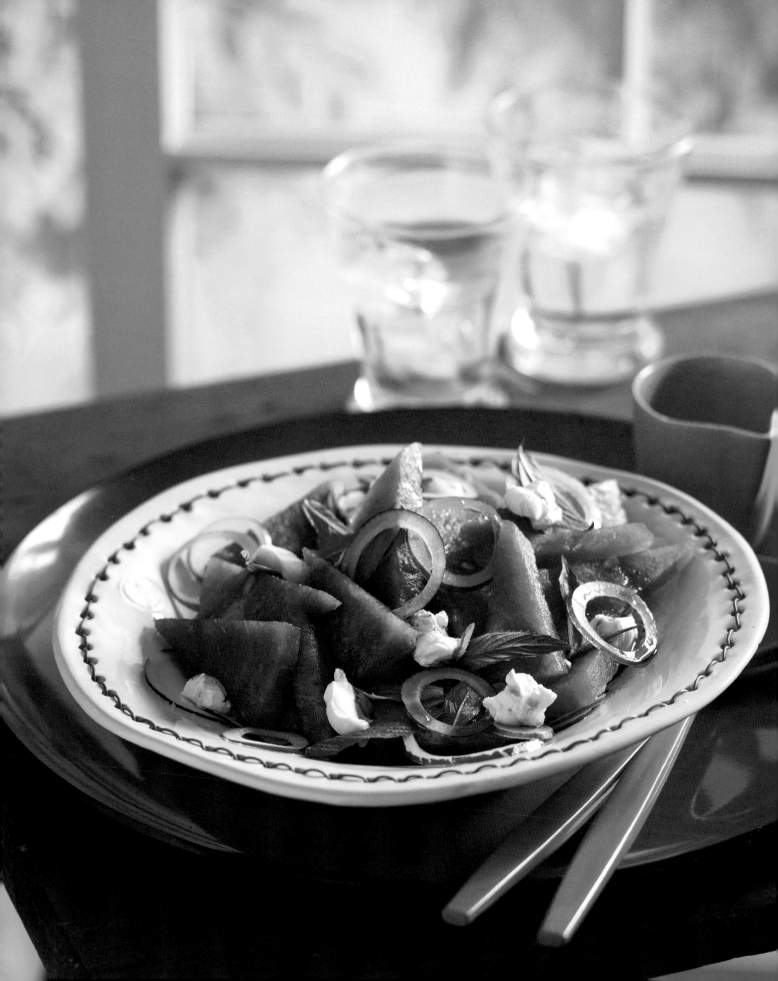

Watermelon, mint, red onion and labna salad

1.5 kg (3 lb) seedless watermelon, rind removed
½ small red onion, very thinly sliced, rings separated
¼ cup (5 g) fresh mint leaves
1 tablespoon extra virgin olive oil
1 tablespoon balsamic vinegar
freshly ground black pepper
100 g (3½ oz) labna or soft goat's cheese

PREPARATION 10 minutes SERVES 4

EACH SERVING PROVIDES 698 kJ, 167 kcal, 3 g protein, 7 g fat (2 g saturated fat), 22 g carbohydrate (22 g sugars), 2 g fibre, 58 mg sodium

This Greek-style salad combines a variety of anti-oxidants from the melon, onion, mint and olive oil, with high-protein, high-calcium labna.

1 Cut watermelon crosswise into 1 cm (½ inch) slices, then cut into wedges about 4 cm (1½ inches) wide. Remove and discard any visible seeds.

2 Arrange watermelon wedges in a large shallow bowl. Scatter onion and all but a few mint leaves over the top. Put oil, vinegar and a good grind of pepper in a jug and whisk to combine. Drizzle over salad.

3 Crumble labna or goat's cheese over salad and season with pepper. Scatter remaining mint leaves over the top and serve.

COOK'S TIP This salad is best assembled close to serving time, although the individual components can be prepared 2 hours beforehand.

You can make your own labna, or yogurt cheese, as described in Yogurt cheese on toast, see pages 42–43.

Baked tofu squares with tomato relish

300 g (10 oz) firm tofu
2 tablespoons plain (all-purpose) flour
freshly ground black pepper
olive oil, for brushing

Tomato relish

1 tablespoon olive oil
1 small brown (yellow) onion, finely chopped
1 teaspoon ground coriander
½ teaspoon ground cumin
½ teaspoon mild paprika
350 g (12 oz) ripe tomatoes, finely chopped
2 teaspoons balsamic vinegar
¼ cup (15 g) chopped fresh coriander
   (cilantro) leaves and stems

PREPARATION 25 minutes
COOKING 25 minutes SERVES 4

EACH SERVING PROVIDES 686 kJ, 164 kcal, 11 g protein,
10 g fat (1 g saturated fat), 8 g carbohydrate
(3 g sugars), 3 g fibre, 16 mg sodium

> This snack of tofu with a richly spiced tomato relish combines the benefits of soy protein with the cancer-protective properties of cooked tomato and the strong anti-oxidant substances in cumin, coriander and paprika.

1 Preheat oven to 220°C (425°F/Gas 7) and line a baking tray with baking paper (baking sheet with parchment paper). Drain tofu on paper towel about 5 minutes to remove surface moisture.

2 Meanwhile, make the tomato relish. Heat oil in a medium saucepan over medium heat. Add onion and cook, stirring, 3 minutes, until soft. Add ground coriander, cumin and paprika and cook, stirring, 30 seconds. Add tomatoes and any tomato juices, along with vinegar. Bring to a simmer, then cook uncovered, stirring frequently, 20 minutes, or until thick. Stir in chopped coriander. Remove from heat and cover to keep warm.

3 Meanwhile, cut tofu into 1 cm (½ inch) slices, then halve each slice crosswise. Combine flour and pepper on a plate and mix together. Toss tofu pieces in flour to coat lightly. Put on prepared tray and brush with olive oil. Bake in oven 25 minutes, or until pale golden on the edges.

4 Serve pieces of warm tofu topped with a spoonful of tomato relish.

COOK'S TIP You can make the relish up to 2 days beforehand, then heat through just before serving. Bake the tofu close to serving time.

Serve with a leafy salad for a light meal.

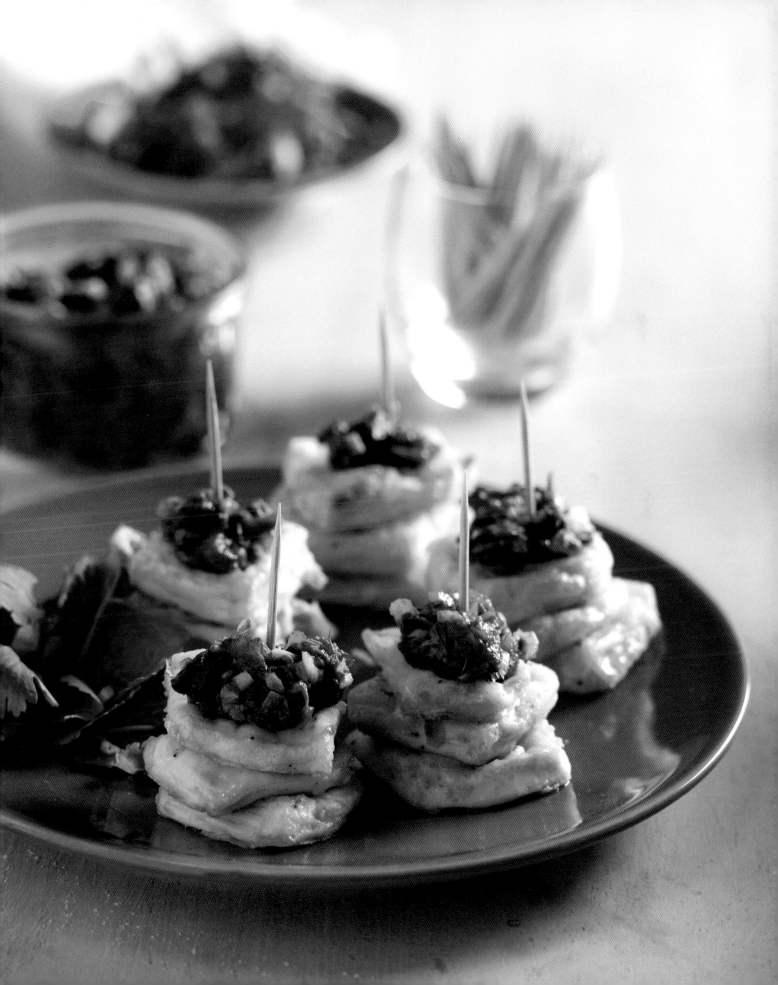

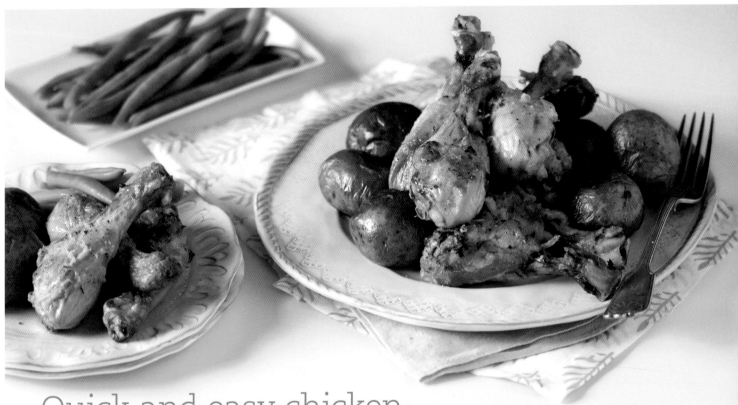

Quick and easy chicken drumsticks

olive oil cooking spray
12 small chicken drumsticks (legs)
    (about 1.5 kg/3 lb), skin removed
1 tablespoon olive oil
3 cloves garlic, crushed
5 cm (2 inch) piece fresh ginger,
    finely grated
juice and finely grated zest of 1 lemon
freshly ground black pepper

PREPARATION 10 minutes
COOKING 40 minutes **SERVES** 4

EACH SERVING PROVIDES 1312 kJ, 313 kcal, 35 g
protein, 17 g fat (4 g saturated fat), 3 g carbohydrate
(1 g sugars), 1 g fibre, 196 mg sodium

1 Preheat oven to 200°C (400°F/Gas 6). Lightly spray a shallow non-stick roasting pan (baking dish) with cooking spray. Put chicken drumsticks in pan.

2 Combine oil, garlic, ginger, lemon zest and juice in a bowl. Pour marinade over chicken and toss until well coated. Season with pepper.

3 Bake chicken 35–40 minutes, or until golden and cooked through. Serve immediately.

COOK'S TIP Serve the chicken drumsticks with roasted small new potatoes and steamed green beans or a green salad.

If you prefer, you could replace lemon zest and juice with orange or lime zest and juice in this recipe.

 This easy high-protein meal is high in anti-oxidants from the garlic, ginger and lemon.

Herby Thai salad

1½ tablespoons light olive oil

500 g (1 lb) lean chicken or beef mince

2 teaspoons finely grated fresh ginger

2 garlic cloves, crushed

2 long green chillies, seeds removed, finely chopped

1 large French shallot (eschalot), halved, thinly sliced

⅓ cup (10 g) fresh coriander (cilantro) leaves

2 tablespoons torn fresh mint

¼ cup (15 g) firmly packed torn fresh basil

1 kaffir lime (makrut) leaf, finely shredded

¼ cup (60 ml) lime juice

2 teaspoons fish sauce

1 tablespoon grated palm sugar, jaggery, dark brown sugar or caster (superfine) sugar

8 lettuce leaves, such as butter or iceberg lettuce, to serve

¼ cup (40 g) chopped unsalted roasted peanuts (groundnuts), to serve

PREPARATION 20 minutes, plus 15 minutes cooling

COOKING 5 minutes SERVES 4

EACH SERVING PROVIDES 1375 kJ, 328 kcal, 27 g protein, 22 g fat (4 g saturated fat), 6 g carbohydrate (4 g sugars), 2 g fibre, 336 mg sodium

1 Heat oil in a wok or large frying pan over high heat. Add chicken or beef, ginger, garlic and chillies, and stir to break up any lumps in the meat. Cook, stirring regularly, 5 minutes, or until just cooked through. Add shallot and mix well. Transfer mixture to a bowl and leave to cool, 15 minutes.

2 Add coriander, mint and basil to meat in bowl. Put kaffir lime leaf, lime juice, fish sauce and sugar in a small bowl and whisk to combine. Pour over meat and herb mixture and toss well.

3 Divide lettuce leaves between four serving plates and fill with meat and herb mixture. Sprinkle with peanuts and serve.

COOK'S TIP If available, use Vietnamese mint and Thai basil instead of regular mint and basil for a more fragrant and authentic flavour. You could replace kaffir lime leaf with 1 teaspoon grated lime zest.

Fish sauce, known as *nam pla* in Thailand and *nuoc nam* in Vietnam, is available from Asian food stores and large supermarkets.

This salad is based on *larb*, a Thai salad that combines minced or shredded chicken or beef, ginger, garlic, lime juice and plenty of herbs to make a high-protein light meal that is also high in anti-oxidants.

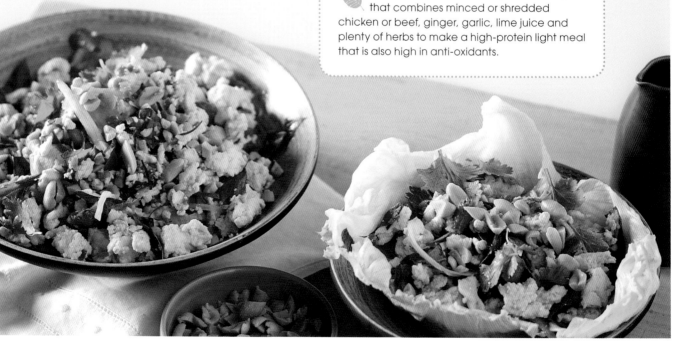

Tuna, chickpea and dill salad

425 g (15 oz) can tuna in springwater,
    well drained, flaked
400 g (14 oz) can chickpeas,
    rinsed and drained
4 gherkins (pickles), finely chopped
4 radishes, finely sliced
1 large celery stalk, thinly sliced
1 tablespoon baby capers, rinsed and
    squeezed dry
1 tablespoon chopped fresh dill
2 large hard-boiled (hard-cooked) eggs,
    halved
2 tablespoons fresh chervil or fresh small
    flat-leaf (Italian) parsley leaves

Dressing

1½ tablespoons extra virgin olive oil
2 tablespoons orange juice
1 tablespoon red wine vinegar
1 teaspoon dijon mustard
freshly ground black pepper

PREPARATION 20 minutes SERVES 4

EACH SERVING PROVIDES 1516 kJ, 362 kcal, 29 g protein,
23 g fat (4 g saturated fat), 10 g carbohydrate
(2 g sugars), 3 g fibre, 704 mg sodium

1 To make the dressing, put oil, orange juice, vinegar and mustard in a small jug. Season with pepper and whisk to combine well. Set aside.

2 Put tuna, chickpeas, gherkins, radishes, celery, capers and dill in a large bowl. Pour dressing over and toss gently to combine.

3 Divide salad among four serving bowls. Top each with an egg half, scatter with chervil or parsley, and serve.

COOK'S TIP The salad can be prepared up to 3 hours in advance, but it is best to toss with the dressing close to serving time.

This high-protein salad is also high in beneficial fats from the tuna and olive oil, as well as providing good amounts of fibre and anti-oxidants.

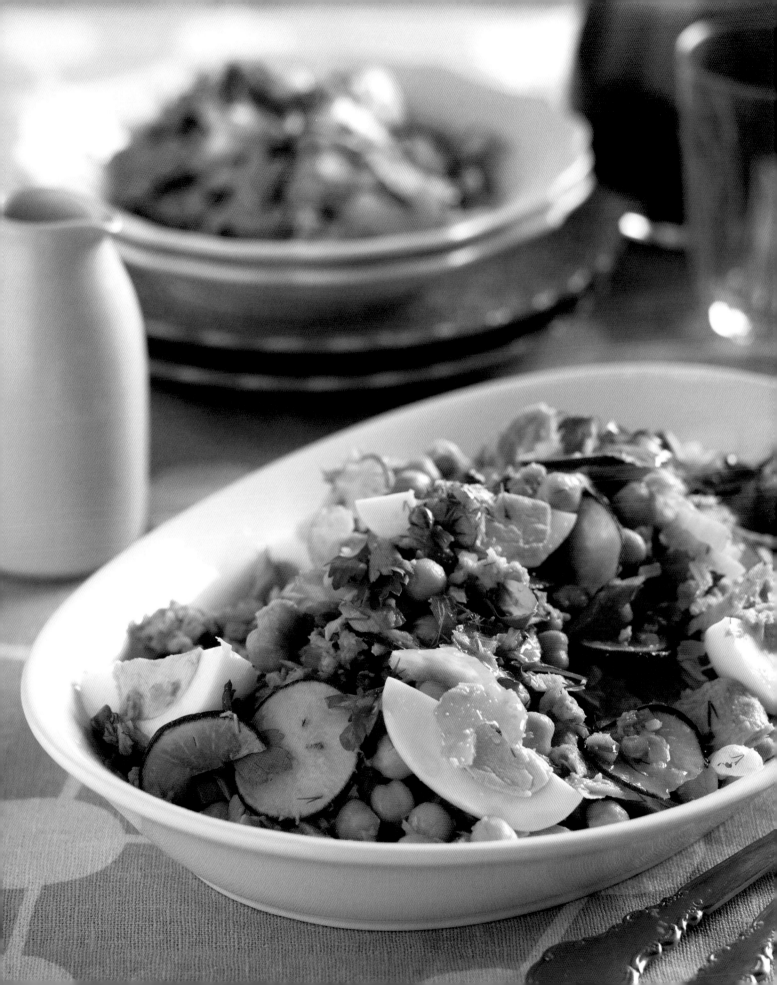

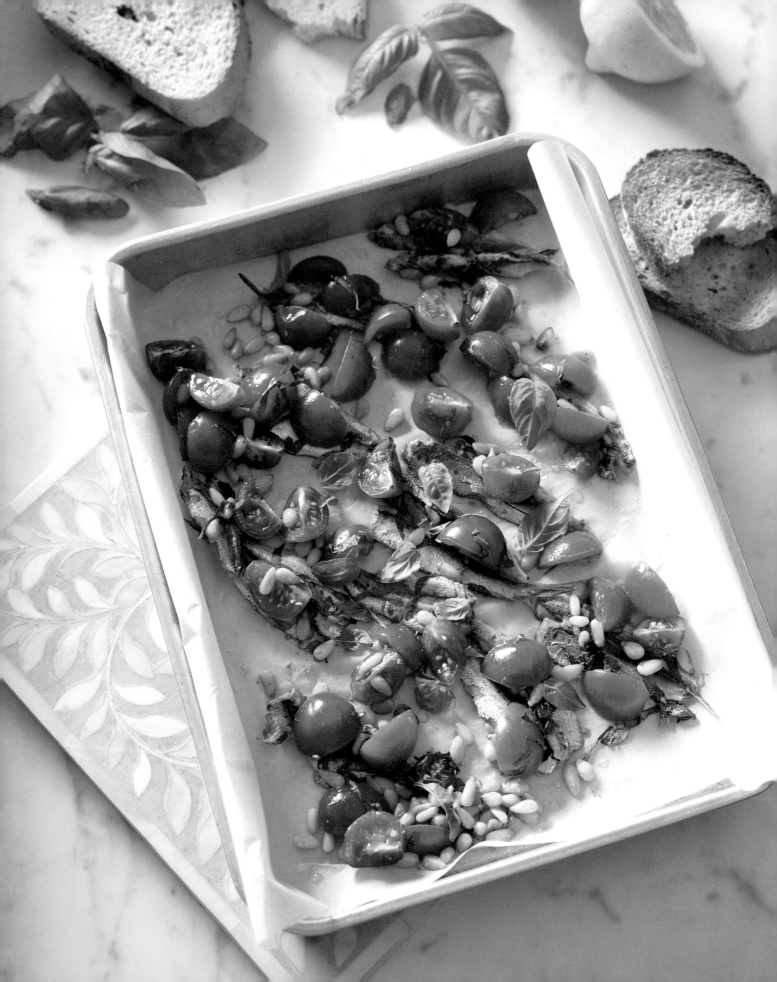

Grilled sardines with cherry tomatoes

12 fresh sardines, butterflied
1 tablespoon extra virgin olive oil
1 tablespoon lemon juice
200 g (7 oz) red cherry tomatoes, quartered
2 tablespoons toasted pine nuts
2 tablespoons shredded fresh basil,
    plus extra small leaves, to serve
4 slices sourdough, toasted
freshly ground black pepper

PREPARATION 15 minutes
COOKING 4 minutes SERVES 4

EACH SERVING PROVIDES 1466 kJ, 350 kcal, 33 g protein,
20 g fat (5 g saturated fat), 8 g carbohydrate (2 g sugars),
2 g fibre, 251 mg sodium

Sardines are one of the richest sources of beneficial omega-3 oils, but the canned version often contains a lot of salt. In this recipe salt is minimised by using fresh sardines. Here, they are combined with anti-oxidants from the tomatoes and basil for a powerfully anti-inflammatory dish that is delicious too.

1 Preheat grill (broiler) to medium–high. Line grill tray with baking (parchment) paper or foil and put sardines on tray. Combine oil and lemon juice in a small bowl, then brush over sardines. Combine tomatoes, pine nuts and shredded basil in a separate bowl and set aside.

2 Grill sardines 2 minutes. Spoon tomato mixture over sardines and grill a further 2 minutes, or until sardines are cooked.

3 Transfer sardines with topping onto toasted sourdough and season with pepper. Sprinkle with extra basil leaves and serve.

COOK'S TIP Ask your fishmonger to butterfly the sardines for you. To do it yourself, put the gutted and cleaned sardine belly side down on a chopping board. Run your thumb along the backbone to press out the backbone. Turn the sardine over, pull out the backbone and discard.

If the sardines are large, cook them a little longer in the first phase of cooking. Add the tomato mixture when the sardines are almost cooked through.

Sardine salad with almonds

juice and grated zest of 1 orange
freshly ground black pepper
2 tablespoons extra virgin olive oil
½ small red onion, thinly sliced
4 cups (180 g) mixed salad leaves, baby
   spinach leaves or rocket (arugula)
1 red and 1 yellow capsicum (bell pepper),
   seeds removed, cut into flat pieces
2 x 110 g (3½ oz) cans sardines in springwater, drained
¼ cup (40 g) raw almonds, sliced

PREPARATION 15 minutes
COOKING 10 minutes SERVES 2

EACH SERVING PROVIDES 1993 kJ, 476 kcal, 24 g
protein, 37 g fat (5 g saturated fat), 12 g carbohydrate
(12 g sugars), 5 g fibre, 111 mg sodium

> High in omega-3 oils from the sardines, this salad is also rich in anti-oxidants, thanks to the orange, almonds and salad greens.

1 Preheat grill (broiler) or chargrill pan to high. Put orange juice, zest and pepper in a salad bowl and whisk together. Continue whisking while gradually adding oil. Add onion and mixed salad leaves, baby spinach leaves or rocket to bowl and toss to coat.

2 Put capsicums on grill rack or chargrill pan and cook 8–10 minutes, turning several times, until skin is charred and flesh is tender.

3 Meanwhile, with a knife, split sardines lengthwise and remove backbones.

4 Allow capsicums to cool, then peel off skin and slice flesh into long strips. Stir capsicums and sardines into salad, scatter over almonds and serve.

COOK'S TIP You could use fresh sardine fillets for this recipe. After the capsicums are cooked in step 2, briefly grill or chargrill 3–4 fillets per person, 2 minutes on one side only.

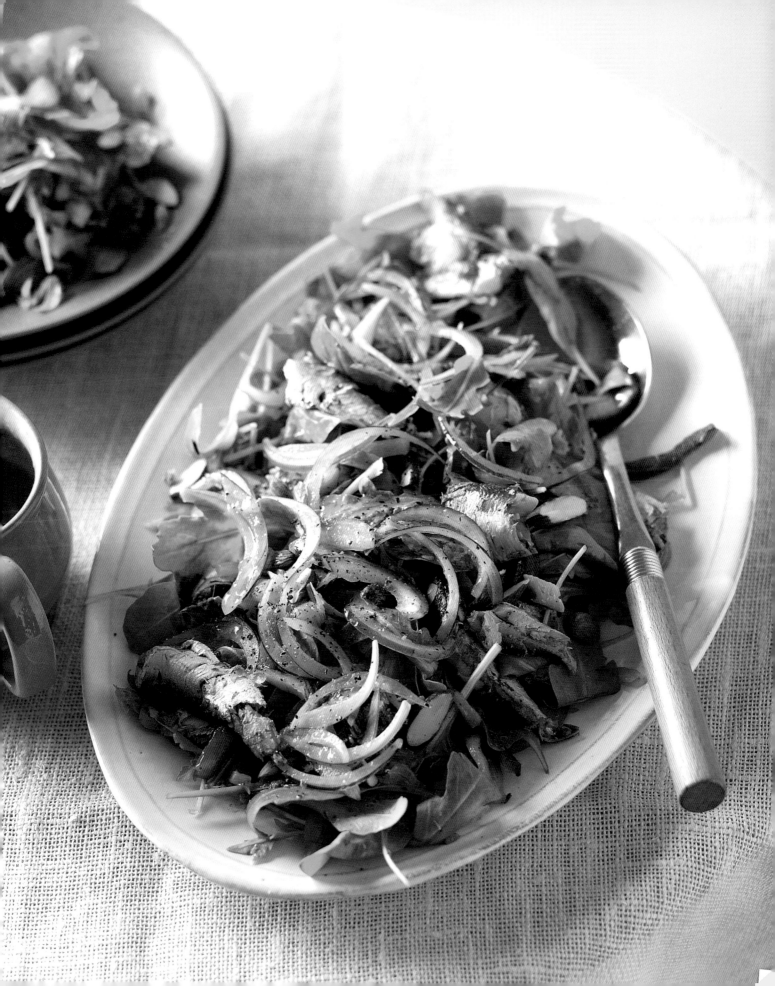

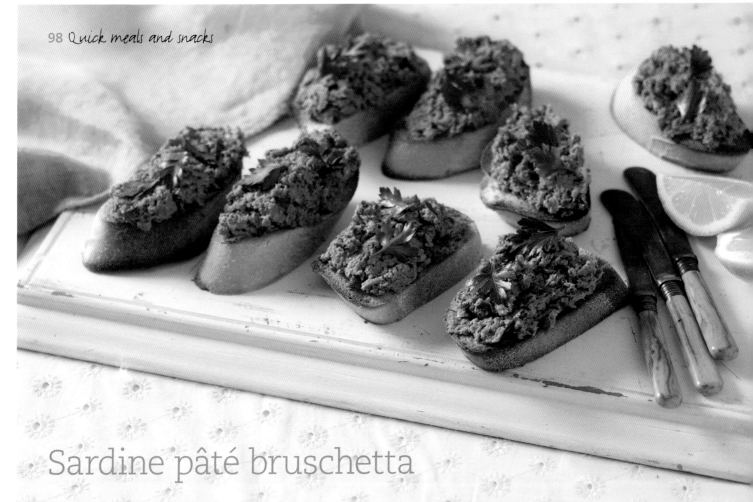

Sardine pâté bruschetta

2 cloves garlic
few grains coarse salt
2 x 210 g (7 oz) cans sardines in oil
    or springwater, drained
⅓ cup (7 g) fresh flat-leaf (Italian) parsley,
    finely chopped, extra leaves for garnish
finely grated zest of 1 lemon
2 tablespoons lemon juice
2 tablespoons extra virgin olive oil
8 thick slices wholegrain or sourdough
    baguette, toasted or grilled
freshly ground black pepper
1 lemon, quartered, to serve

PREPARATION 10 minutes   **SERVES** 4

EACH SERVING PROVIDES 1838 kJ, 439 kcal, 27 g protein,
25 g fat (6 g saturated fat), 21 g carbohydrate (2 g sugars),
11 g fibre, 725 mg sodium

1 Pound garlic with salt in a mortar, until smooth. Add sardines, parsley, lemon zest and juice and continue to pound until it forms a spreadable consistency. Gradually drizzle in oil while mixing the pâté briskly until oil is fully incorporated.

2 Spread pâté on slices of toast. Top with parsley. Season with pepper and serve with lemon quarters on the side.

COOK'S TIP If you like spicy food, add 1 long red chilli, finely chopped, to the sardine mixture after pounding. Depending on how hot you like it, either remove the seeds or leave them in.

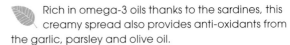 Rich in omega-3 oils thanks to the sardines, this creamy spread also provides anti-oxidants from the garlic, parsley and olive oil.

Broad bean bruschetta

1 kg (2 lb) broad (fava) bean pods, shelled,
   or 500 g (1 lb) frozen
3 tablespoons extra virgin olive oil
3 large cloves garlic, crushed
1/4 cup (5 g) fresh flat-leaf (Italian) parsley,
   finely chopped
10 fresh mint leaves, finely chopped
8 thick slices wholegrain or sourdough
   baguette, toasted or grilled
freshly ground black pepper
fresh or dried oregano leaves, to serve

PREPARATION 10 minutes
COOKING 5 minutes **SERVES** 4

EACH SERVING PROVIDES 2060 kJ, 492 kcal, 25 g protein,
20 g fat (3 g saturated fat), 50 g carbohydrate
(1 g sugars), 22 g fibre, 335 mg sodium

> Broad beans are high in protein and
> heart-protective fibre. In this recipe they
> are combined with garlic, herbs and olive oil,
> which are all rich in anti-oxidants.

1 Bring a medium saucepan of water to boil. Add broad beans and cook 4–5 minutes (2–3 minutes if frozen), until tender. Drain, cover with cold water and stand until cool enough to handle.

2 Meanwhile, add 1 tablespoon oil to a large saucepan and gently fry garlic 1 minute, or until translucent. Remove from heat and allow to cool.

3 Peel skins off broad beans and add to garlic in the pan. Add parsley, mint and remaining oil and mash roughly with a fork until beans are broken up and all ingredients are well combined.

4 Spread mixture thickly on slices of toast. Season with pepper and scatter over oregano.

COOK'S TIP Traditionally called riganatha, this is a Greek version of bruschetta, and it is named after the oregano (*rigani* in Greek) that is always part of this dish – the other ingredients can be varied according to the season. Try 400 g (14 oz) can cannellini beans or chickpeas, rinsed and drained, instead of the broad beans, or use a different combination of herbs.

All except young tender broad beans need to be double-podded: that is, they are shelled (the outer pod is removed), then after blanching the individual beans are peeled to remove the tough grey membrane.

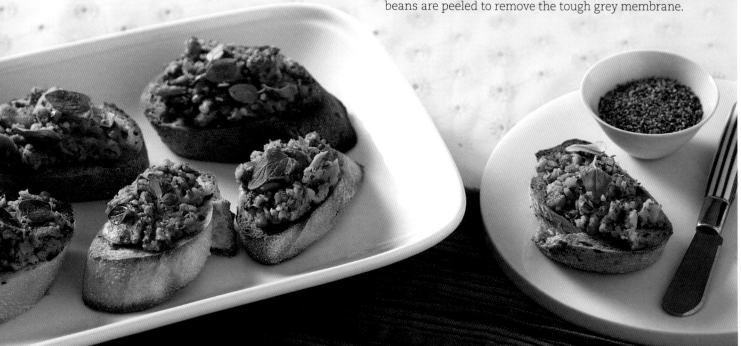

Quinoa cranberry salad

1½ cups (300 g) quinoa, rinsed and drained,
    or brown rice
½ cup (60 g) dried cranberries
½ cup (75 g) mixed seeds, such as pepitas
    (pumpkin seeds) and sunflower seeds
400 g (14 oz) can mixed beans,
    rinsed and drained
½ cup (15 g) roughly chopped fresh flat-leaf
    (Italian) parsley
1½ tablespoons balsamic vinegar
2 tablespoons extra virgin olive oil
freshly ground black pepper

PREPARATION 10 minutes
COOKING 15 minutes SERVES 4

EACH SERVING PROVIDES 1942 kJ, 464 kcal, 17 g protein,
13 g fat (2 g saturated fat), 71 g carbohydrate (5 g sugars),
13 g fibre, 289 mg sodium

Quinoa is a high-protein grain that originated in South America. The Incas recognised its nutritional value, calling it 'the mother of all grains'. Unlike most other plant proteins, quinoa contains 'complete' protein, meaning that it does not need to be combined with other foods in order to be useful as a building block in the body. White, red and black quinoa are available, so use a mixture for added colour.

1 Put quinoa or brown rice and 3 cups (750 ml) water in a small saucepan over high heat and bring to a boil. Reduce heat to low, then cover and simmer until all the water is absorbed, about 15 minutes (or 30 minutes if using brown rice).

2 Meanwhile, put cranberries in a small heatproof bowl, cover with boiling water and soak 10 minutes. Put mixed seeds in a frying pan over medium heat and cook, stirring occasionally, 3–4 minutes, or until they start to brown. Tip into a salad bowl.

3 Drain cranberries. Add to salad bowl with mixed beans, parsley and quinoa or rice, and stir to mix well.

4 Put vinegar, oil and pepper to taste in a small bowl and whisk together, then stir dressing through salad. Serve immediately, or refrigerate until required.

COOK'S TIP You can use couscous instead of quinoa and replace the mixed seeds with toasted walnuts or pine nuts. Add mint or spring onions (scallions).

Rinse quinoa well before use, to remove the bitter-tasting saponin layer from the surface of the grains.

If time permits, reserve the liquid from the soaking cranberries and add it to the quinoa during cooking.

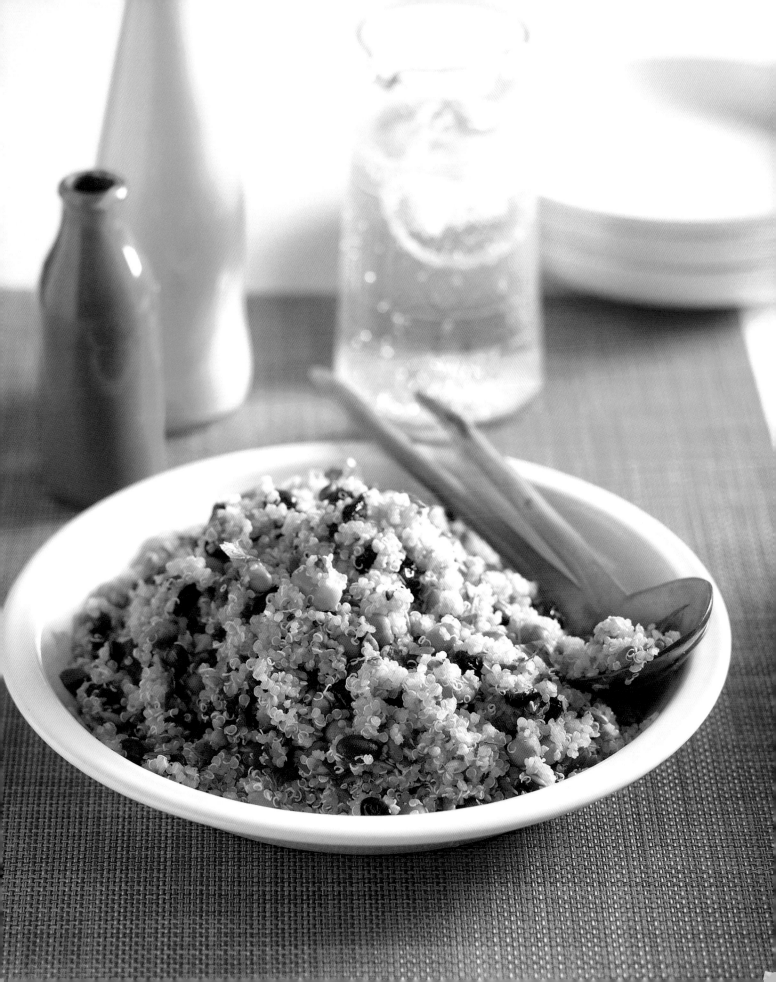

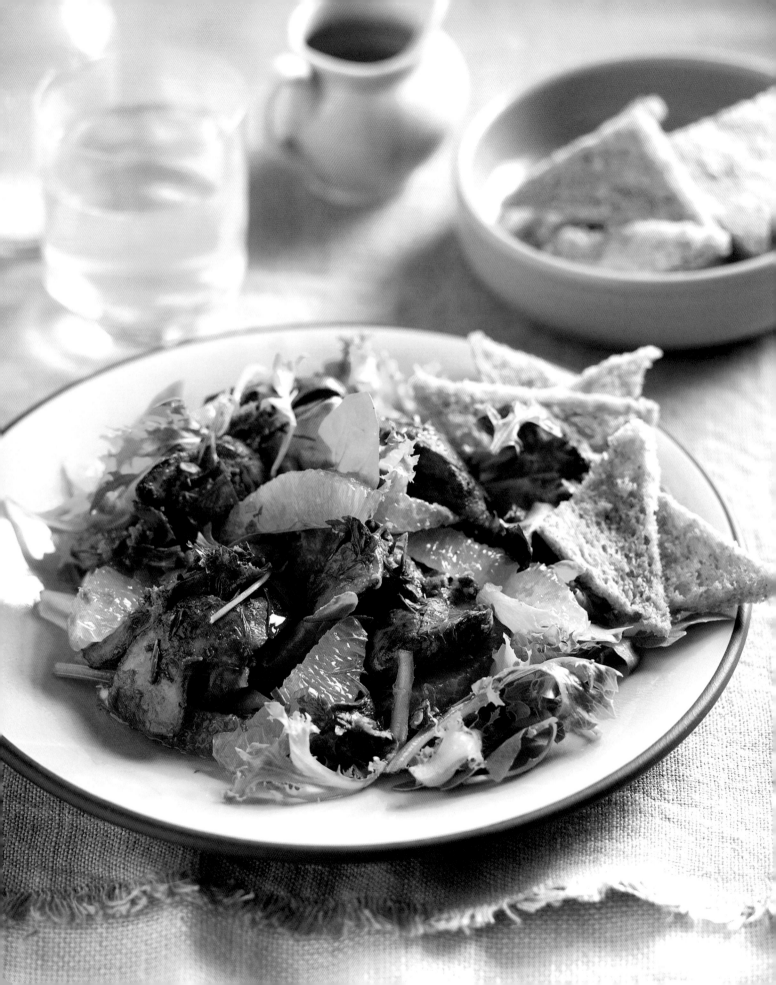

Chicken liver salad

8 thin slices wholemeal (whole-wheat)
   bread, crusts removed
olive oil cooking spray
2 large oranges
1 tablespoon olive oil
500 g (1 lb) chicken livers, sinew discarded,
   halved if large
½ cup (15 g) roughly chopped fresh
   flat-leaf (Italian) parsley
freshly ground black pepper
125 g (4 oz) mixed salad leaves

PREPARATION 15 minutes
COOKING 20 minutes SERVES 4

EACH SERVING PROVIDES 2188 kJ, 523 kcal, 35 g protein,
17 g fat (3 g saturated fat), 56 g carbohydrate
(12 g sugars), 10 g fibre, 695 mg sodium

> This dish provides the nutrient-rich benefits
> of liver, combined with the high levels of
> anti-oxidants found in oranges, parsley and
> many salad greens.

1 Preheat oven to 200°C (400°F/Gas 6). Line a large baking tray with baking paper (baking sheet with parchment paper). Cut each slice of bread into 4 small triangles. Put on prepared tray and spray with cooking spray. Bake 10–15 minutes, or until crisp and golden. Leave to cool.

2 Meanwhile, finely grate zest of oranges and set aside. Remove all skin and pith from oranges. Using a small sharp knife, remove segments from oranges, working over a bowl to catch the juice. Put segments on a plate and set juice aside.

3 Heat 1 teaspoon oil in a non-stick frying pan over medium heat. Add a quarter of the livers and cook 1–2 minutes on each side, or until browned and almost cooked through. Transfer to a plate, cover and keep warm. Repeat with remaining livers, cooking a quarter at a time.

4 Return all livers to pan. Add orange zest and parsley and toss until combined and heated through, 1–2 minutes. Season with pepper, stir through and remove from heat.

5 Arrange salad leaves and orange segments on four serving plates. Top with chicken livers and put toast triangles alongside. Whisk remaining oil and reserved orange juice in a jug. Drizzle over individual salads just before serving.

COOK'S TIP You can buy different combinations of mixed salad leaves in packets at supermarkets and greengrocers.

Seafood salad

¼ cup (35 g) currants
¼ cup (60 ml) lemon juice
2 red capsicums (bell peppers), seeds
    removed, cut into flat pieces
2 teaspoons olive oil
2 stalks celery, leaves reserved, stalks diced
½ cup (60 g) pitted green olives, sliced
2 tablespoons salt-reduced tomato paste
    (concentrated purée)
1 tablespoon capers, rinsed and squeezed
    dry
4 ocean trout fillets (about 150 g/5 oz each)
    or 4 small mackerel or other small oily fish
    (about 200 g/7 oz each), cleaned
olive oil cooking spray
freshly ground black pepper
¼ cup (40 g) raw almonds, toasted,
    roughly chopped

PREPARATION 15 minutes, plus 15 minutes cooling
COOKING 30 minutes SERVES 4

EACH SERVING PROVIDES 1387 kJ, 331 kcal, 44 g protein,
14 g fat (3 g saturated fat), 7 g carbohydrate (5 g sugars),
2 g fibre, 199 mg sodium

This tangy Italian-style sweet–sour vegetable salad is rich in anti-oxidants from the olives, capsicums, almonds and currants, as well as cancer-protective lycopene from the tomato paste. The fish contains omega-3 oils.

1 Soak the currants in lemon juice in a small bowl 20 minutes.

2 Meanwhile, preheat grill (broiler) to high. Put capsicums on a baking tray (sheet) or grill tray and put under grill. Alternatively, put on a chargrill pan preheated to high. Cook 20 minutes, turning often, until skin is blackened and blistered. Transfer to a bowl, cover and stand 15 minutes. When cool enough to handle, peel skin from capsicums and remove seeds and pulp. Roughly chop capsicum flesh.

3 Heat oil in a saucepan over medium heat. Add diced celery and cook 3 minutes, or until softened. Add currants and soaking liquid, capsicums, olives, tomato paste, capers and ¾ cup (180 ml) water. Stir until well combined and mixture comes to a boil. Reduce heat and simmer 10 minutes, or until mixture has thickened.

4 Meanwhile, preheat grill (broiler) or chargrill pan to high. If using the grill, cover grill rack with foil and put mackerel or trout fillets, skin side up first, on rack. Spray with cooking spray and season with pepper. Grill or chargrill 4–5 minutes on each side, or until cooked through.

5 Spoon vegetable mixture onto four serving plates. Top with a grilled trout fillet or mackerel. Sprinkle over almonds, garnish with reserved celery leaves and serve.

COOK'S TIP If you prefer, ask your fishmonger to fillet the mackerel. Cook fillets under a hot grill or on a hot chargrill pan 2–3 minutes on each side, or until cooked through.

These quantities make about 3½ cups of the vegetable mixture.

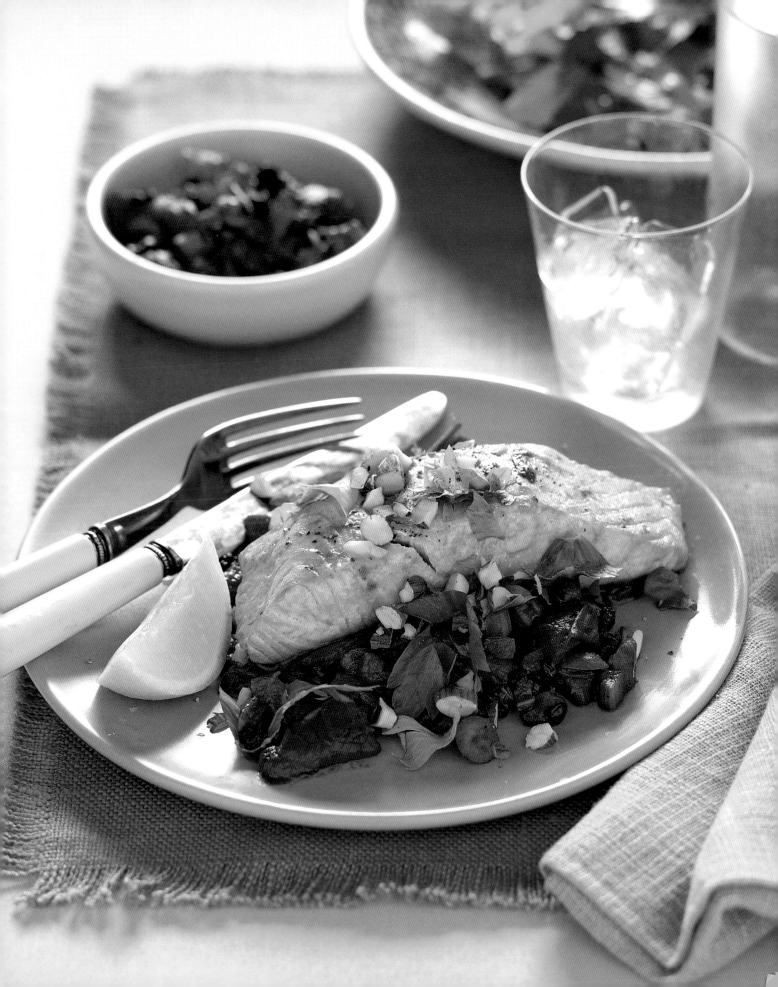

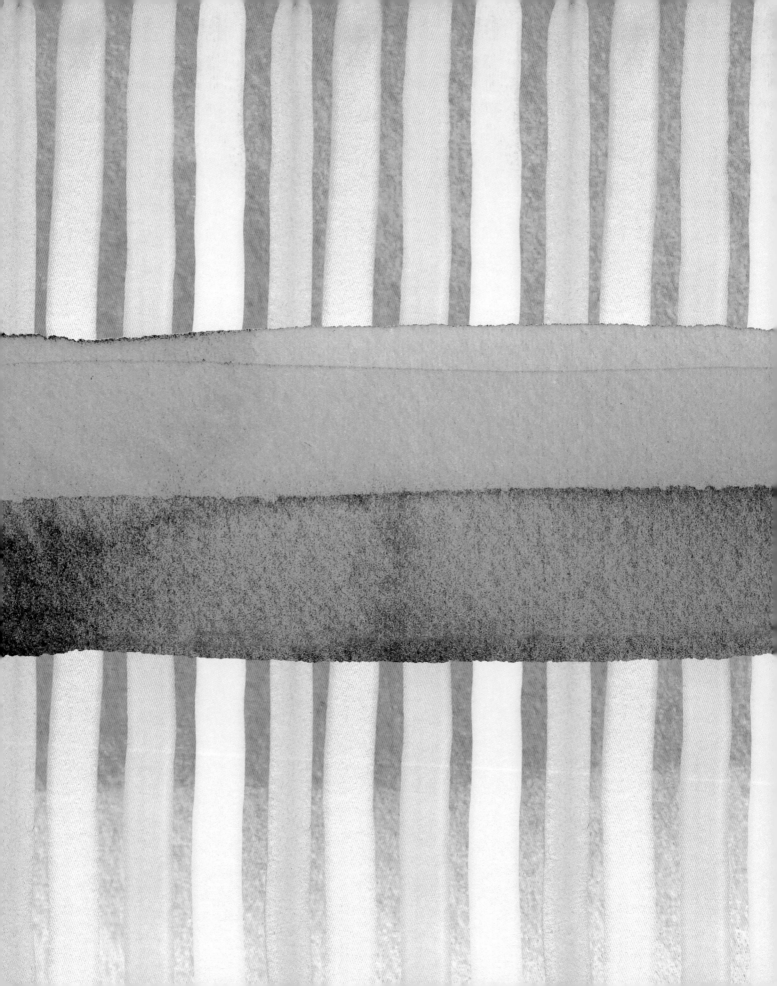

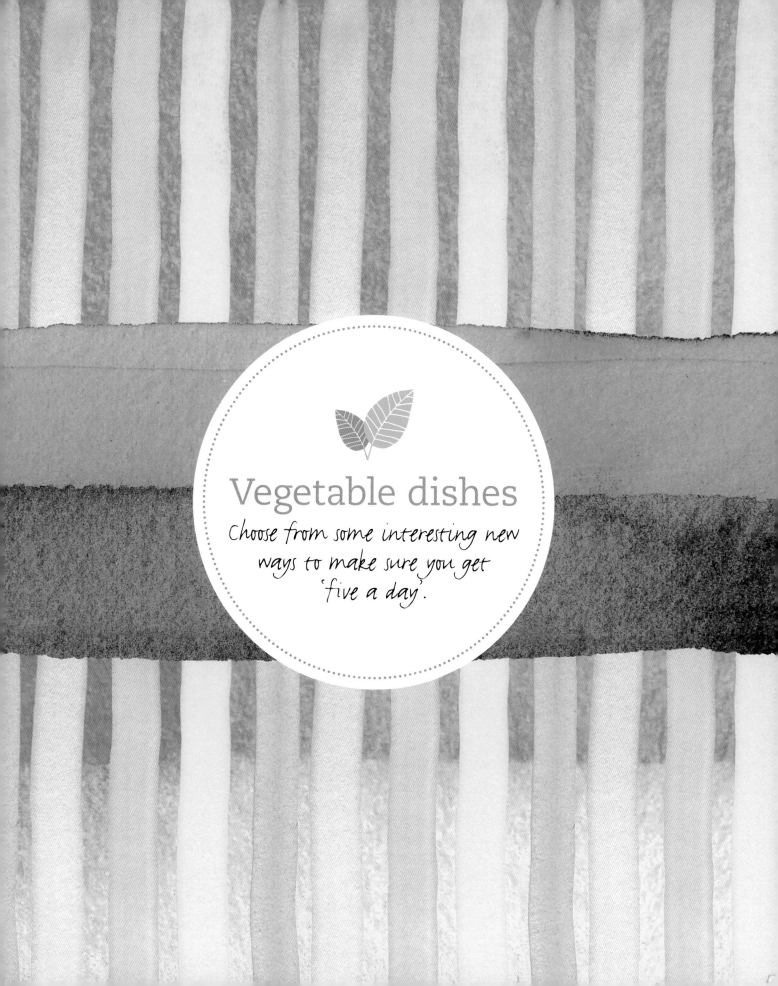

Vegetable dishes

Choose from some interesting new
ways to make sure you get
'five a day'.

Ricotta and spinach gnocchi

2¾ cups (120 g) baby spinach leaves
1¼ cups (300 g) low-fat ricotta
½ cup (50 g) finely grated parmesan
1 egg, lightly beaten
½ cup (75 g) plain (all-purpose) flour
2 teaspoons olive oil
1 brown (yellow) onion, finely chopped
2 cloves garlic, crushed
5 tomatoes (about 750 g/1½ lb), or 800 g
   (28 oz) can tomatoes, roughly chopped
freshly ground black pepper

PREPARATION 20 minutes
COOKING 20 minutes SERVES 4

EACH SERVING PROVIDES 1220 kJ, 291 kcal, 19 g protein,
15 g fat (7 g saturated fat), 21 g carbohydrate
(6 g sugars), 4 g fibre, 362 mg sodium

> This is a great high-protein vegetarian main dish that contains good amounts of calcium from the ricotta and anti-oxidants from the spinach.

1 Put spinach in a heatproof bowl. Cover with boiling water and stand 1 minute. Drain and rinse under cold running water. Using your hands, squeeze as much water as possible out of spinach. Finely chop, then put in a large bowl.

2 Add ricotta, half the parmesan, egg and flour to spinach. Stir until well combined.

3 Heat oil in a non-stick frying pan over medium heat. Add onion and garlic and cook 3 minutes, or until tender. Add tomatoes and ½ cup (125 ml) water. Stir until well combined and mixture comes to a boil. Simmer 15 minutes, or until it forms a thick sauce.

4 Meanwhile, bring a large saucepan of water to a boil. Drop tablespoons of ricotta mixture into boiling water, 8 at a time, and cook 3 minutes, or until gnocchi float to the surface. Remove with a slotted spoon and transfer to a plate. Cover and keep warm while cooking remaining gnocchi.

5 Spoon gnocchi into four serving bowls. Top with tomato sauce and sprinkle over remaining parmesan. Season with pepper and serve.

COOK'S TIP Making your own ricotta is easy, and produces a firmer-textured cheese that works better in this recipe. Simply bring 4 cups (1 litre) low-fat milk to a boil, add 1 tablespoon epsom salts and ¼ cup (60 ml) white vinegar. Stir 3 seconds, then gently simmer 10 minutes. Turn off heat and leave to stand 15 minutes, then pour mixture into a large mesh sieve lined with muslin (cheesecloth) to drain 1–2 hours, or until it reaches the desired consistency.

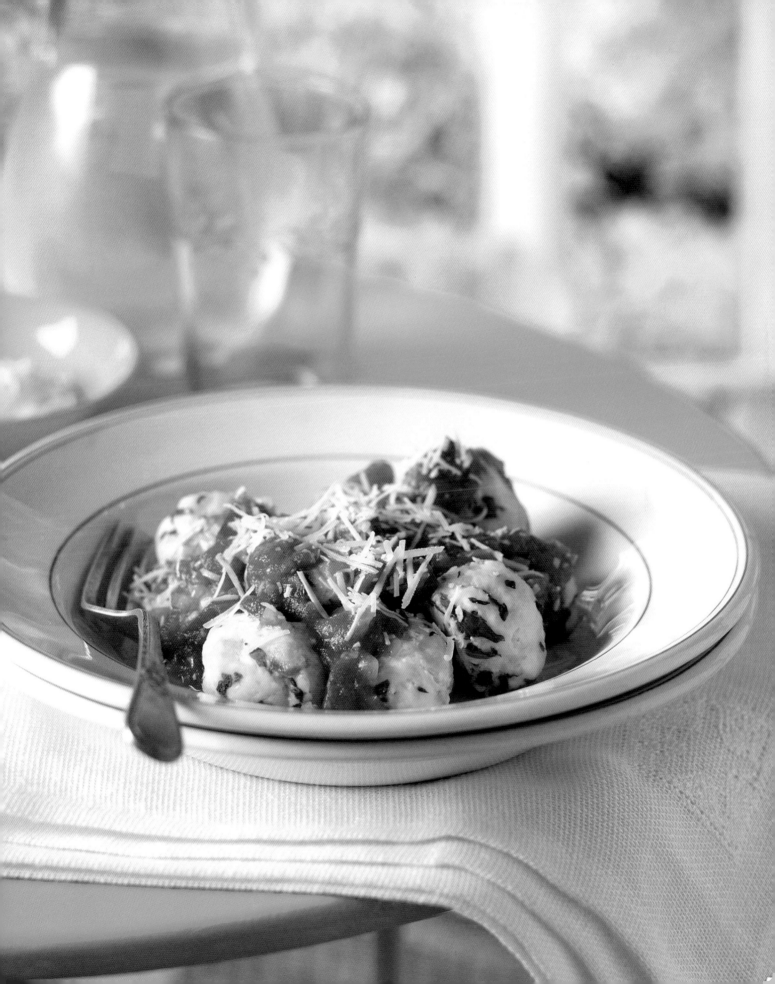

Baby spinach and asparagus mornay

30 g (1 oz) olive oil spread
2 tablespoons plain (all-purpose) flour
¾ cup (180 ml) light evaporated milk
½ cup (125 ml) low-fat milk
⅓ cup (40 g) grated low-fat cheddar
½ cup (60 g) finely grated parmesan
3½ cups (160 g) baby spinach leaves
2 bunches asparagus (300 g/10 oz), trimmed,
   cut into 3 cm (1¼ inch) pieces
4 hard-boiled (hard-cooked) eggs,
   sliced 1 cm (½ inch) thick
freshly ground black pepper

PREPARATION 20 minutes
COOKING 25 minutes SERVES 4

EACH SERVING PROVIDES 1169 kJ, 279 kcal, 22 g protein,
17 g fat (6 g saturated fat), 10 g carbohydrate
(6 g sugars), 2 g fibre, 431 mg sodium

The light evaporated milk and low-fat cheese help to make this a high-protein, low-fat version of the comfort food classic. Both spinach and asparagus are excellent sources of folate, fibre and anti-oxidants, and this dish is also rich in calcium due to the milk and cheeses.

1 Preheat oven to 200°C (400°C/Gas 6). Melt oil spread in a saucepan over medium heat. When melted and foaming, stir in flour. Cook 2 minutes, or until mixture is bubbly. Remove from heat and slowly add evaporated milk and low-fat milk, stirring constantly. Return pan to heat and whisk constantly until mixture comes to a boil. Reduce heat and simmer 2 minutes, still whisking continuously. Add cheddar and half the parmesan and stir until melted, then remove from heat.

2 Put spinach in a large heatproof bowl. Cover with boiling water and stand 1 minute. Drain and rinse under cold running water. Using your hands, squeeze as much water as possible out of spinach. Roughly chop, then put in a separate bowl.

3 Put asparagus in the large heatproof bowl and cover with boiling water. Stand 1 minute. Drain well. Add asparagus and hard-boiled eggs to spinach, and gently mix together to combine well.

4 Transfer mixture to a 6 cup (1.5 litre) shallow gratin dish or ovenproof dish. Spoon cheese sauce over top, sprinkle with remaining parmesan and season with pepper. Bake 20 minutes, or until parmesan is golden on top. Serve immediately.

COOK'S TIP Light evaporated milk gives this dish a creamy effect without adding fat. Replace with low-fat milk if light evaporated milk is not available.

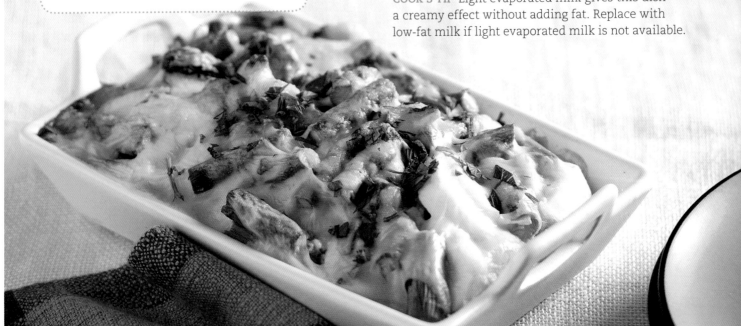

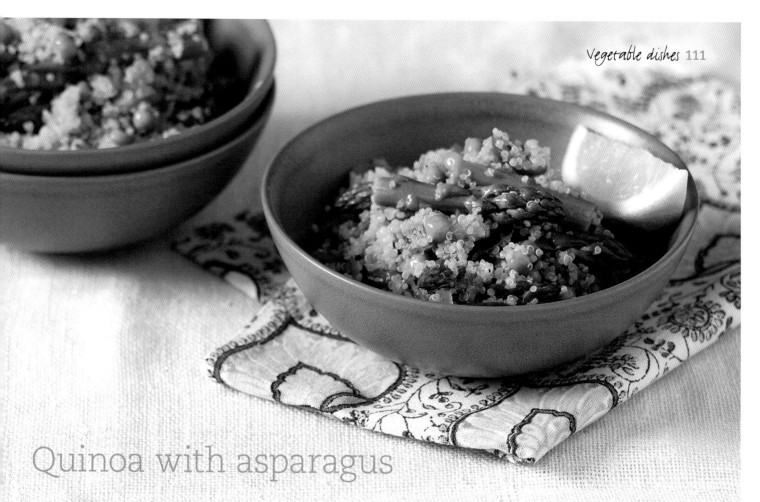

Quinoa with asparagus

1 cup (200 g) quinoa, rinsed and drained,
    or brown rice
1 tablespoon olive oil
1 small red onion, thinly sliced
½ cup (125 ml) homemade or salt-reduced
    vegetable or chicken stock
400 g (14 oz) asparagus spears, trimmed and
    cut into 5 cm (2 inch) pieces
1 cup (150 g) fresh or thawed frozen peas
lemon wedges, to serve

PREPARATION 10 minutes
COOKING 15 minutes **SERVES** 6

EACH SERVING PROVIDES 748 kJ, 179 kcal, 8 g protein,
5 g fat (<1 g saturated fat), 26 g carbohydrate
(2 g sugars), 3 g fibre, 87 mg sodium

1 Put quinoa or brown rice and 2 cups (500 ml) water in a small saucepan over high heat and bring to a boil. Reduce heat to low, then cover and simmer until all water is absorbed, about 15 minutes (or 30 minutes if using brown rice).

2 Meanwhile, heat oil in a large non-stick frying pan over medium heat. Add onion and cook until lightly browned, about 4 minutes. Add stock, asparagus and peas, and cook until crisp but tender, about 5 minutes.

3 Add quinoa and stir to mix well. Serve immediately with lemon wedges on the side.

Quinoa contains more protein than any of the other grains. Unlike many other plant foods, the protein in quinoa is good-quality 'complete' protein that can be readily used by the body without needing to be combined with other foods.

White bean stew

1 tablespoon olive oil
1 brown (yellow) onion, finely chopped
1 large carrot, diced
1 head celeriac (celery root)
(about 1 kg/2 lb), peeled and diced
2 teaspoons mixed dried herbs
3 bay leaves
2 x 400 g (14 oz) cans butterbeans
(lima beans), rinsed and drained
½ cup (15 g) roughly chopped fresh
flat-leaf (Italian) parsley
freshly ground black pepper

PREPARATION 10 minutes
COOKING 1 hour SERVES 4

EACH SERVING PROVIDES 952 kJ, 227 kcal, 11 g protein,
10 g fat (<1 g saturated fat), 24 g carbohydrate
(10 g sugars), 19 g fibre, 568 mg sodium

1 Heat oil in a large deep heavy-based saucepan over medium–high heat. Add onion, carrot and celeriac, and cook, stirring occasionally, 10 minutes, or until soft and golden.

2 Add 3 cups (750 ml) water and stir to mix through. Bring to a boil, then add mixed dried herbs and bay leaves and stir. Reduce heat to medium and simmer, uncovered, 25 minutes, or until vegetables are tender.

3 Add butterbeans and cook 20 minutes, or until beans are soft and mixture has thickened. Add three-quarters of the parsley and stir to combine.

4 Serve seasoned with pepper and sprinkled with remaining parsley.

COOK'S TIP You could replace the celeriac with celery or parsnips.

Serve this stew with steamed basmati or brown rice, or baked or mashed potatoes.

Celeriac is high in fibre and minerals and creates a great savoury celery flavour and a creamy texture without the stringy effect that celery can have.

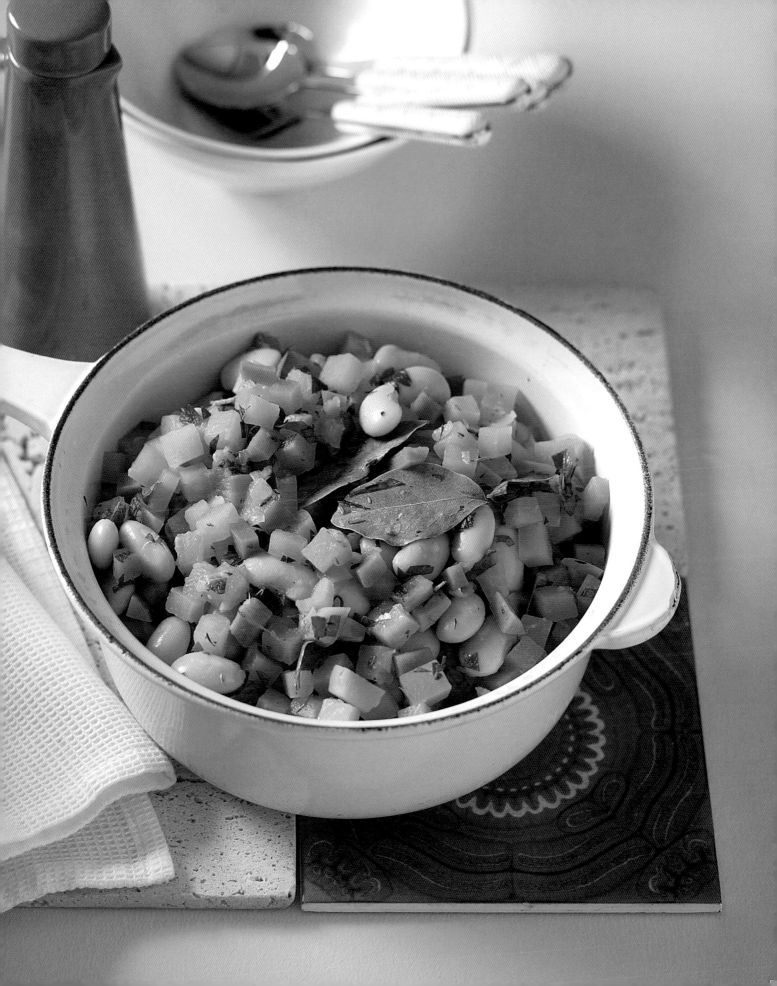

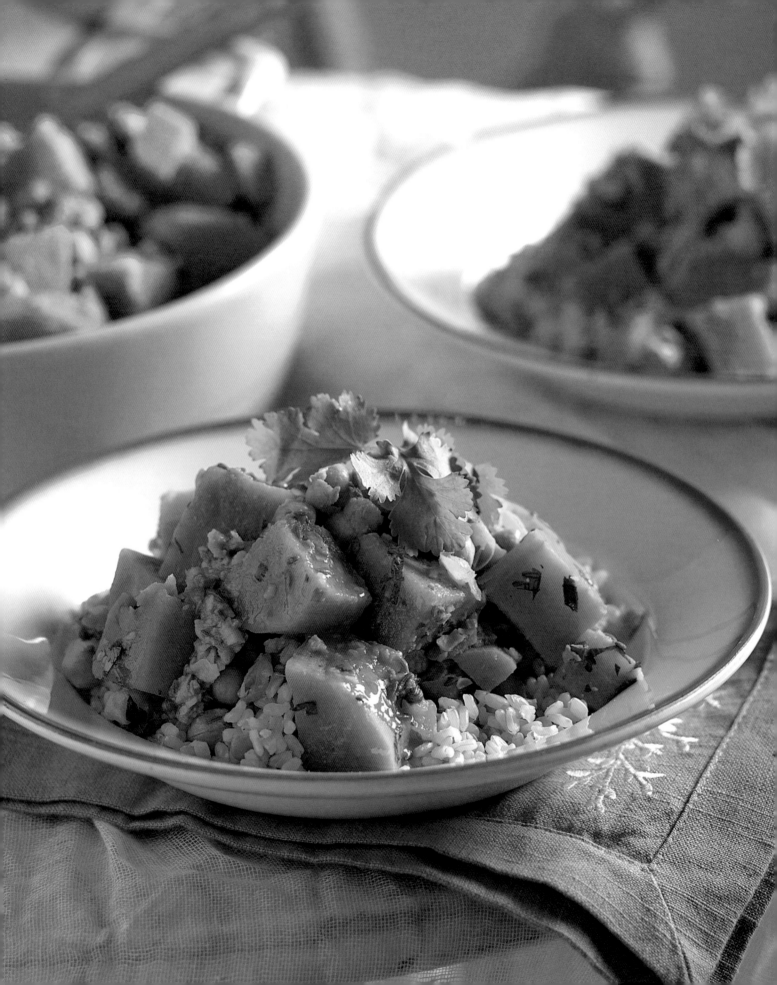

Chickpea, sweet potato and carrot stew

2 cups (450 g) dried chickpeas or 2 x 400 g
(14 oz) cans chickpeas, rinsed and
drained
1 tablespoon olive oil
3 teaspoons cumin seeds
2 teaspoons coriander seeds
3 cm (1¼ inch) piece fresh turmeric, peeled
and finely grated, or 3 teaspoons ground
dried turmeric
roots and stems of 1 bunch (125 g/4 oz) fresh
coriander (cilantro), finely chopped,
plus 4 sprigs fresh coriander, to garnish
2 orange sweet potatoes (kumara)
(about 800 g/1¾ lb), peeled,
cut into small chunks
2 large carrots, cut into small chunks
2 cloves garlic, crushed
finely grated zest of 1 lemon
¼ cup (60 ml) lemon juice

PREPARATION 15 minutes, plus overnight soaking if using
dried beans COOKING 1 hour SERVES 4

EACH SERVING PROVIDES 1391 kJ, 332 kcal, 13 g protein,
8 g fat (1 g saturated fat), 51 g carbohydrate
(14 g sugars), 12 g fibre, 358 mg sodium

1 Put dried beans, if using, in a large bowl and cover well with water. Soak overnight.

2 Drain soaked beans. Put in a large saucepan or pressure cooker, cover with plenty of fresh water and the lid, and boil until tender – about 30 minutes in a saucepan, or 10 minutes in a pressure cooker.

3 Meanwhile, heat oil in a large deep heavy-based saucepan over medium–high heat. Add cumin seeds, coriander seeds, turmeric and fresh coriander roots and stems. Cook 2 minutes, or until aromatic.

4 Add sweet potatoes, carrots and garlic, and stir until combined. Cook 10 minutes, or until softened. Add lemon zest, lemon juice and 2½ cups (625 ml) water. Stir, then bring to a boil. Reduce heat and simmer 25 minutes, or until vegetables are tender.

5 Add cooked or canned chickpeas. Cook 20 minutes, or until chickpeas are very soft and mixture has thickened. Serve garnished with coriander sprigs.

COOK'S TIP Serve with steamed basmati or brown rice, wholegrain quinoa or toasted sourdough.

Fresh turmeric is available from larger supermarkets or Asian food stores.

This stew is rich in anti-oxidants, particularly from the turmeric, and is also high in fibre. Low glycaemic index carbohydrate foods, such as sweet potato and chickpeas, release their energy slowly to keep you feeling satisfied for longer and your blood glucose level stable.

Borscht with caramelised onion toasts

1 tablespoon olive oil
1 brown (yellow) onion, finely chopped
1 carrot, diced
2 large beetroot (beets) (about 500 g/1 lb),
    trimmed and peeled, cut into chunks
2 tomatoes, roughly chopped
2 teaspoons fennel seeds
1 cup (250 g) low-fat thick Greek-style yogurt
1 tablespoon finely chopped fresh dill
3 tablespoons finely snipped fresh chives
freshly ground black pepper

Caramelised onion toasts

1 tablespoon olive oil
2 brown (yellow) onions, thinly sliced
1 tablespoon soft brown sugar
freshly ground black pepper
4 slices wholegrain or rye bread, toasted

PREPARATION 30 minutes
COOKING 1 hour 25 minutes SERVES 4

EACH SERVING PROVIDES 1482 kJ, 354 kcal, 15 g protein,
14 g fat (3 g saturated fat), 39 g carbohydrate
(25 g sugars), 12 g fibre, 289 mg sodium

Beetroot has powerful anti-oxidant
properties as well as being a good source
of folate. Whole rye breads such as pumpernickel
are great for this recipe, and bring extra fibre and
low glycaemic index carbohydrate to the meal.

1 Heat oil in a large deep heavy-based saucepan over medium heat. Add onion, carrot and beetroot, and stir until well combined. Cook, stirring occasionally, 10 minutes, or until onion is softened.

2 Add tomatoes and fennel seeds. Cook, stirring occasionally, 10 minutes, or until tomatoes are soft. Add 6 cups (1.5 litres) water and bring to a boil. Reduce heat and simmer 1 hour, or until the beetroot is tender.

3 Meanwhile, combine yogurt, dill, 2 tablespoons chives and pepper to taste in a small bowl. Cover and refrigerate the herb yogurt until required.

4 While soup is cooking, make the caramelised onion toasts. Heat oil in a non-stick frying pan over medium heat. When hot, add onions and stir. Reduce heat to low and cook, stirring occasionally, 20–25 minutes, or until onions are a rich golden brown. Add sugar and pepper to taste. Stir until well combined and sugar has melted.

5 When beetroot is tender and soup is cooked, use a hand-held stick blender to purée soup until smooth. Alternatively, allow soup to cool a little, then process in a food processor or blender until smooth. Return to pan and heat until boiling.

6 Ladle soup into bowls. Top each with a dollop of herb yogurt and remaining chives. Cut toast into fingers, top with caramelised onions and serve with the soup.

COOK'S TIP Wear disposable gloves when peeling beetroot to prevent your hands turning pink.

You could top the caramelised onion toasts with a little grated cheddar and grill (broil) before serving.

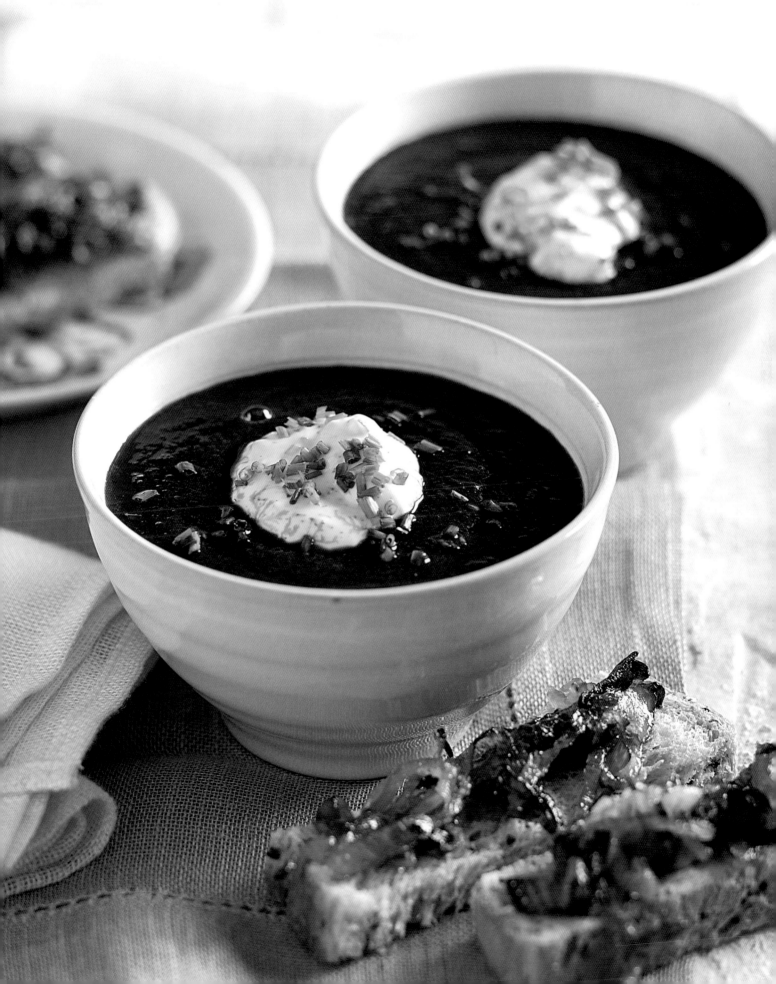

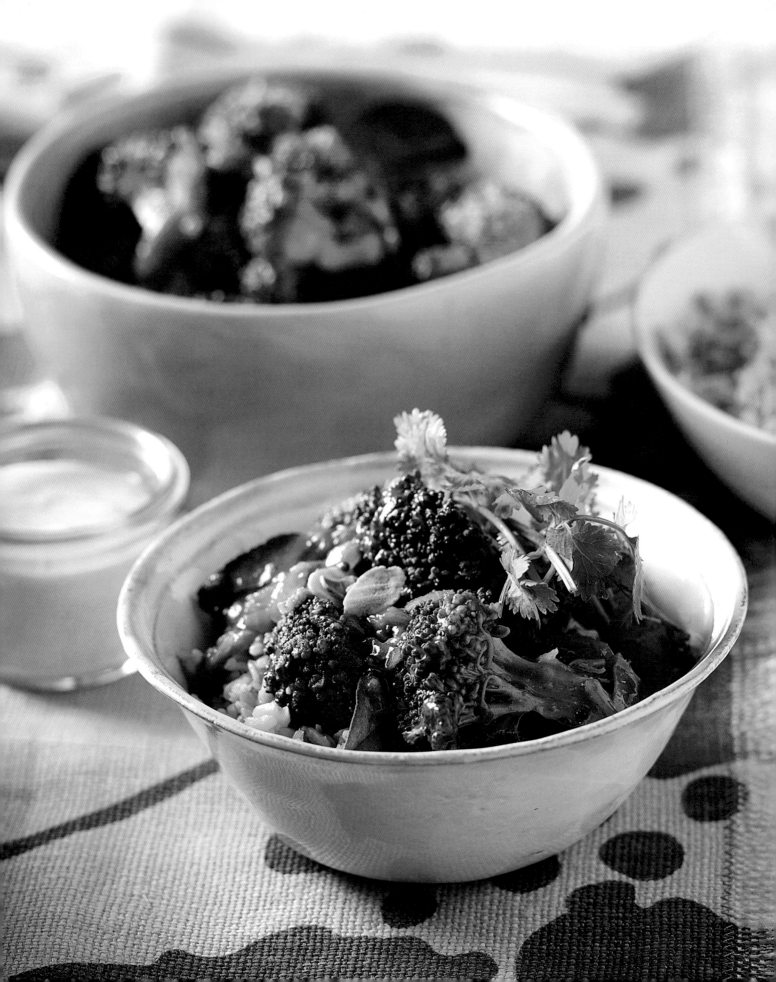

Broccoli curry with turmeric yogurt and almonds

2 teaspoons vegetable oil

1 brown (yellow) onion, finely chopped

3 teaspoons ground cumin

2 teaspoons ground coriander

1 teaspoon brown or yellow mustard seeds

1½ teaspoons ground turmeric

4 cardamom pods, bruised

10 fresh or dried curry leaves

1 tablespoon tamarind purée

6 cups (500 g) broccoli florets

200 g (7 oz) tub low-fat thick Greek-style yogurt

1 tablespoon cornflour (cornstarch)

½ cup (45 g) toasted flaked almonds, to garnish

2 tablespoons chopped coriander (cilantro), to garnish (optional)

PREPARATION 15 minutes

COOKING 15 minutes **SERVES** 4

EACH SERVING PROVIDES 862 kJ, 206 kcal, 26 g protein, 11 g fat (2 g saturated fat), 15 g carbohydrate (7 g sugars), 7 g fibre, 305 mg sodium

> In this South Indian–style dish, folate-rich broccoli is cooked gently with many spices high in anti-oxidants, such as curry leaves, mustard seeds, cumin, cardamom and tamarind.

1 Heat oil in a non-stick frying pan over medium heat. Add onion and cook 3 minutes, or until soft. Add cumin, coriander, mustard seeds, 1 teaspoon turmeric, cardamom and curry leaves, and stir to combine. Cook 1 minute, or until aromatic.

2 Add tamarind purée, broccoli and 1½ cups (375 ml) water. Stir until combined and mixture comes to a boil. Reduce heat, cover and simmer 4–5 minutes, or until broccoli is just tender and still bright green.

3 Meanwhile, combine yogurt and remaining turmeric in a small bowl

4 When broccoli is tender, combine cornflour and 1 tablespoon cold water in a small bowl. Add to curry and cook, stirring, 1–2 minutes, until sauce thickens.

5 Spoon curry into bowls. Top each with a spoonful of turmeric yogurt and sprinkle over almonds. Garnish with coriander if using. Serve immediately. This dish goes well with brown rice.

COOK'S TIP Tamarind purée is used in Asian and Indian cooking to give a tangy flavour. The purée can be found in the Asian food section of supermarkets or in Asian food stores. If you can't obtain it, use a squeeze of lime juice instead.

Curry leaves provide a characteristic flavour in Southern Indian cooking. They are available in specialty greengrocers and Asian and Indian food stores and can be frozen in an airtight container for later use. If you can't find them, just omit them as there is no real substitute.

Spinach pasta with walnuts and garlic yogurt

400 g (14 oz) spinach fettuccine
¼ cup (60 ml) olive oil
½ cup (50 g) walnuts, roughly chopped

Garlic yogurt

1 cup (250 g) low-fat thick Greek-style yogurt
1 clove garlic, crushed
⅓ cup (20 g) finely chopped fresh dill
freshly ground black pepper

PREPARATION 20 minutes, plus overnight draining
COOKING 20 minutes SERVES 4

EACH SERVING PROVIDES 2719 kJ, 650 kcal, 21 g protein,
26 g fat (5 g saturated fat), 83 g carbohydrate
(7 g sugars), 5 g fibre, 124 mg sodium

> In this recipe folate-rich spinach fettuccine is combined with walnuts, which are high in omega-3 oils, and dollops of garlic yogurt, or labna, which provide extra protein and calcium.

1 To make the garlic yogurt, put a fine mesh strainer over a bowl. Rinse a 25 cm (10 inch) piece of muslin (cheesecloth) in hot water. Wring out, then line strainer with muslin. Combine yogurt and garlic in a medium bowl. Spoon yogurt mixture into strainer and cover with plastic wrap. Refrigerate overnight and preferably at least 24 hours to drain.

2 Transfer drained thickened yogurt from strainer to a bowl. Add dill, season with pepper and stir to combine. Set aside.

3 Cook fettuccine in a large saucepan of boiling water, following packet instructions, until just tender.

4 When pasta is almost cooked, heat oil in a non-stick frying pan over medium heat. Add walnuts and cook 3 minutes, or until golden.

5 Drain pasta and return to saucepan. Toss walnuts and oil through pasta until well combined. Divide pasta among warmed bowls, top with a generous dollop of garlic yogurt and serve.

COOK'S TIP Fine muslin or cheesecloth is available from fabric stores and kitchenware stores, or you can use a new clean tea towel or kitchen cloth instead.

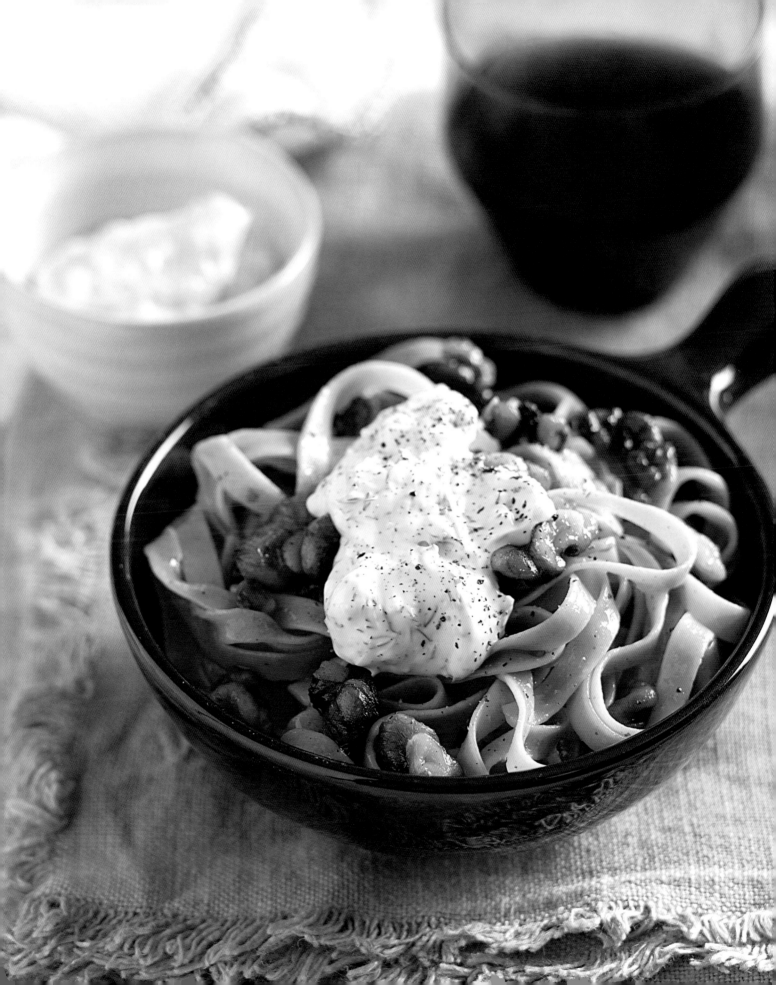

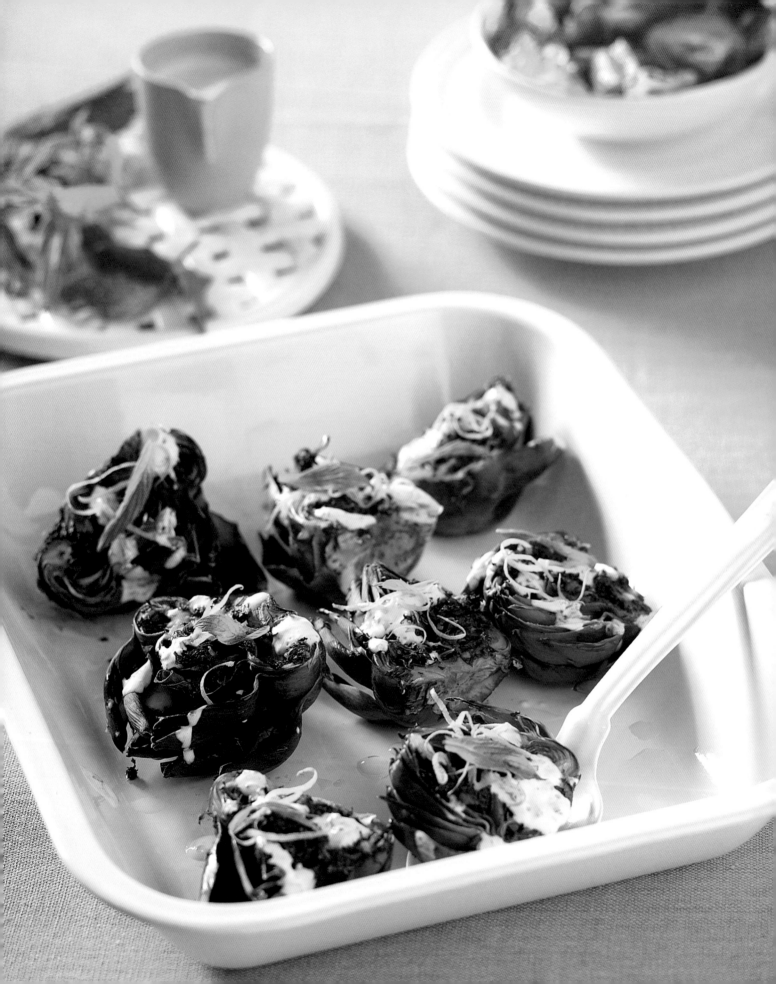

Artichokes stuffed with garlic and mint

1 bunch (125 g/4 oz) fresh mint
finely grated zest of 1 large lemon
3 cloves garlic, crushed
¼ cup (60 ml) lemon juice
4 globe artichokes (about 800 g/1¾ lb)
¼ cup (60 ml) olive oil
2 tablespoons balsamic vinegar
1 cup (250 g) low-fat thick Greek-style yogurt
2 tablespoons milk
freshly ground black pepper

PREPARATION 20 minutes
COOKING 30 minutes SERVES 2

EACH SERVING PROVIDES 2259 kJ, 540 kcal, 19 g protein,
33 g fat (7 g saturated fat), 44 g carbohydrate
(15 g sugars), 16 g fibre, 397 mg sodium

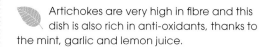
Artichokes are very high in fibre and this dish is also rich in anti-oxidants, thanks to the mint, garlic and lemon juice.

1 Set aside a few mint leaves and some lemon zest for garnish. Finely chop the remaining mint. Put three-quarters of chopped mint in a bowl. Add remaining lemon zest and garlic and stir until well combined.

2 Fill a large bowl with cold water and add lemon juice. Trim stalk from artichokes, leaving about 5 cm (2 inches) of stalk. Trim 2 cm (¾ inch) from top of artichokes. Remove outer leaves until you reach the softer, light green leaves. Trim hard base where leaves have been removed. Cut artichokes in half lengthwise and remove furry 'choke' from the centres. Put the trimmed artichokes in the bowl of lemon water while preparing remaining artichokes.

3 Preheat oven to 200°C (400°F/Gas 6). Drain artichokes and put in a large roasting pan (baking dish). Stuff mint, garlic and lemon mixture between artichoke leaves. Combine 2 tablespoons oil and vinegar in a jug, and drizzle over artichokes. Cover roasting pan tightly with foil and put in oven. Bake 30 minutes, or until artichokes are tender.

4 Meanwhile, whisk together yogurt, milk, remaining oil and mint in a jug. To serve the cooked artichokes, drizzle with yogurt dressing, season with pepper and top with lemon zest and a sprinkling of mint leaves.

COOK'S TIP Serve this dish with bread, cheese and salad as a light springtime meal.

It is very important that all the 'choke' is removed from the artichokes. It is tough and inedible.

Wholemeal penne with borlotti beans

2 cups (450 g) dried borlotti (cranberry)
    beans or 2 x 400 g (14 oz) cans borlotti
    beans, rinsed and drained
1 tablespoon olive oil
1 brown (yellow) onion, finely chopped
1 large carrot, diced
2 cloves garlic, crushed
200 g (7 oz) wholemeal (whole-wheat) penne
1 bunch silverbeet (Swiss chard), thick stalks
    discarded, leaves thinly sliced
½ cup (15 g) roughly chopped fresh flat-leaf
    (Italian) parsley
freshly ground black pepper
½ cup (50 g) finely grated parmesan

PREPARATION 20 minutes, plus overnight soaking if using
dried beans COOKING 30 minutes SERVES 4

EACH SERVING PROVIDES 2297 kJ, 548 kcal, 28 g protein,
12 g fat (3 g saturated fat), 81 g carbohydrate
(5 g sugars), 19 g fibre, 768 mg sodium

> This delicious high-protein, high-fibre
> vegetarian dish is also high in anti-oxidants
> from the onion, carrot, garlic and parsley.

1 Put dried beans, if using, in a large bowl and cover well with water. Soak overnight.

2 Drain soaked beans. Put in a large saucepan or pressure cooker, cover with plenty of fresh water and the lid, and boil until tender – about 30 minutes in a saucepan, or 10 minutes in a pressure cooker.

3 Meanwhile, heat oil in a non-stick frying pan over medium heat. Add onion, carrot and garlic, and cook, stirring occasionally, 8 minutes, or until vegetables are soft.

4 Add cooked or canned borlotti beans and 1 cup (250 ml) water and stir to combine. Cook, uncovered, 20 minutes, or until beans are soft and mixture has thickened.

5 Meanwhile, cook pasta in a large saucepan of boiling water, following packet instructions, until just tender.

6 Add silverbeet to borlotti beans and stir to combine. Cook, 1–2 minutes, or until silverbeet has just wilted. Stir in parsley and season with pepper.

7 Drain pasta and return to saucepan. Add borlotti bean mixture and toss through gently to combine well. Spoon into four serving bowls, scatter with parmesan and serve.

COOK'S TIP This pasta would go well with a salad of mixed green leaves for a complete meal.

You could use English spinach instead of silverbeet.

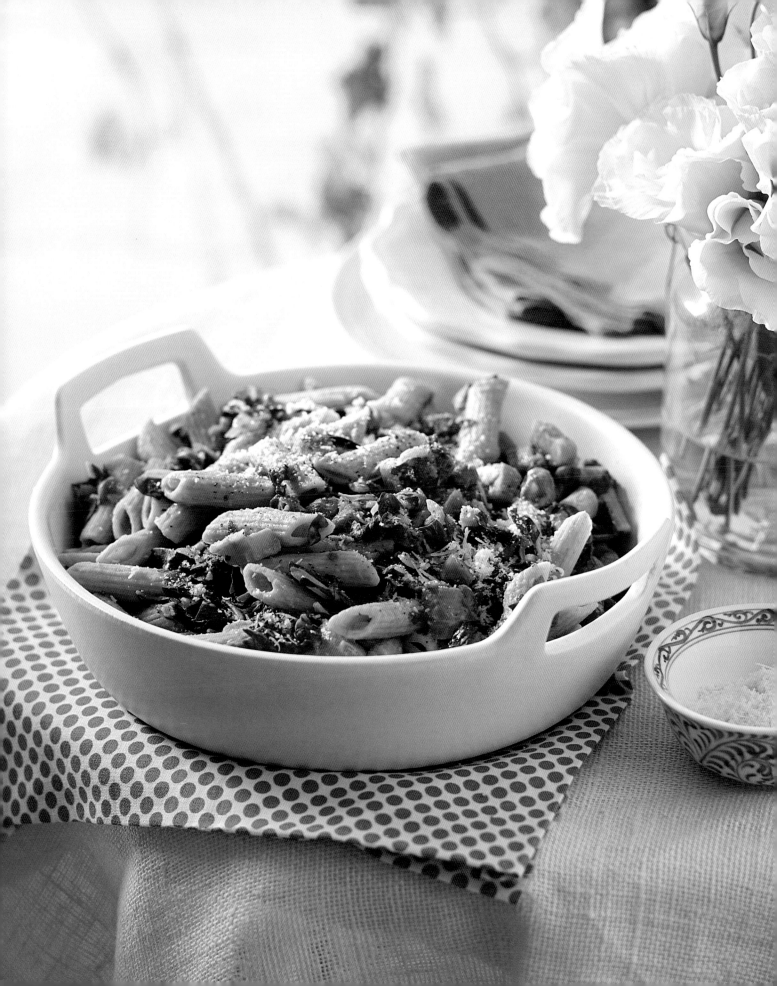

Zucchini rice slice

1 cup (200 g) brown rice
olive oil cooking spray
2 teaspoons olive oil
1 brown (yellow) onion, finely chopped
2 cloves garlic, crushed
5 zucchini (courgettes) (about 600 g/1¼ lb),
   coarsely grated
2 eggs, lightly beaten
1¼ cups (155 g) grated reduced-fat cheddar
½ cup (50 g) finely grated parmesan
½ cup (10 g) fresh mint leaves,
   roughly chopped

PREPARATION 20 minutes, plus 10 minutes standing
COOKING 1 hour SERVES 4

EACH SERVING PROVIDES 1722 kJ, 411 kcal, 27 g protein,
15 g fat (6 g saturated fat), 42 g carbohydrate
(3 g sugars), 4 g fibre, 476 mg sodium

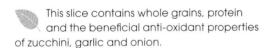 This slice contains whole grains, protein
and the beneficial anti-oxidant properties
of zucchini, garlic and onion.

1 Put rice and 2½ cups (625 ml) water in a large saucepan over high heat. Bring to a boil, then reduce heat to low and simmer, covered, 25–30 minutes, or until rice is tender and all water has been absorbed. Transfer to a large bowl.

2 Meanwhile, preheat oven to 200°C (400°F/Gas 6). Spray an 8 cup (2 litre) ovenproof dish with cooking spray. Heat oil in a non-stick frying pan over medium heat. Add onion and garlic and cook 3 minutes, or until onion is softened. Leave to cool.

3 Tip grated zucchini into a colander. With your hands, press and squeeze out as much liquid as possible.

4 Add zucchini and onion to rice in the bowl. Add eggs, 1 cup (125 g) cheddar, half the parmesan and the mint and stir until well combined. Spoon mixture into prepared ovenproof dish. Sprinkle remaining cheddar and parmesan over the top.

5 Bake 25–30 minutes, or until set and firm. Leave to stand 10 minutes before cutting into squares. Serve.

COOK'S TIP This delicious slice can be served warm or cold, accompanied by steamed vegetables, a tossed green salad, or a tomato, red onion and parsley salad.

A cup of uncooked brown rice gives about 2½ cups (470 g) of cooked rice.

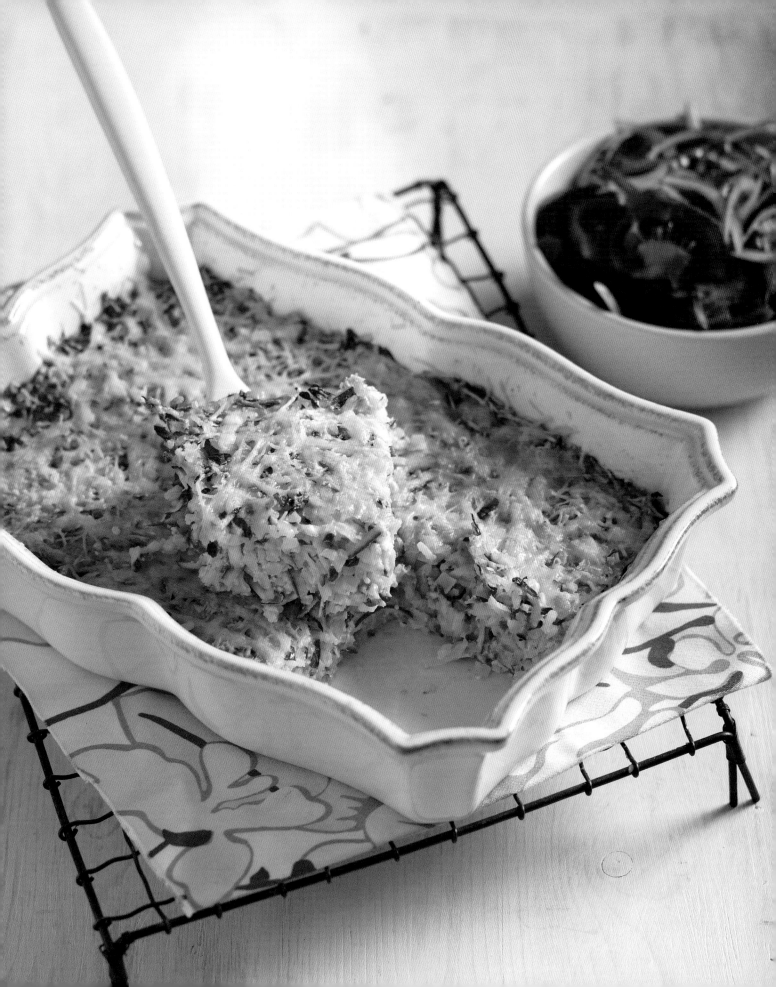

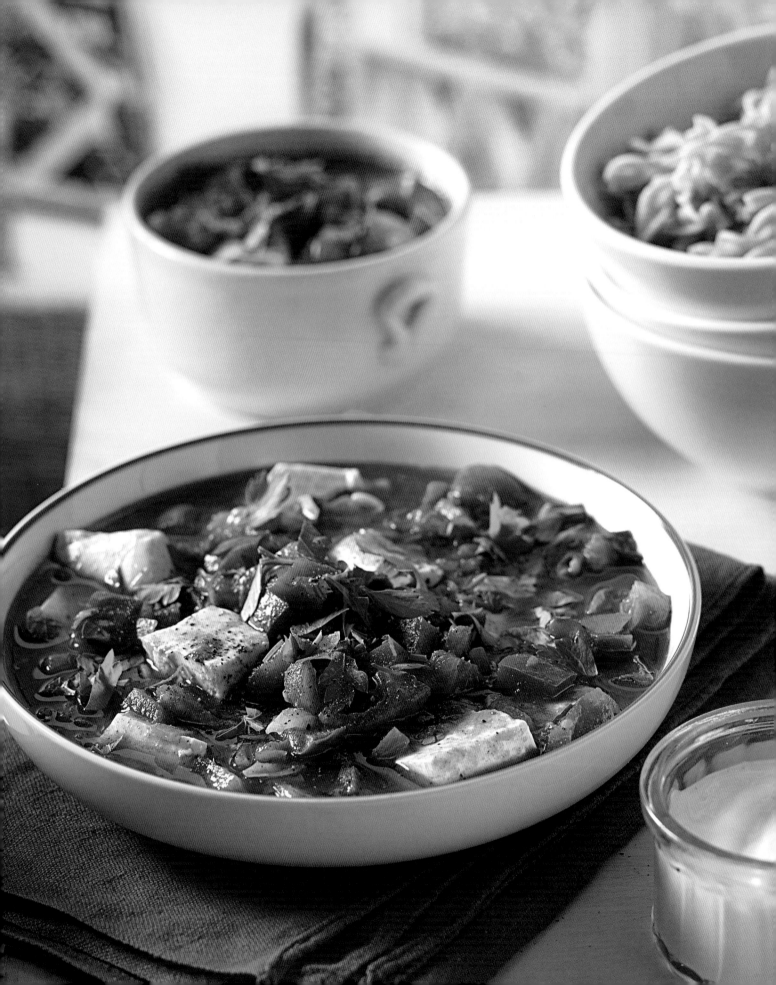

'Goulash'-style tofu

1 tablespoon olive oil
1 red onion, finely chopped
2 red capsicums (bell peppers),
    seeds removed, diced
2 cloves garlic, crushed
2 teaspoons sweet paprika
2 tablespoons salt-reduced tomato paste
    (concentrated purée)
5 ripe tomatoes (about 750 g/1½ lb),
    skins removed, diced
2 x 300 g (10 oz) packets firm tofu, drained,
    cut into 1.5 cm (³/₄ inch) slices
½ cup (15 g) roughly chopped fresh flat-leaf
    (Italian) parsley
4 tablespoons low-fat thick Greek-style yogurt
freshly ground black pepper

PREPARATION 15 minutes
COOKING 15 minutes SERVES 4

EACH SERVING PROVIDES 1118 kJ, 267 kcal, 21 g protein,
15 g fat (3 g saturated fat), 12 g carbohydrate
(9 g sugars), 7 g fibre, 64 mg sodium

Tofu is a great source of soy protein, and it has special heart- and bone-protective benefits. Here, it is combined with a rich-tasting Hungarian-style sauce of tomato, paprika, parsley and capsicum, high in anti-oxidants.

1 Heat oil in a large non-stick frying pan over medium heat. Add onion, capsicums and garlic, and cook 5 minutes, or until onion and capsicums are softened. Sprinkle paprika over the mixture and stir to combine.

2 Stir in tomato paste and 1⅓ cups (330 ml) water. Add tomatoes, stir and bring mixture to a boil. Reduce heat and simmer 5 minutes, or until thickened.

3 Stir in tofu and cook 2 minutes, or until heated through. Stir through half the parsley.

4 Spoon goulash onto four serving plates. Top each with a dollop of yogurt, sprinkle over remaining parsley, season with pepper and serve.

COOK'S TIP Serve this dish with a green salad.

When tomatoes are expensive and not in season, use an 800 g (28 oz) can chopped tomatoes instead.

To remove skin from tomatoes, use a small sharp knife to mark a small cross on the base of each tomato. Put in a large heatproof bowl, cover with boiling water and stand 2 minutes. Drain, then plunge into icy cold water. Drain again and peel off the skin.

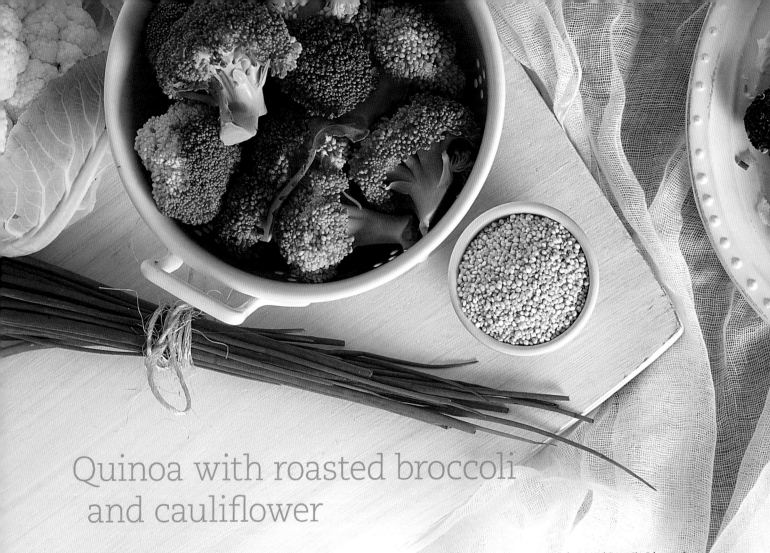

Quinoa with roasted broccoli and cauliflower

2 heads broccoli, thick stalks discarded,
  cut into florets
1 small cauliflower (about 750 g/1½ lb),
  thick stalks discarded, cut into florets
2 tablespoons olive oil
1½ cups (300 g) quinoa
½ cup (80 g) sesame seeds
1 tablespoon finely chopped fresh parsley
1 tablespoon finely snipped fresh chives
freshly ground black pepper
125 g (4 oz) goat's cheese, plain or ashed,
  crumbled

PREPARATION 15 minutes
COOKING 30 minutes SERVES 4

EACH SERVING PROVIDES 2946 kJ, 704 kcal, 39 g protein,
35 g fat (9 g saturated fat), 58 g carbohydrate
(6 g sugars), 22 g fibre, 258 mg sodium

1 Preheat oven to 200°C (400°F/Gas 6). Line a large baking tray with baking paper (baking sheet with parchment paper).

2 Put broccoli and cauliflower in a large bowl. Add oil and toss to coat vegetables. Spread on prepared tray and roast 25–30 minutes, or until vegetables are soft and beginning to turn golden at the edges.

3 Meanwhile, bring 3 cups (750 ml) water to a boil in a medium saucepan over high heat. Add quinoa and return to a boil. Reduce heat to medium and simmer, uncovered, 10 minutes, or until tender. Drain well and transfer to a large bowl.

4 Toss sesame seeds in a non-stick frying pan over high heat until light brown. Tip over quinoa and stir through. Add parsley and chives, season with pepper and stir to combine.

5 When broccoli and cauliflower are cooked, add to quinoa and toss until well combined. Gently stir goat's cheese through just before serving.

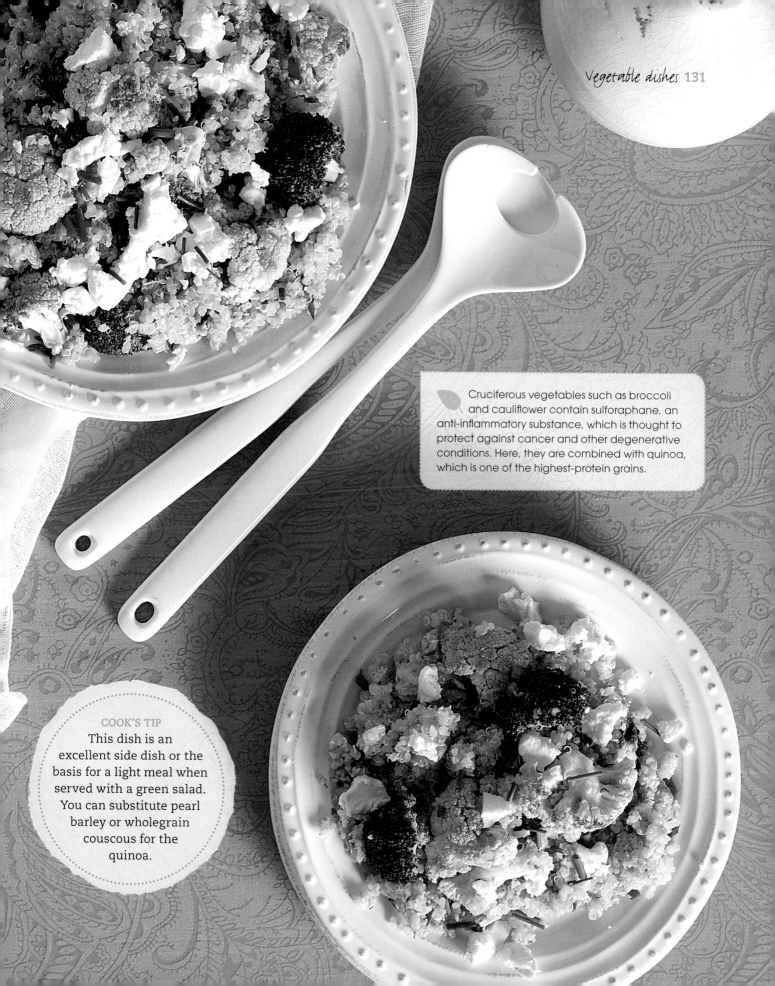

Cruciferous vegetables such as broccoli and cauliflower contain sulforaphane, an anti-inflammatory substance, which is thought to protect against cancer and other degenerative conditions. Here, they are combined with quinoa, which is one of the highest-protein grains.

COOK'S TIP
This dish is an excellent side dish or the basis for a light meal when served with a green salad. You can substitute pearl barley or wholegrain couscous for the quinoa.

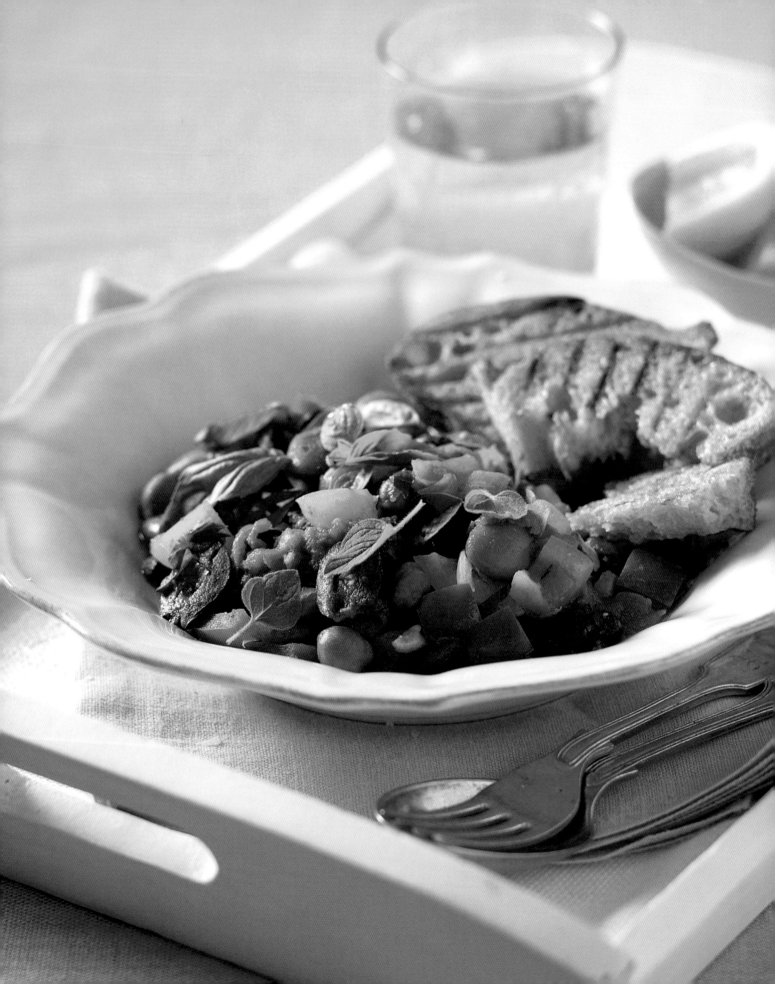

Provençal bean hotpot

2 cups (450 g) dried mixed beans, such as
  chickpeas, red kidney beans, cannellini
  beans and butterbeans (lima beans), or
  2 x 400 g (14 oz) cans mixed beans
1 tablespoon olive oil
1 brown (yellow) onion, chopped
2 cloves garlic, crushed
1 red and 1 yellow capsicum (bell pepper),
  seeds removed, diced
5 ripe tomatoes (about 750 g/1½ lb),
  skins removed, diced
finely grated zest of 1 lemon
2 tablespoons lemon juice
¼ cup (30 g) pitted black olives
½ cup (10 g) fresh flat-leaf (Italian) parsley,
  roughly chopped
¼ cup (8 g) fresh oregano, roughly chopped
freshly ground black pepper
¼ cup (8 g) fresh basil, roughly chopped
4 thick slices sourdough, toasted, to serve

PREPARATION 20 minutes, plus overnight soaking if using
dried beans **COOKING** 30 minutes **SERVES** 4

EACH SERVING PROVIDES 1836 kJ, 439 kcal, 29 g protein,
8 g fat (1 g saturated fat), 49 g carbohydrate
(11 g sugars), 28 g fibre, 103 mg sodium

> A mix of legumes simmered with onion,
> capsicums, garlic, parsley, tomatoes, basil,
> oregano and black olives gives a hearty and
> filling dish that is high in fibre and anti-oxidants.

1 Put dried mixed beans, if using, in a large bowl
and cover well with water. Soak overnight.

2 Drain soaked beans. Put in a large saucepan or
pressure cooker, cover with plenty of fresh water and
the lid, and boil until tender – about 30 minutes in
a saucepan, or 10 minutes in a pressure cooker.

3 Meanwhile, heat oil in a large non-stick frying pan
over medium heat. Add onion, garlic and capsicums,
and stir to combine. Cook, stirring occasionally,
8 minutes, or until softened.

4 Add tomatoes, lemon zest and juice and ½ cup
(125 ml) water, and stir to combine. Bring to a boil.
Add cooked or canned mixed beans, olives, half the
parsley and half the oregano. Season with pepper
and stir, then simmer 10 minutes, or until beans are
soft and mixture has thickened.

5 Spoon bean hotpot into serving bowls. Sprinkle
with remaining parsley, remaining oregano and the
basil, and serve with sourdough toast.

COOK'S TIP Dried beans are easy to cook, but acidic
ingredients, such as tomatoes, can slow the cooking
time and cause the beans to harden. For best results
always make sure dried beans and lentils are cooked
to your liking before you combine them with the
remaining ingredients.

Lentil macaroni cheese

2 tablespoons olive oil
1 brown (yellow) onion, finely chopped
2 cloves garlic, crushed
5 ripe tomatoes (about 750 g/1½ lb),
    skins removed, diced
400 g (14 oz) can brown lentils,
    rinsed and drained
½ cup (15 g) roughly chopped fresh flat-leaf
    (Italian) parsley
400 g (14 oz) macaroni
20 g (²/₃ oz) olive oil spread
¼ cup (35 g) plain (all-purpose) flour
1¾ cups (435 ml) skim milk
1 cup (125 g) grated reduced-fat cheddar
½ cup (50 g) grated parmesan
freshly ground black pepper

PREPARATION 25 minutes
COOKING 50 minutes SERVES 4

EACH SERVING PROVIDES 2962 kJ, 708 kcal, 37 g protein,
21 g fat (6 g saturated fat), 90 g carbohydrate
(11 g sugars), 8 g fibre, 654 mg sodium

> Macaroni cheese made with low-fat cheese and milk, served on top of a thick tomato and lentil sauce, makes for a low-fat, high-fibre version of this comfort food classic.

1 Heat 1 tablespoon olive oil in a large non-stick frying pan over medium heat. Add onion and cook 3 minutes, or until softened. Add garlic and cook 1 minute. Stir in tomatoes and 1 cup (250 ml) water and bring mixture to a boil. Reduce heat and simmer 10 minutes, or until thickened. Add lentils and half the parsley and stir to combine. Simmer 10 minutes. Spoon into a shallow 6 cup (1.5 litre) ovenproof dish.

2 Meanwhile, cook macaroni in a large saucepan of boiling water, following packet instructions, until just tender. Drain well and return to the saucepan.

3 Preheat oven to 200°C (400°F/Gas 6). Heat spread and remaining oil in a non-stick medium saucepan over medium heat. When sizzling, add flour and stir until well combined. Cook, stirring continuously, 1 minute, or until mixture is bubbling. Remove from heat and slowly pour in milk, whisking continuously until well combined. Return to heat and continue whisking until mixture comes to a boil. Reduce heat and simmer 2 minutes. Add half the cheddar and half the parmesan and stir until melted.

4 Add cheese sauce to pasta, season with pepper and stir until well combined. Spoon macaroni cheese mixture over lentil mixture in the ovenproof dish. Sprinkle remaining cheddar and parmesan over the top and bake 20–25 minutes, or until cheese on top is melted and golden.

5 Carefully spoon macaroni cheese onto serving plates. Sprinkle with remaining parsley and serve.

COOK'S TIP Serve macaroni cheese with a green salad or steamed vegetables for a balanced meal.

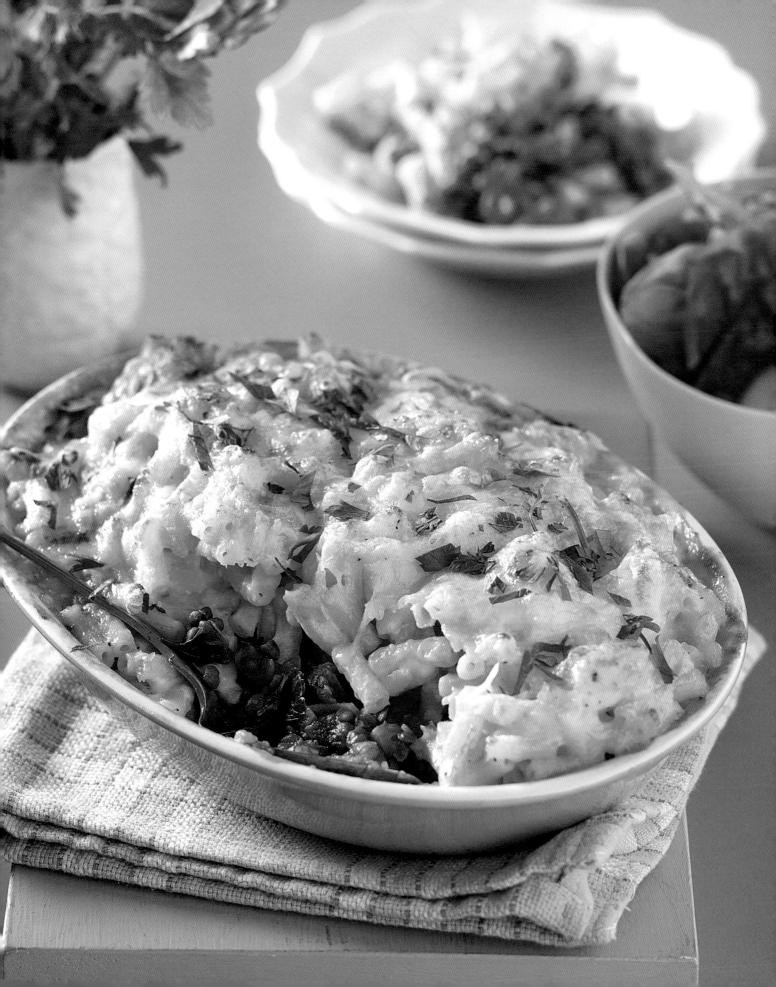

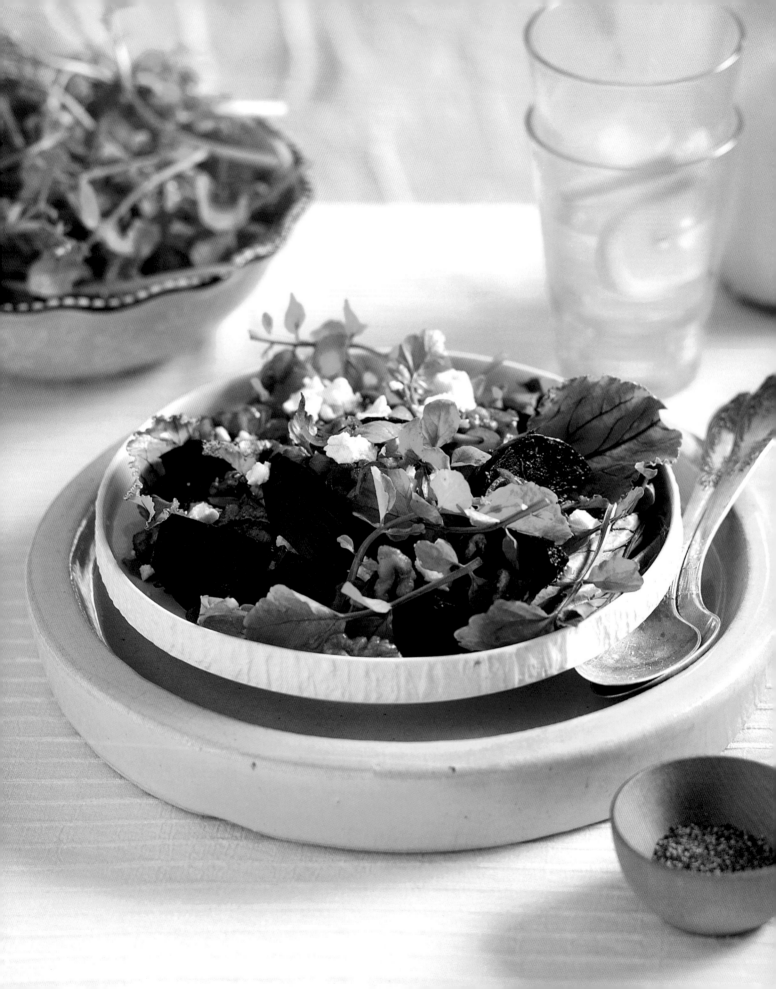

Beetroot and goat's cheese salad

4 large beetroot (beets) (about 800 g/1¾ lb),
  with leaves
2 teaspoons olive oil
6 French shallots (eschalots), thinly sliced
3 tablespoons red wine vinegar
1 teaspoon soft brown sugar or light
  muscovado sugar
½ cup (50 g) toasted walnut halves
1 bunch (250 g/8 oz) watercress,
  thick stems discarded
125 g (4 oz) goat's cheese, ashed or plain
freshly ground black pepper

PREPARATION 20 minutes, plus 15 minutes standing
COOKING 1 hour 15 minutes SERVES 4

EACH SERVING PROVIDES 1345 kJ, 321 kcal, 14 g protein,
21 g fat (7 g saturated fat), 20 g carbohydrate
(19 g sugars), 9 g fibre, 309 mg sodium

This salad is high in omega-3 oils from
the walnuts, and lots of anti-oxidants
from the beetroot, French shallots and greens.

1 Preheat oven to 200°C (400°F/Gas 6). Set aside small leaves from beetroot stalks. Trim beetroot and scrub clean. Wrap each beetroot in a piece of foil and put on a baking tray (sheet). Bake 1–1¼ hours, or until soft. Stand 15 minutes, or until cool enough to handle. Remove foil, peel skin from beetroot and cut beetroot into large cubes or wedges.

2 While beetroot is cooking, heat oil in a non-stick frying pan over medium heat. Add French shallots and cook gently, stirring occasionally, 8 minutes, or until golden. Add vinegar and sugar and cook, stirring, 1–2 minutes, until liquid has thickened. Add walnuts and stir to coat well with shallot mixture. Remove from heat and allow to cool.

3 Put small beetroot leaves, watercress and walnut and French shallot mixture in a large bowl and toss to combine. Transfer to a large serving platter and scatter over beetroot.

4 Crumble goat's cheese over the salad, season with pepper and serve.

COOK'S TIP Whole beetroot wrapped in foil and baked in the oven gives a sweet flavour that is absent from boiled beetroot.

To peel shallots easily, put them in a heatproof bowl and cover with boiling water. Stand 2 minutes, then drain. The skins will come off easily.

Pasta with lentils and spinach

2 tablespoons olive oil
1 small onion, diced
1 small carrot, diced
3 cloves garlic, crushed
¾ cup (140 g) brown lentils,
    rinsed and picked over
5 sprigs thyme, leaves removed, or
    1 teaspoon dried thyme
4 cups (1 litre) homemade or salt-reduced
    chicken or vegetable stock
1 bay leaf
1¼ cups (115 g) wholemeal (whole-wheat)
    pasta spirals or shells
410 g (15 oz) can chopped tomatoes
4 cups (180 g) baby spinach leaves
2 tablespoons lemon juice
freshly ground black pepper
4 tablespoons finely grated parmesan

PREPARATION 10 minutes
COOKING 1 hour SERVES 4

EACH SERVING PROVIDES 1501 kJ, 358 kcal, 21 g protein,
13 g fat (1 g saturated fat), 40 g carbohydrate
(8 g sugars), 10 g fibre, 831 mg sodium

This pasta recipe makes a balanced meal,
with heart-protective vegetable protein,
low glycaemic index carbohydrates, and plenty
of fibre and anti-oxidants.

1 Heat oil in a large saucepan over medium heat.
Add onion and carrot and cook, stirring frequently,
until softened and starting to caramelise, about
10 minutes. Add garlic and cook, stirring, 1 minute.
Add lentils and thyme and stir to coat, then add
stock and bay leaf and bring to a simmer. Reduce
heat to low, cover and simmer 20 minutes, until
lentils are almost tender.

2 Add pasta shells and simmer, covered, stirring
occasionally, until almost tender, 10–15 minutes.

3 Add tomatoes and simmer, covered, until lentils
and pasta are tender and the mixture has thickened,
5–10 minutes. Discard bay leaf. Add spinach and
cook, stirring, until just wilted, about 1 minute. Stir
in lemon juice and season with pepper.

4 Spoon into four serving bowls, scatter over
parmesan and serve.

COOK'S TIP Make sure the lentils are tender before
adding the tomatoes. Acidic foods such as tomatoes
can slow the cooking process and make legumes
become hard.

This warm, hearty dish will keep, covered, in the
refrigerator for up to 2 days.

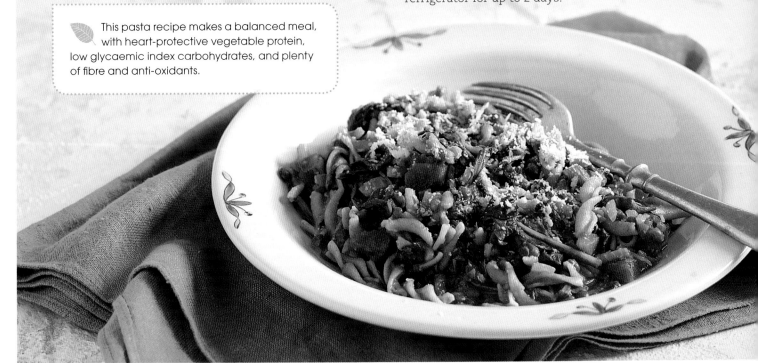

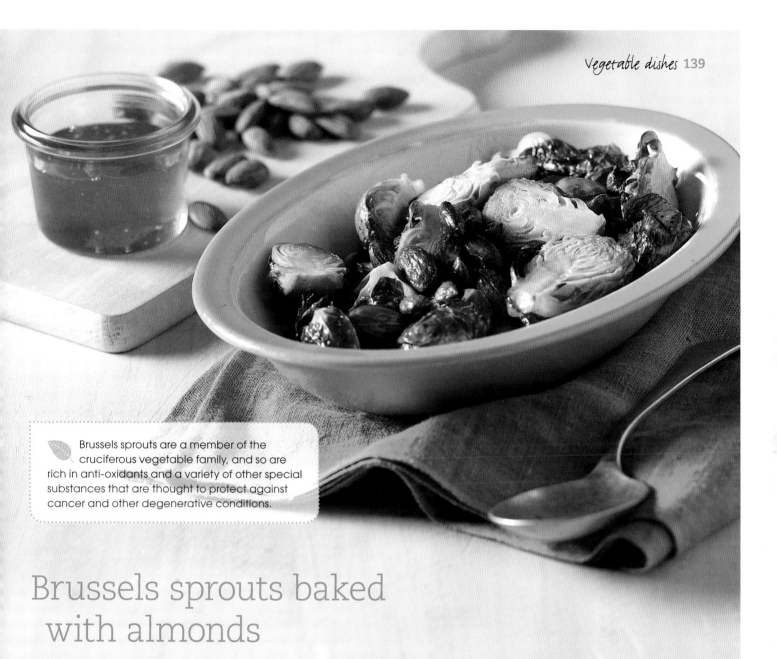

Brussels sprouts are a member of the cruciferous vegetable family, and so are rich in anti-oxidants and a variety of other special substances that are thought to protect against cancer and other degenerative conditions.

Brussels sprouts baked with almonds

2 tablespoons olive oil
2 tablespoons honey
500 g (1 lb) brussels sprouts, trimmed, halved lengthwise
½ cup (80 g) raw almonds

PREPARATION 5 minutes
COOKING 20 minutes **SERVES** 4

EACH SERVING PROVIDES 1162 kJ, 278 kcal, 9 g protein, 20 g fat (2 g saturated fat), 15 g carbohydrate (15 g sugars), 6 g fibre, 40 mg sodium

1 Preheat oven to 200°C (400°F/Gas 6). Line a baking tray with baking paper (baking sheet with parchment paper).

2 Put oil and honey in a large bowl and whisk together. Add brussels sprouts and almonds and toss to coat well. Transfer to prepared tray and bake 15–20 minutes, or until golden. Serve.

COOK'S TIP This recipe will convert anyone who thinks they dislike brussels sprouts, as it brings out their sweetness, making a deliciously different side dish to accompany a grill or roast.

Filo bake with tofu and pumpkin

1 kg (2 lb) butternut pumpkin (squash),
    peeled, seeds removed
1¹/₂ tablespoons olive oil
300 g (10 oz) silken tofu, drained,
    roughly chopped
¹/₂ cup (50 g) grated parmesan
4 spring onions (scallions), thinly sliced
5 sprigs fresh dill, finely chopped
freshly ground black pepper
6 sheets filo pastry
olive oil cooking spray

PREPARATION 25 minutes, plus 5 minutes standing
COOKING 50 minutes SERVES 4

EACH SERVING PROVIDES 1383 kJ, 330 kcal, 16 g protein,
16 g fat (5 g saturated fat), 30 g carbohydrate
(12 g sugars), 4 g fibre, 338 mg sodium

 This is a very good vegetarian dish, high in protein, fibre and anti-oxidants, and low in fat, as well as providing the benefits of soy.

1 Preheat oven to 200°C (400°F/Gas 6). Line a large baking tray with baking paper (baking sheet with parchment paper). Cut pumpkin into 2 cm (³/₄ inch) chunks. Put in a large bowl, add 1 tablespoon olive oil and toss to combine well. Spread pumpkin out over prepared tray. Roast 20–25 minutes, or until golden and tender.

2 Put half the cooked pumpkin, tofu and half the parmesan in a food processor or blender and pulse until smooth and well combined. Transfer to a large bowl. Add remaining pumpkin, spring onions and dill, season with pepper and gently stir to combine.

3 Line a large baking tray with baking paper. Put 1 sheet filo pastry on a flat surface and spray with cooking spray. Cover with another sheet of filo pastry and spray with cooking spray. Repeat to use up remaining sheets of filo pastry. Spoon pumpkin mixture along a long edge of the pastry, leaving a 5 cm (2 inch) border at the sides. Carefully roll over once, then fold in sides of pastry and continue rolling to enclose pumpkin filling.

4 Transfer roll to prepared baking tray. Brush with remaining olive oil and sprinkle with remaining parmesan. Bake 20–25 minutes, or until pastry is golden and crisp. Transfer to a serving platter and stand 5 minutes, then slice with a sharp knife and serve.

COOK'S TIP When working with filo pastry, cover the sheets of pastry with a damp clean tea towel (dish towel) to prevent it from drying out and cracking.

This recipe is delicious served with green vegetables or a salad. You can also make individual mini rolls, using 1 sheet of filo per roll. You will need 8 sheets of filo for this.

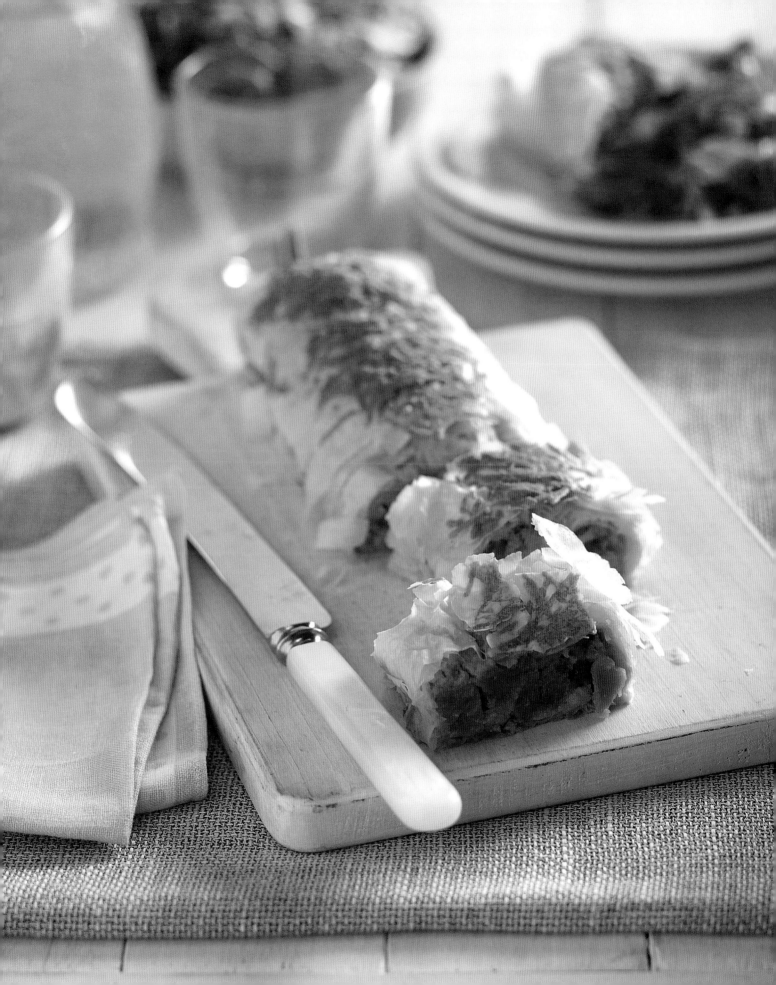

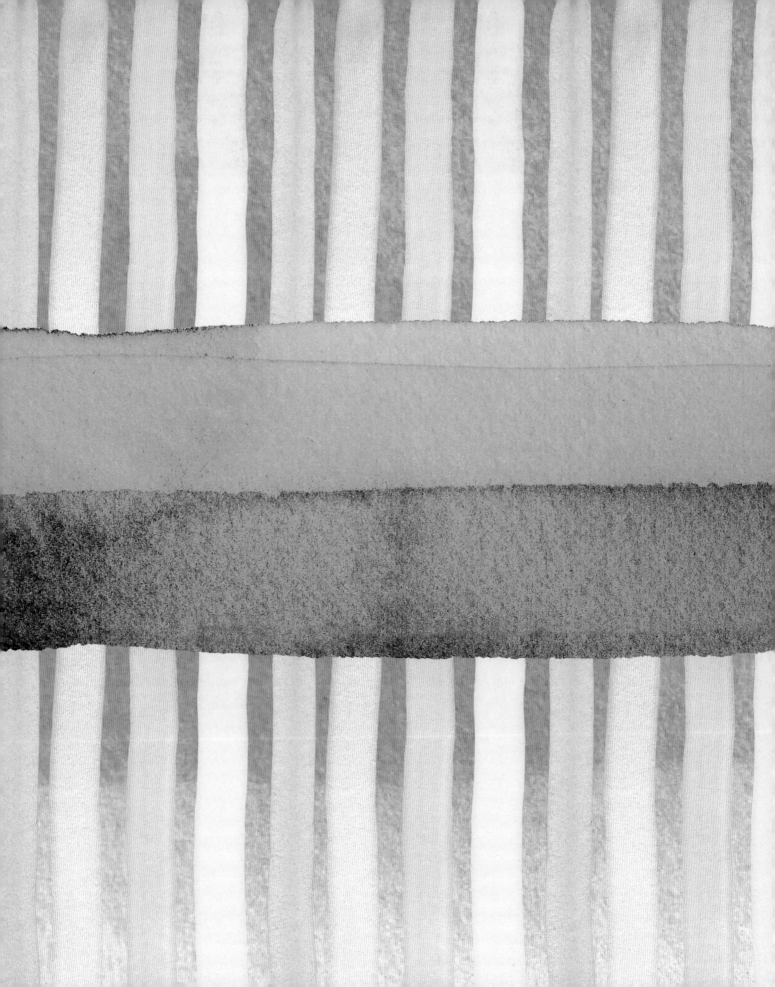

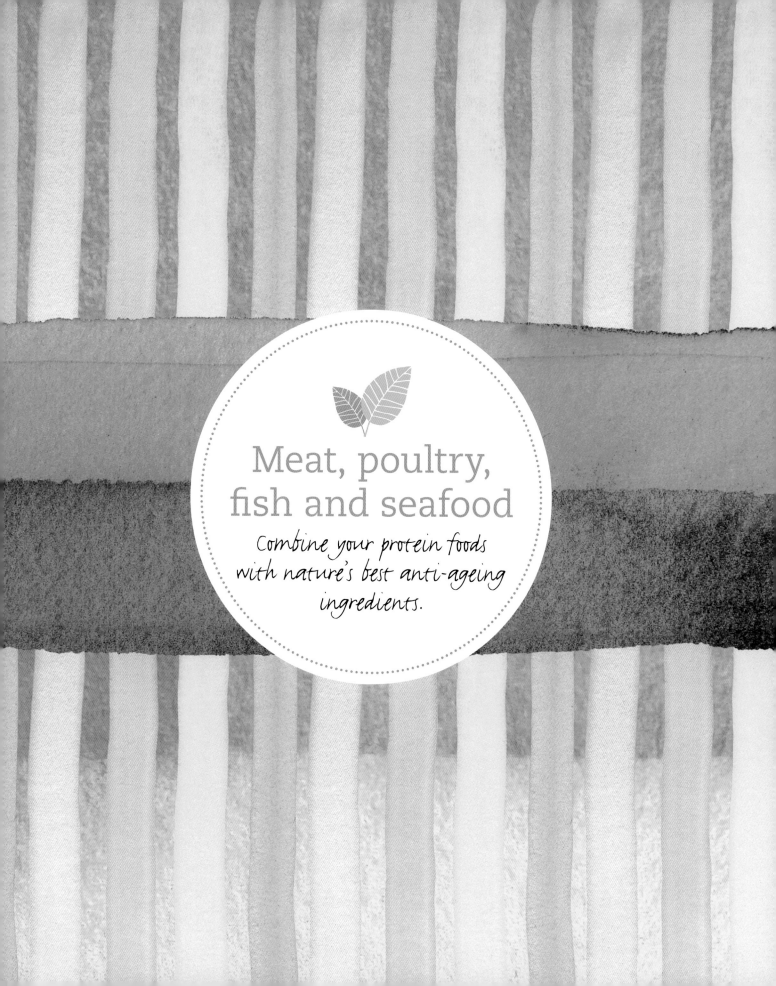

Meat, poultry, fish and seafood

Combine your protein foods with nature's best anti-ageing ingredients.

Oyster omelette with mushrooms

250 g (8 oz) mixed mushrooms, such as
    shiitake, cup, enoki and oyster mushrooms
4 eggs
freshly ground black pepper
2 teaspoons extra virgin olive oil
½ cup (45 g) bean sprouts, trimmed
extra virgin olive oil cooking spray
12 fresh oysters, drained, patted dry
1 cup (30 g) fresh coriander (cilantro) leaves,
    to serve

PREPARATION 15 minutes
COOKING 8 minutes **SERVES** 2

EACH SERVING PROVIDES 1441 kJ, 344 kcal, 34 g protein,
22 g fat (6 g saturated fat), 3 g carbohydrate (1 g sugars),
7 g fibre, 572 mg sodium

> Mushrooms, particularly shiitake
> mushrooms, contain good amounts
> of selenium and iron, as well as beneficial
> anti-inflammatory substances. Oysters have
> an excellent zinc content.

1 Trim shiitake mushrooms, if using, and discard
tough stalks. Slice cup mushrooms. Trim stem end
of enoki and oyster mushrooms.

2 Place eggs and 2 tablespoons water in a bowl and
season with pepper. Beat quickly with a fork until
whites and yolks are just blended. (Don't overbeat;
just beat to combine.)

3 Heat a 23 cm (9 inch) non-stick frying pan over
medium–high heat. Heat oil, then add mushrooms
and cook until just tender, about 2–3 minutes.
Add bean sprouts and cook until just wilted, about
30 seconds. Put mixture in a bowl and set aside.

4 Reduce heat to medium. Lightly spray pan with
cooking spray and heat. Pour half the egg mixture
into pan and tilt to coat the base evenly. (It should
begin to set immediately.) Using a small spatula, draw
edges of omelette into the centre of the pan. The
liquid egg will flow into the space this creates. While
the egg still looks wet on top, scatter half the oysters
and half the mushroom mixture over one side of
the omelette and cook about a further 20 seconds.
Fold the omelette over to enclose the oysters and
mushrooms. Slide onto a plate, scatter with half the
coriander and serve immediately. Repeat with
remaining ingredients to make a second omelette.

COOK'S TIP You can purchase oysters in a jar to make
this recipe – use a small jar (about 18 small oysters).

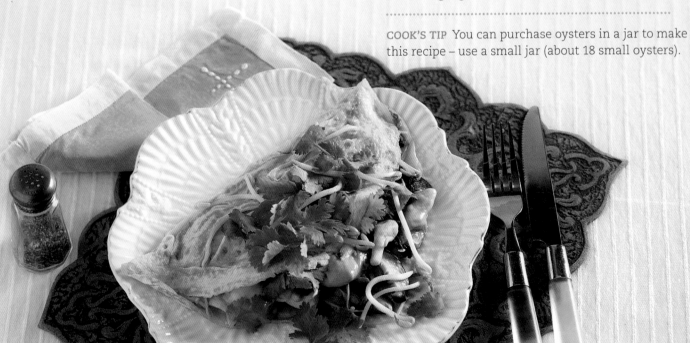

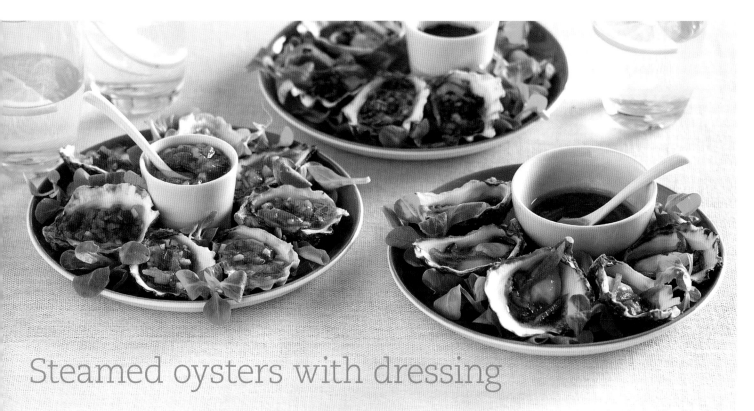

Steamed oysters with dressing

24 large fresh oysters, on the half shell

Orange and sesame dressing

1 tablespoon orange juice
2 teaspoons salt-reduced soy sauce
2 teaspoons sesame oil
2 teaspoons mirin or rice wine vinegar
1 tablespoon shredded spring onion
    (scallion)

Balsamic and chive dressing

⅓ cup (80 ml) balsamic vinegar
1 tablespoon extra virgin olive oil
1 small French shallot (eschalot),
    very finely chopped
2 teaspoons finely snipped fresh chives

Bloody Mary dressing

½ small ripe tomato, very finely diced
½ small celery stalk, very finely diced
¼ small red onion, very finely diced
¼ teaspoon worcestershire sauce
¼ teaspoon Tabasco sauce
¼ cup (60 ml) salt-reduced tomato juice
1 tablespoon vodka (optional)

1 Preheat oven to 200°C (400°C/Gas 6).

2 Combine the ingredients for each dressing in three separate small bowls.

3 Arrange oysters on two large plates. Divide the three dressings among the oysters, drizzling each oyster with 1 teaspoon dressing. Put a wire rack in each of two large roasting pans (baking dishes) and place a plate of oysters on each rack.

4 Carefully pour boiling water into the roasting pans so that it comes to just under the racks. Cover pans with foil, tucking it around or under the rims to trap steam during cooking. Put pans in oven to steam oysters, 3–6 minutes, depending on size of oysters and how cooked you prefer them. Carefully remove foil and serve oysters immediately.

PREPARATION 20 minutes
COOKING 6 minutes **SERVES** 4 as a starter

EACH SERVING PROVIDES 643 kJ, 154 kcal, 11 g protein, 9 g fat (2 g saturated fat), 5 g carbohydrate (4 g sugars), <1 g fibre, 388 mg sodium

Gravlax-style marinated salmon or ocean trout

800 g–1 kg (1¾–2 lb) side of salmon or
   ocean trout, with skin on
60 g (2 oz) sea salt
60 g (2 oz) sugar
3 teaspoons coriander seeds, toasted,
   crushed
¼ cup (60 ml) vodka
1 bunch (90 g/3 oz) fresh dill, chopped
2 small or 1 large beetroot (beet),
   coarsely grated

PREPARATION 30 minutes, plus 24–36 hours curing
SERVES 10 as a starter

EACH SERVING PROVIDES 580 kJ, 138 kcal, 16 g protein,
6 g fat (1 g saturated fat), 5 g carbohydrate (3 g sugars),
<1 g fibre, 1202 mg sodium

> Salmon and ocean trout are examples of oily fish that are the world's best source of beneficial omega-3 oils. In this recipe salmon or trout is sliced finely and used as a healthful alternative to smoked salmon.

1 Remove small pin bones in salmon with tweezers. Put salmon or trout skin side up in a wide, shallow glass or ceramic dish.

2 Combine salt, sugar, coriander seeds, vodka, dill and beetroot in a small bowl. Spoon half the mixture over salmon or trout to cover well, then turn fish over and spoon over remaining mixture. Cover fish with 2 layers of plastic wrap. Place a plate or tray on top of fish and weight the tray down with several unopened cans of food or a large bag of rice. (The weighted tray or plate should be pressing down heavily on the fish.) Refrigerate 24–36 hours.

3 Wipe all the dill and beetroot mixture off the fish, then pat dry with paper towel. With a long-bladed knife, cut marinated salmon or trout into very thin slices to serve.

COOK'S TIP To make less mess when applying the marinade, place the fish with the dill and beetroot mixture in a large ziplock plastic bag. Close the bag and massage the mixture into the fish.

Make hors d'oeuvres for a party by piling slices of the fish on top of thick cucumber rounds, or rounds of pumpernickel or rye bread, then sprinkle with fresh dill.

For a stylish salad, toss the sliced fish with mixed lettuce leaves and thinly sliced radishes, and dress with a mustard vinaigrette.

Serve with a tomato and basil salad. Use red and yellow cherry tomatoes for variety.

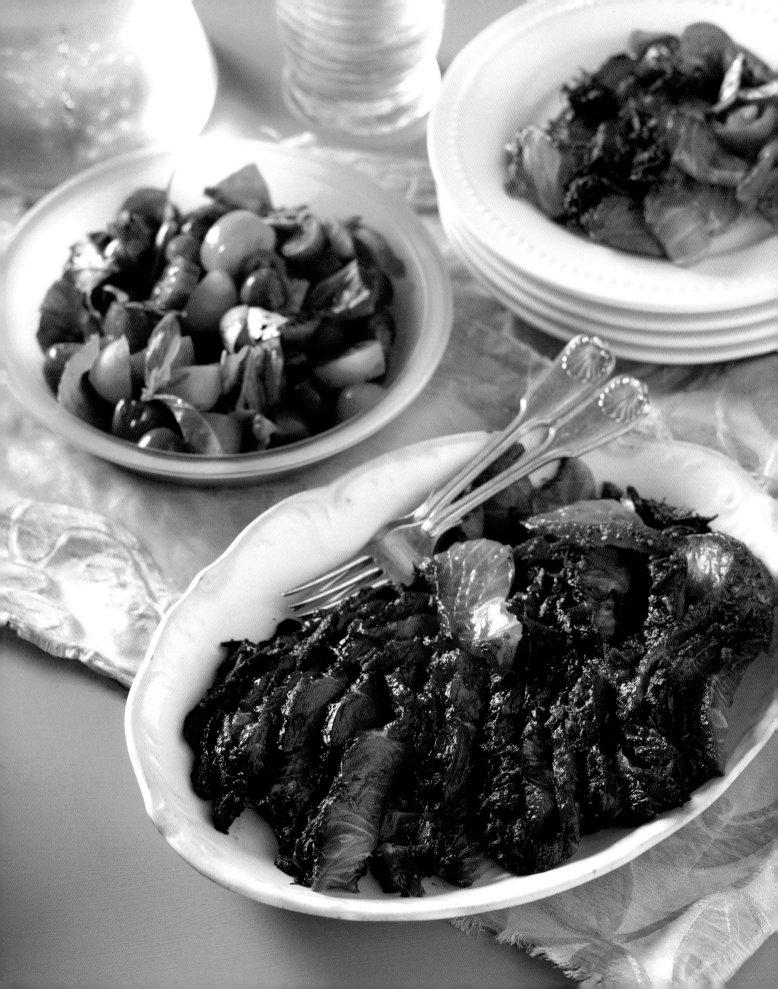

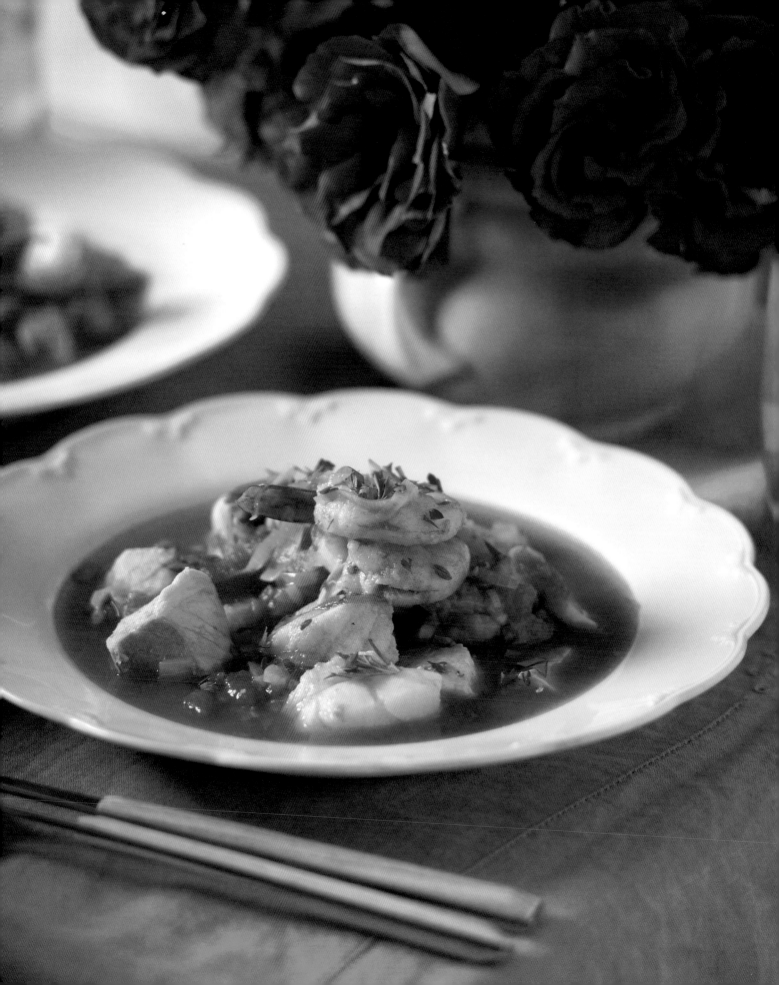

Seafood in a saffron tomato broth

1 kg (2 lb) assorted fish fillets and fish steaks,
    such as ling, sea bream, salmon,
    red mullet, whiting, hake and cod,
    and raw prawns (uncooked shrimp)
4–5 saffron threads
2 tablespoons extra virgin olive oil
1 small leek, thinly sliced
1 small red onion, very finely chopped
2 large cloves garlic, crushed
1 teaspoon fennel seeds
1 teaspoon cumin seeds
2 strips orange zest, all white pith discarded,
    finely shredded
1 kg (2 lb) ripe tomatoes, skins removed,
    chopped
1 cup (250 ml) tomato passata
    (puréed tomatoes)
4 cups (1 litre) salt-reduced fish or
    vegetable stock
freshly ground black pepper
chopped fresh parsley, to garnish
4 slices sourdough, toasted, to serve

PREPARATION 25 minutes
COOKING 20 minutes SERVES 6

EACH SERVING PROVIDES 1181 kJ, 282 kcal, 39 g protein,
10 g fat (2 g saturated fat), 8 g carbohydrate (6 g sugars),
3 g fibre, 246 mg sodium

> Saffron, garlic and tomato contain high
> levels of anti-oxidants and make a tasty
> base for this traditional seafood stew. Make sure
> you include some oily fish, such as salmon,
> ocean trout or mackerel, to get the benefits of
> their high levels of omega-3 oils.

1 Cut fish into 2.5 cm–5 cm (1–2 inch) pieces. Peel and devein prawns. Set aside.

2 Toast saffron threads in a dry pan over medium heat for just 30 seconds, until threads become a little dry. Remove from heat and crush lightly with back of a spoon. Set aside.

3 Heat oil in a large heavy-based saucepan. Add leek, onion and garlic, and cook over low heat, stirring frequently, about 5 minutes. Add fennel and cumin seeds and orange zest, and continue to cook a further 3–4 minutes. Add tomatoes and saffron, and cook, stirring, a further 3–4 minutes. Add tomato passata and stock. Bring to a boil, then reduce heat and simmer gently 5 minutes. Season well with pepper.

4 Add fish pieces, beginning with those that have the firmest flesh, then adding the softer, thinner-fleshed pieces of fish and the prawns a little later. Simmer until seafood is just cooked, then use a slotted spoon to remove seafood and arrange in a warmed serving bowl. Increase heat until the broth boils, then ladle over seafood in the bowl.

5 Scatter over parsley. Serve hot, accompanied by slices of toasted sourdough.

COOK'S TIP Using different types of fish, along with prawns, will give a range of textures and flavours. Well-cleaned fresh mussels or clams are also good additions. Cook the firmer-fleshed fish slightly longer than the delicate pieces and the prawns. Make sure the broth simmers gently; if it cooks too robustly, the fish will overcook very quickly.

You could rub the slices of sourdough with 1 clove garlic, halved, before toasting, if you prefer.

Citrus-marinated scallops

1 lime
1 small lemon
2 small oranges
2 tablespoons extra virgin olive oil
12 large fresh scallops, without roe
1 cup (30 g) fresh coriander (cilantro) leaves
1 cup (30 g) watercress sprigs, trimmed
freshly ground black pepper

PREPARATION 15 minutes
COOKING 5 minutes SERVES 4 as a starter

EACH SERVING PROVIDES 539 kJ, 129 kcal, 5 g protein,
9 g fat (1 g saturated fat), 6 g carbohydrate (4 g sugars),
2 g fibre, 72 mg sodium

This quick and easy dish is a delicious source of omega-3 oils, as well as being high in anti-oxidants thanks to the citrus and herbs.

1 Finely grate zest of lime, lemon and 1 orange. Put citrus zest and 1 tablespoon olive oil in a bowl and combine. Add scallops and stir to coat well with marinade.

2 Discard white pith from lemon and both oranges, then carefully cut out the segments with a sharp knife. Slice each lemon segment into 2 or 3 pieces. Leave orange segments whole. Put lemon and orange segments in a serving bowl. Add coriander leaves and watercress sprigs.

3 Juice the lime. Whisk together with remaining oil and a little pepper in a small bowl. Set dressing aside.

4 Heat a large non-stick frying pan over medium–high heat. Add scallops and cook 1–2 minutes on each side. Remove from heat and toss warm scallops with lemon and orange segments, coriander and watercress in the serving bowl. Pour over dressing and toss through carefully. Serve immediately.

COOK'S TIP Frozen scallops can be used for this recipe. Defrost overnight in the refrigerator, then pat dry with paper towel and marinate as in step 1.

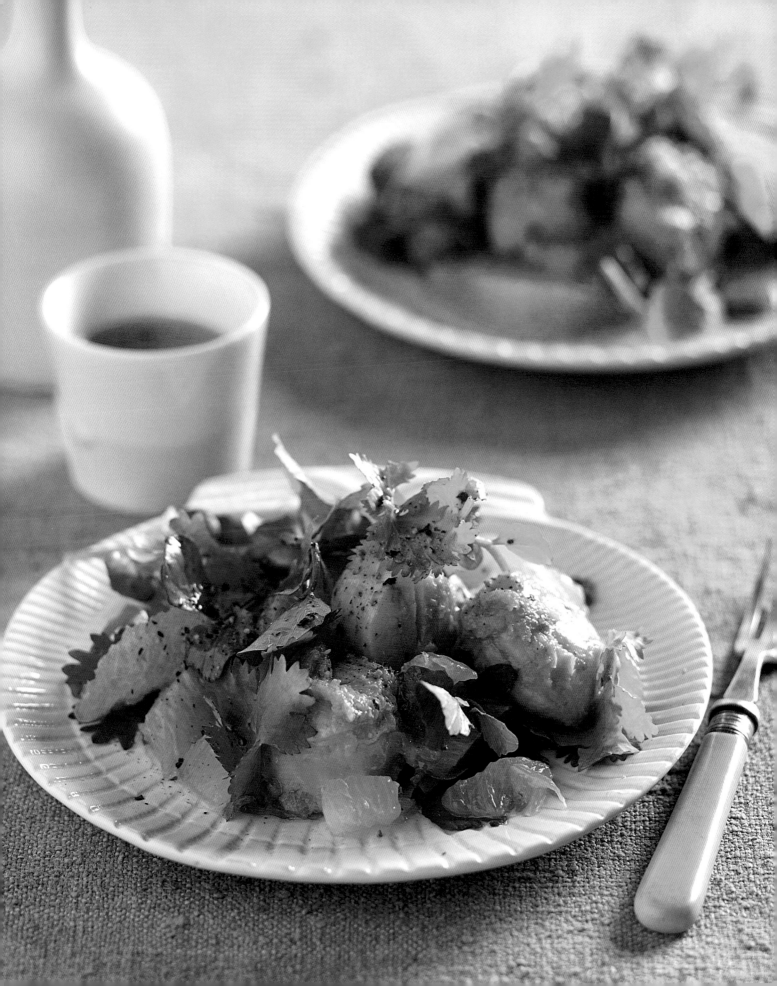

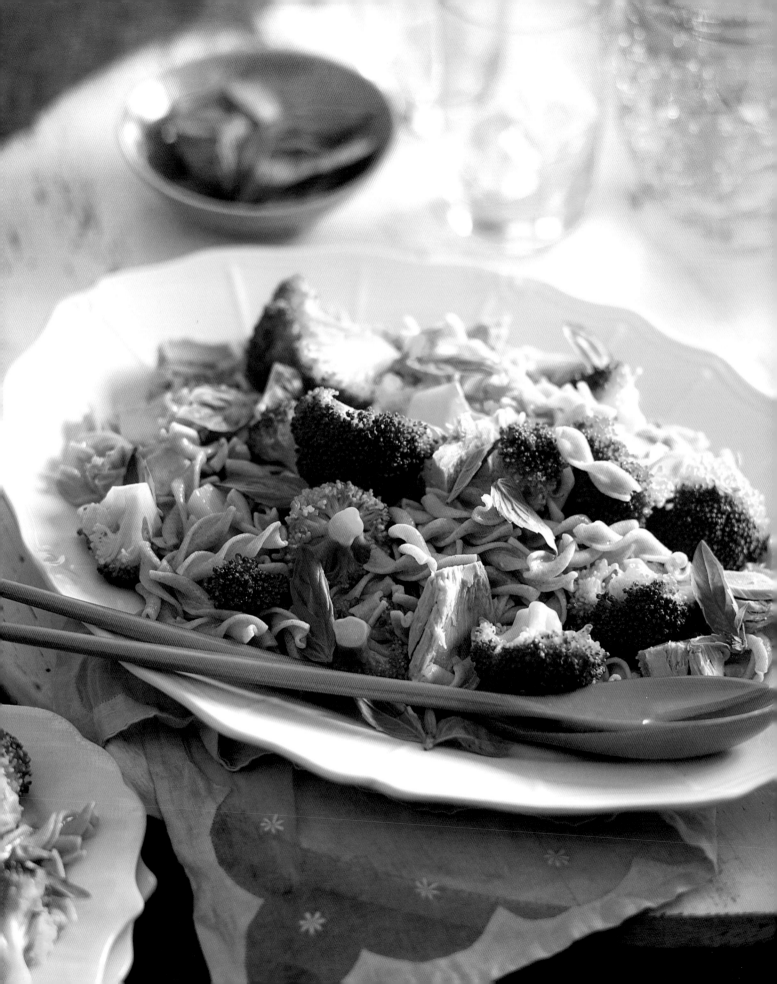

Wholemeal pasta with broccoli, tuna and basil

300 g (10 oz) wholemeal (whole-wheat)
   pasta spirals
500 g (1 lb) broccoli, cut into florets
2 tablespoons red wine vinegar
2 tablespoons extra virgin olive oil
425 g (15 oz) can tuna in olive oil
1/3 cup (10 g) fresh basil, torn
freshly ground black pepper
1/2 lemon, for juice

PREPARATION 10 minutes
COOKING 15 minutes SERVES 4

EACH SERVING PROVIDES 2263 kJ, 541 kcal, 36 g protein,
22 g fat (3 g saturated fat), 47 g carbohydrate (<1 g sugars),
13 g fibre, 410 mg sodium

A meal of wholemeal pasta tossed with basil, canned tuna and broccoli makes a high-protein and high-fibre light meal, with a good amount of folate and omega-3 oils from the tuna.

1 Cook pasta in a large saucepan of boiling water, 10–12 minutes, or until just tender, following packet instructions. Add broccoli for final 2 minutes of cooking time. Drain, then return pasta and broccoli to the pan.

2 Meanwhile, put vinegar and extra virgin olive oil in a small bowl and mix to combine well.

3 Drain tuna of excess oil, reserving 2 tablespoons oil. Break up tuna with a fork, then add to saucepan with reserved oil, basil and vinegar and oil mixture. Gently toss through pasta and broccoli, season with pepper and a squeeze of lemon juice, and serve.

COOK'S TIP You can replace the broccoli with asparagus and broad (fava) beans. Or try artichoke hearts in brine (from a jar), rinsed, along with halved red cherry tomatoes, chopped fresh parsley, finely chopped chilli and grated lemon zest.

White fish ceviche with avocado, capsicum, onion and tomato

500 g (1 lb) firm white fish, such as blue-eye, snapper, hake or cod
3 large limes
1 red capsicum (bell pepper), finely diced
1 small red onion, finely diced
1 small clove garlic, crushed (optional)
2 ripe tomatoes, skins removed, diced
1 small cucumber, peeled and seeded, diced
1 tablespoon chopped fresh coriander (cilantro) leaves, plus extra leaves, to garnish
1/4 teaspoon ground cumin
1/2 teaspoon dried oregano
1 small pinch white pepper
1 firm ripe avocado, diced
1 lime, quartered, to serve

PREPARATION 20 minutes, plus 3–6 hours marinating
SERVES 4

EACH SERVING PROVIDES 1244 kJ, 297 kcal, 29 g protein, 17 g fat (4 g saturated fat), 11 g carbohydrate (5 g sugars), 5 g fibre, 122 mg sodium

In this recipe, chunks of white fish are 'cooked' by being marinated in lime juice. This is the ultimate in anti-inflammatory recipes with its combination of high anti-oxidant foods and omega-3 oils from the fish.

1 Pat fish dry with paper towel. Cut into 2 cm (3/4 inch) cubes and remove any bones. Put in a glass dish with a lid.

2 Finely grate zest of 1 lime and juice all 3 limes. Add lime zest and juice to fish and stir to coat. Cover with lid or plastic wrap and refrigerate 3–6 hours. The fish is 'cooked' and ready to eat when it is firm and opaque.

3 Drain off any liquid from fish. Transfer fish to a large bowl. Add capsicum, onion, garlic if using, tomatoes, cucumber, chopped coriander, cumin, oregano and white pepper and stir to combine. Gently fold in avocado.

4 Spoon fish mixture onto serving plates. Garnish with extra coriander leaves and serve with lime.

COOK'S TIP The amount of marinating time the fish will need so that it is 'cooked' and ready to eat will depend on the type and thickness of the fish. Fresh salmon or tuna also work very well for the ceviche.

Finely chopped chilli will add a little spice to this recipe. If you want to tone down the heat, split the chilli in half with a sharp knife and use the knife tip to rub the seeds and membrane away. Or use jalapeño chilli in brine, rinsed, drained and finely chopped.

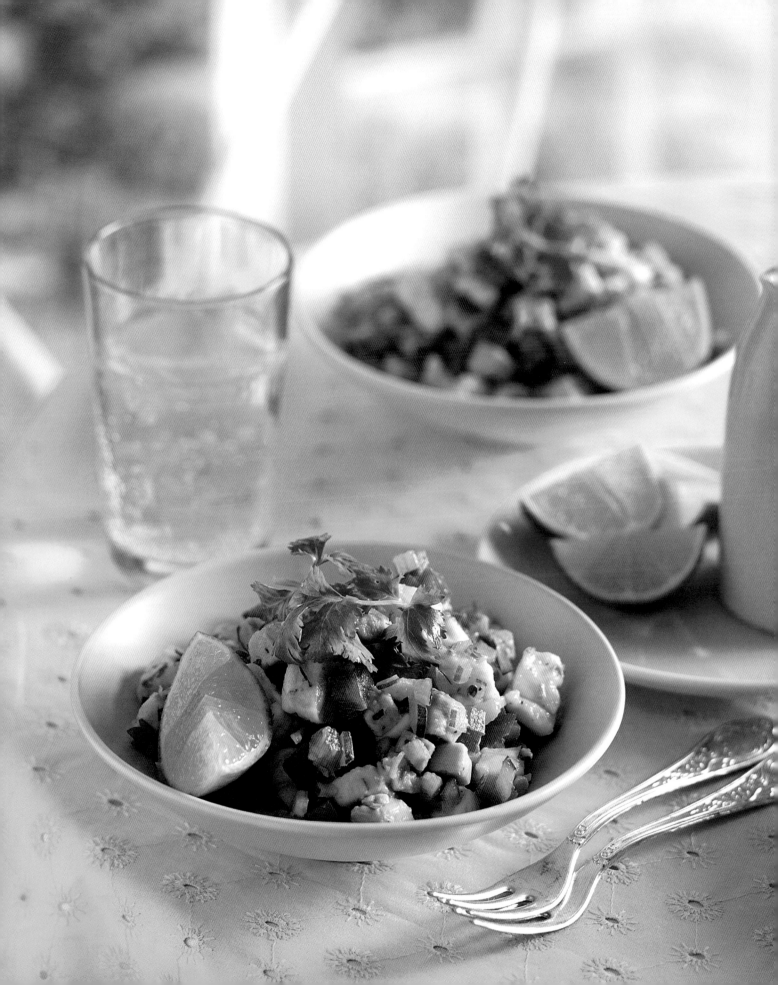

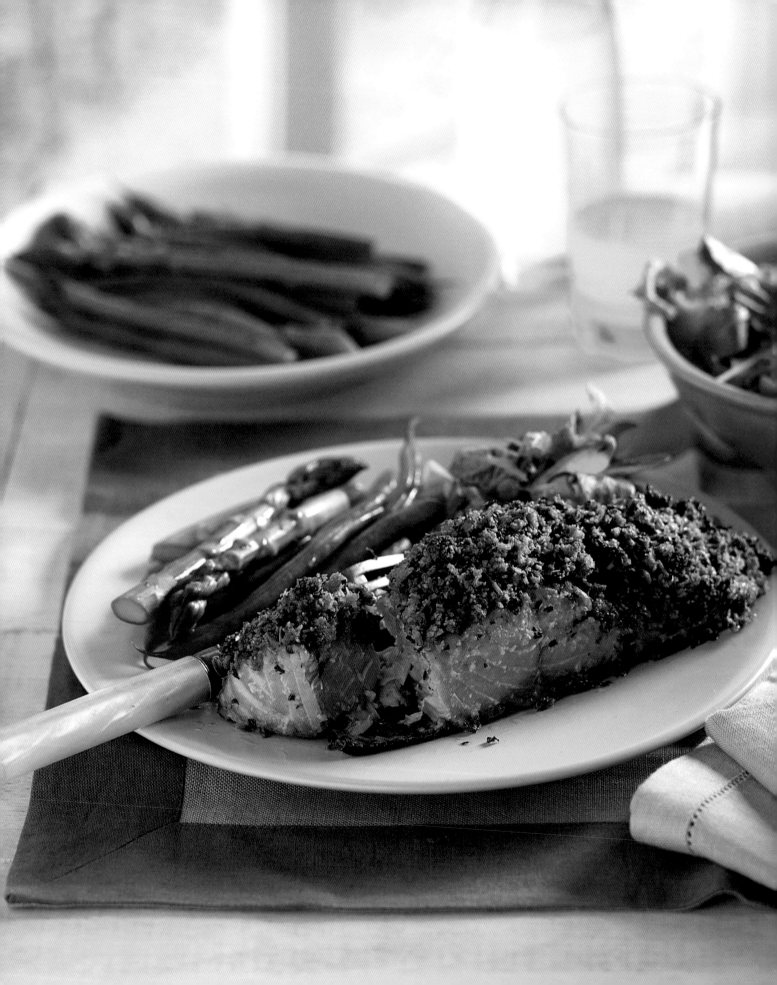

Salmon with pesto crust

4 salmon fillets, with skin on
4 slices wholemeal (whole-wheat) bread
extra virgin olive oil cooking spray
2 cloves garlic, peeled
2 cups (60 g) fresh basil
2 tablespoons pine nuts, toasted
1/3 cup (80 ml) extra virgin olive oil
3 tablespoons grated parmesan

PREPARATION 15 minutes
COOKING 35 minutes SERVES 4

EACH SERVING PROVIDES 2351 kJ, 562 kcal, 38 g protein,
39 g fat (7 g saturated fat), 16 g carbohydrate (1 g sugars),
4 g fibre, 340 mg sodium

> In this recipe salmon, high in omega-3
> oils, is baked with a crust, combining the
> benefits of the fish oil and the anti-oxidants
> from the basil.

1 Preheat oven to 200°C (400°F/Gas 6). Remove any bones from salmon with tweezers. Put salmon skin side down in a shallow non-stick roasting pan (baking dish) or a roasting pan lined with baking (parchment) paper. Set aside.

2 Put bread slices on a baking tray, spray with cooking spray and bake 5 minutes on each side, or until lightly golden and crisp. Leave to cool. Put toasted bread in a food processor or blender and process to form breadcrumbs. Remove and put in a bowl.

3 Put garlic, basil and pine nuts in food processor and process until finely chopped. Add oil and process until combined. Add pesto mixture and parmesan to breadcrumbs in bowl and stir to combine.

4 Spoon pesto crumb mixture over the top of each salmon fillet. Bake 20–25 minutes, depending on the thickness of the fish. Test with the tip of a knife; the fish should be translucent in the centre and the pesto crumb mixture should be crusty. Serve immediately.

COOK'S TIP When purchasing the fish, ask for salmon fillets that are all of a similar thickness, cut from the centre, so that the fish cooks evenly.

The salmon would go well with steamed green vegetables such as beans or asparagus.

Parmesan-crumbed baked fish

1 cup (150 g) plain (all-purpose) flour

1 egg

2 tablespoons low-fat milk

2 cups (170 g) wholemeal (whole-wheat)
    dry breadcrumbs

grated zest of 2 small limes

3 tablespoons grated parmesan

500 g (1 lb) small white fish fillets,
    such as whiting or mirror dory, patted dry,
    sliced into long thin strips

extra virgin olive oil cooking spray

PREPARATION 20 minutes, plus 10 minutes chilling
COOKING 15 minutes SERVES 4

EACH SERVING PROVIDES 2046 kJ, 488 kcal, 40 g protein,
12 g fat (3 g saturated fat), 53 g carbohydrate (3 g sugars),
4 g fibre, 461 mg sodium

 This is a great low-fat alternative to
deep-fried crumbed fish.

1 Preheat oven to 200°C (400°C/Gas 6). Line a large baking tray with baking paper (baking sheet with parchment paper).

2 Put flour on a plate. Beat egg and milk together in a bowl. Combine breadcrumbs, lime zest and parmesan in a separate bowl.

3 Coat each piece of fish in flour, shaking off any excess. Dip each piece into egg mixture, then into breadcrumb mixture. Put crumbed fish in a single layer on a tray or plate and chill in refrigerator about 10 minutes.

4 Put fish on the prepared baking tray. Generously spray one side of fish with cooking spray, then turn and spray the other side. Bake 12–15 minutes, or until crumbs are golden and fish is cooked.

COOK'S TIP Serve with a green salad.

Cut the fish into thin strips rather than large pieces; the fish will cook more quickly and the crumb coating will become crisp more easily. For a crispier crumb coating, use a mixture of half fresh breadcrumbs and half dried breadcrumbs.

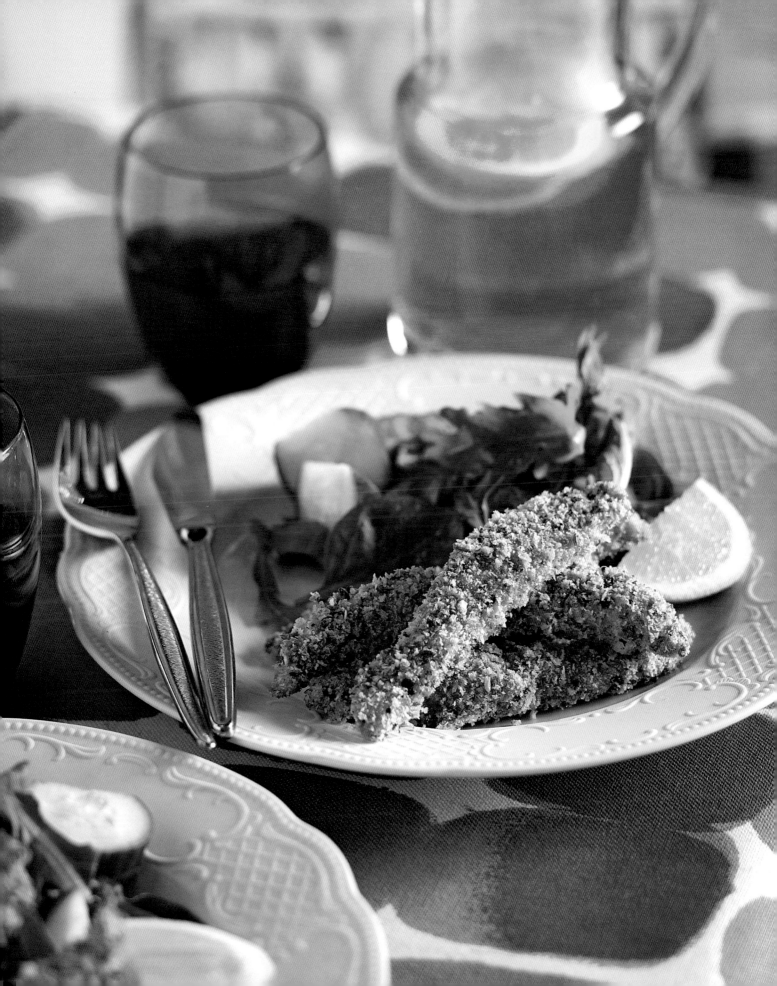

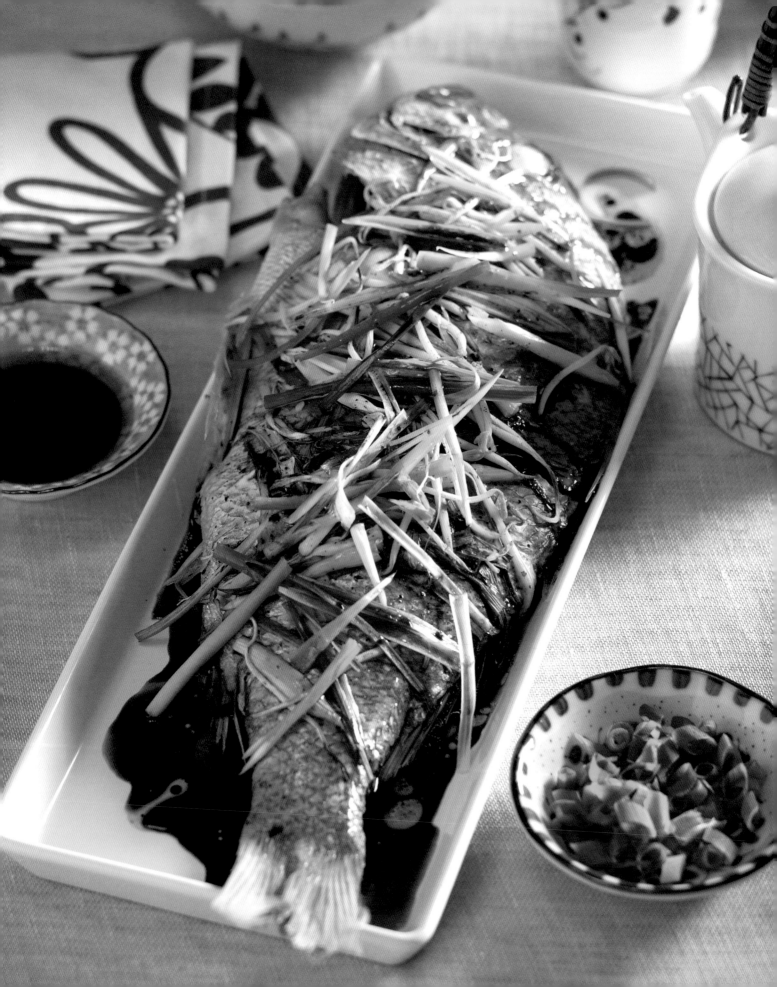

Steamed fish with bean sprouts, ginger and spring onions

1 large whole fish (about 1 kg/2 lb),
    such as snapper, bream, mackerel or cod,
    cleaned by fishmonger
1/2 cup (45 g) bean sprouts, trimmed
4 spring onions (scallions), finely shredded
6 cm (2 1/2 inch) piece fresh ginger, peeled
    and finely shredded
juice of 1 lemon
freshly ground black pepper
1/3 cup (80 ml) salt-reduced soy sauce
1 tablespoon sesame oil

PREPARATION 10 minutes
COOKING 20 minutes SERVES 4

EACH SERVING PROVIDES 1777 kJ, 424 kcal, 73 g protein,
12 g fat (3 g saturated fat), 4 g carbohydrate (2 g sugars),
1 g fibre, 1043 mg sodium

> This traditional Chinese way of serving a large whole fish is rich in anti-oxidants from the ginger and spring onions. Both the fish and the sesame oil are rich in beneficial minerals.

1 Rinse fish and pat dry with paper towel. With a sharp knife, make three or four diagonal cuts down to the bone on each side of fish.

2 Half-fill a large wok, saucepan or steamer base with water and bring to a boil, then reduce heat so that water is at a simmer. Line a large bamboo or metal steamer with a circle of baking (parchment) paper. Snip paper in a few places to allow steam to come through.

3 Put fish on baking paper in the steamer. Scatter bean sprouts, spring onions and ginger over fish. Drizzle with lemon juice and season with pepper.

4 Carefully put steamer above simmering water – the water should not touch the base of the steamer. Cover and steam about 20 minutes, until fish is just cooked.

5 Meanwhile, put soy sauce and sesame oil in a small bowl and whisk with a fork to combine. Transfer fish to warmed serving plates, pour over the soy mixture and serve.

COOK'S TIP You could make this recipe with four evenly sized fish fillets. Reduce the steaming time to about 10 minutes, depending on the thickness of the fillets – check them carefully to avoid overcooking.

Shredding is a technique where the food is cut into fine matchstick-like shreds. You first cut the food into slices, then stack a few slices on top of each other and cut them lengthwise into very fine strips. This technique is often used for preparing ginger.

Serve the fish with extra shredded spring onions (scallions) on the side, if desired.

Fish parcels with pomegranate dressing

1 cup (250 ml) fresh or bottled
   pomegranate juice
¼ cup (90 g) honey
4 firm fish fillets, such as salmon,
   ocean trout or blue-eye trevalla
½ small red onion, very finely chopped
1 small clove garlic, crushed
1 tablespoon chopped fresh basil
1 tablespoon chopped fresh parsley
1 tablespoon chopped fresh coriander
   (cilantro) leaves

PREPARATION 20 minutes
COOKING 20 minutes SERVES 4

EACH SERVING PROVIDES 1122 kJ, 268 kcal, 31 g protein,
3 g fat (1 g saturated fat), 29 g carbohydrate (28 g sugars),
<1 g fibre, 138 mg sodium

> This recipe combines the healthy fats of the fish with the powerful anti-oxidant properties of pomegranate, onion, garlic and herbs. For a healthy meal, serve with couscous and a fresh salad.

1 Preheat oven to 200°C (400°F/Gas 6). Put pomegranate juice and honey in a small saucepan. Bring to a boil, reduce heat to low and simmer 8–10 minutes, or until reduced and slightly syrupy. Leave to cool.

2 Meanwhile, cut four 40 cm (16 inch) circles of foil and four 40 cm circles of baking (parchment) paper. Put a baking paper circle on top of each foil circle. Put 1 fish fillet in the centre of each circle and tuck thin ends of fish under itself. Join foil and paper sides together, pleating to close the parcel securely. Put fish parcels on a baking tray (sheet). Cook 12–15 minutes, or until parcels puff up.

3 Meanwhile, put cooled pomegranate syrup, onion, garlic, basil, parsley and coriander in a bowl and stir to combine.

4 To serve, transfer each fish parcel to a serving plate. Carefully open parcels and spoon pomegranate dressing over each.

COOK'S TIP To make fresh pomegranate juice, put pomegranate seeds in a food processor or blender and process to obtain the juice. (To obtain the seeds from a pomegranate, see page 29.) Strain before using. A medium pomegranate gives about 100 ml (3½ fl oz) of juice. Alternatively, you can buy bottled pomegranate juice in the fresh juice or fresh produce section of many large supermarkets.

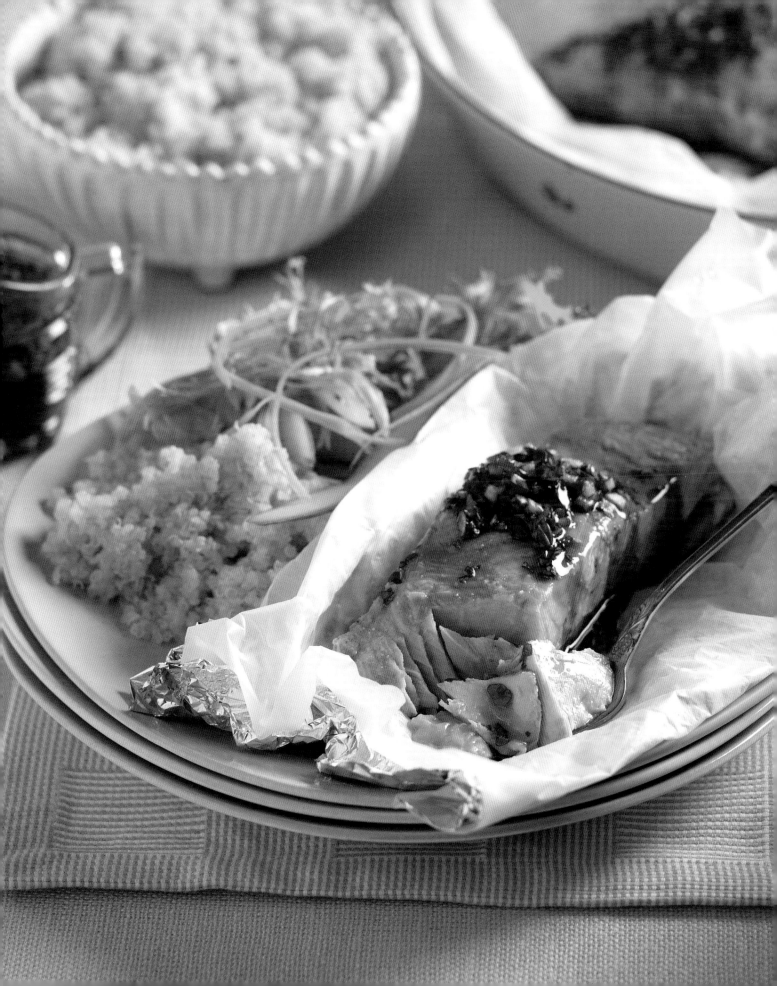

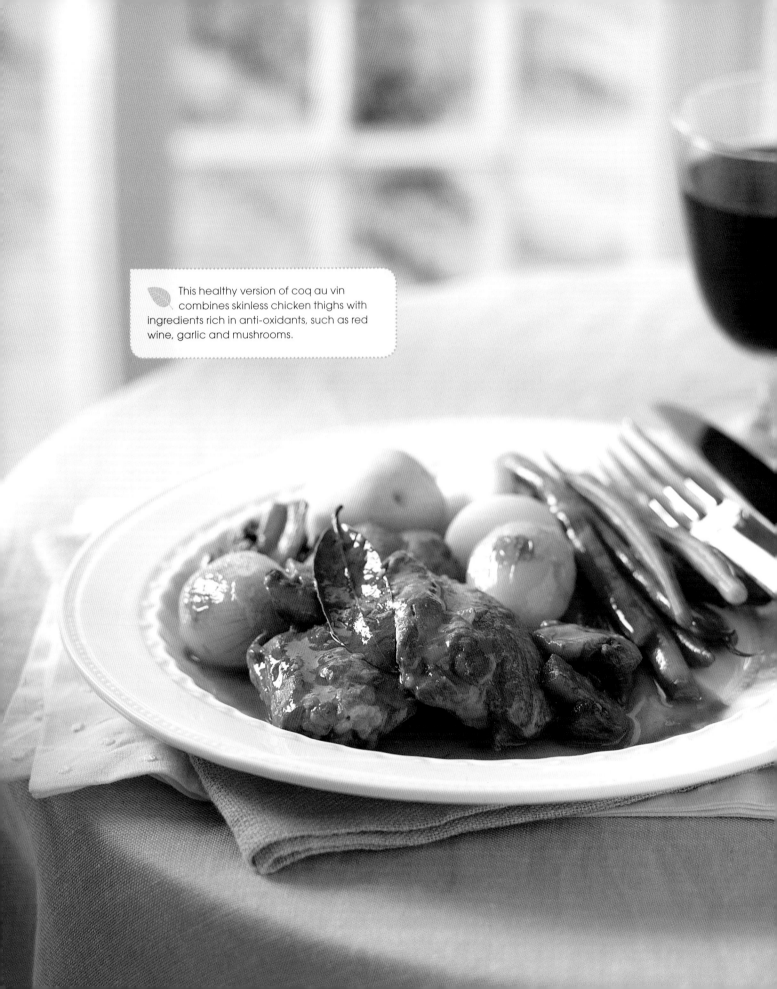

This healthy version of coq au vin combines skinless chicken thighs with ingredients rich in anti-oxidants, such as red wine, garlic and mushrooms.

Red wine braised chicken

1 kg (2 lb) boneless, skinless chicken thighs,
   halved and trimmed of fat
olive oil cooking spray
freshly ground black pepper
1 tablespoon extra virgin olive oil
8 baby onions or small white onions, peeled
15 button mushrooms (about 175 g/6 oz),
   trimmed, halved if large
3 cloves garlic, finely chopped
1 tablespoon plain (all-purpose) flour
1 cup (250 ml) red wine
1 cup (250 ml) homemade or salt-reduced
   chicken stock
1 bay leaf
3 sprigs fresh thyme or 1 teaspoon dried
   thyme or marjoram
2 strips orange zest

PREPARATION 20 minutes
COOKING 1 hour SERVES 4

EACH SERVING PROVIDES 1994 kJ, 476 kcal, 51 g protein,
23 g fat (6 g saturated fat), 7 g carbohydrate (3 g sugars),
3 g fibre, 399 mg sodium

1 Preheat oven to 180°C (350°F/Gas 4).

2 Lightly spray chicken thighs with cooking spray
and season with pepper. Heat a non-stick frying pan
over medium heat, then add chicken in batches and
cook 4–5 minutes, until golden brown. Transfer
chicken to a casserole dish or ovenproof dish with
a tight-fitting lid. Repeat to cook remaining chicken.

3 Reduce heat to medium–low, add oil and onions
and cook, stirring, 2 minutes. Transfer onions to
casserole dish. Add mushrooms to pan and cook,
stirring occasionally, 2–3 minutes, or until mushrooms
are tender. Add garlic and cook a further 30 seconds.

4 Sprinkle in flour and cook, stirring, 1–2 minutes,
until flour coats the mushrooms and is light brown.
Stir in wine and stock and scrape up any residue
from the bottom of the pan. Cook, stirring
constantly, until mixture boils. Pour over chicken
and onions in casserole dish and add bay leaf, thyme
or marjoram and orange zest.

5 Cover dish and cook in oven 45 minutes, or until
chicken is tender. Stir once or twice during cooking,
and add a little more stock or some water if needed
so that chicken remains just covered with liquid.

COOK'S TIP Serve this chicken dish with steamed
small new potatoes and green beans.

You can make this casserole 2–3 days beforehand.
Refrigerate it as soon as the steam has evaporated,
then reheat gently just before it is needed.

Chicken, almond and brown rice pilaf

1 bay leaf
4–5 black peppercorns
1–2 star anise, crushed (optional)
2 skinless, boneless chicken breasts
    (about 200 g/7 oz each)
2 tablespoons extra virgin olive oil
1 small onion, finely chopped
2 cloves garlic, crushed
2 teaspoons ground coriander
2 teaspoons ground cumin
1 cup (210 g) medium-grain brown rice
2½ cups (625 ml) homemade or salt-reduced
    chicken stock
½ cup (45 g) flaked almonds, toasted
2 tablespoons currants
1 cup (30 g) fresh coriander (cilantro) leaves
    or flat-leaf (Italian) parsley

PREPARATION 20 minutes, plus 5 minutes standing
COOKING 50 minutes SERVES 4

EACH SERVING PROVIDES 2739 kJ, 654 kcal, 53 g protein,
28 g fat (5 g saturated fat), 48 g carbohydrate (3 g sugars),
4 g fibre, 530 mg sodium

Shredded chicken, almonds and brown
rice, together with anti-oxidant-rich
spice, combine to make a dish that provides
whole grains and complete protein.

1 Half-fill a medium saucepan with water and add
the bay leaf, peppercorns and star anise. Cover and
simmer 5 minutes. Add chicken, cover and simmer
10 minutes, or until just cooked. Remove chicken
from pan, finely shred and refrigerate until needed.

2 Heat oil in a medium frying pan over medium–low
heat. Add onion and garlic and cook, stirring,
1–2 minutes. Add coriander, cumin and rice, and
cook, stirring, about 2 minutes, or until grains just
begin to colour to a light golden brown.

3 Add stock and bring to a boil, stirring occasionally.
Reduce heat to low and cook, covered, 40–45 minutes,
or until rice is tender. Remove from heat and leave to
stand, covered, 5 minutes.

4 Separate and fluff up rice with a fork or spatula.
Stir in almonds, currants, coriander or parsley and
shredded chicken, and serve.

COOK'S TIP The chicken can be poached and
shredded 2–3 hours ahead of time, or even the day
before if you prefer.

This tasty rice dish makes a great lunch for the office
or for a picnic.

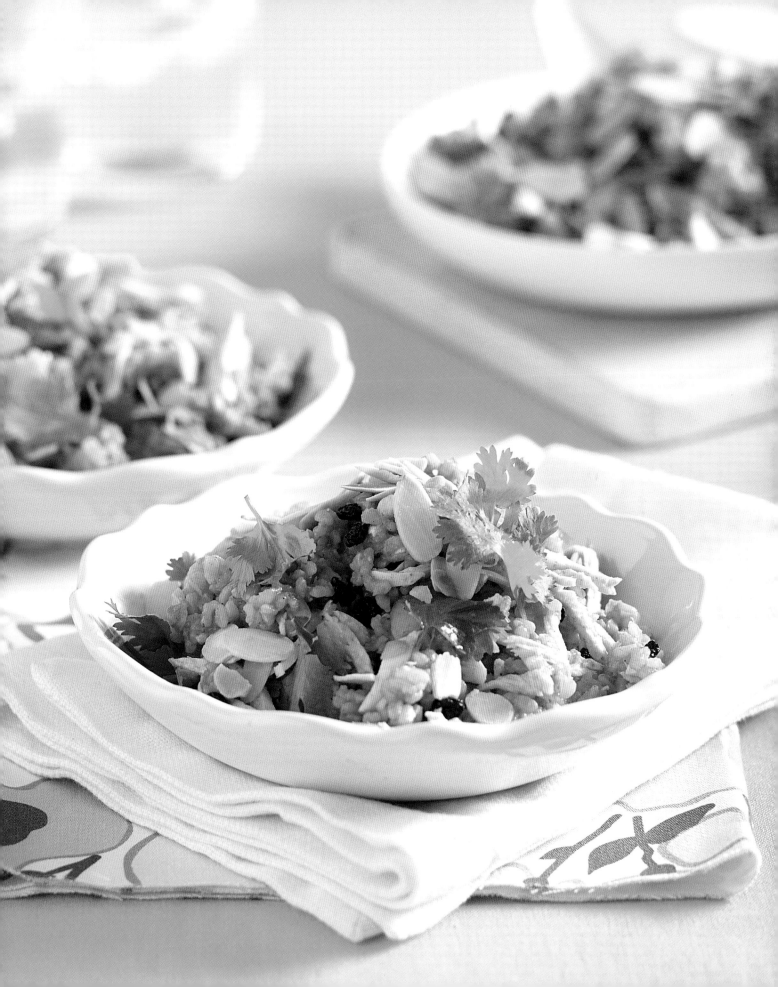

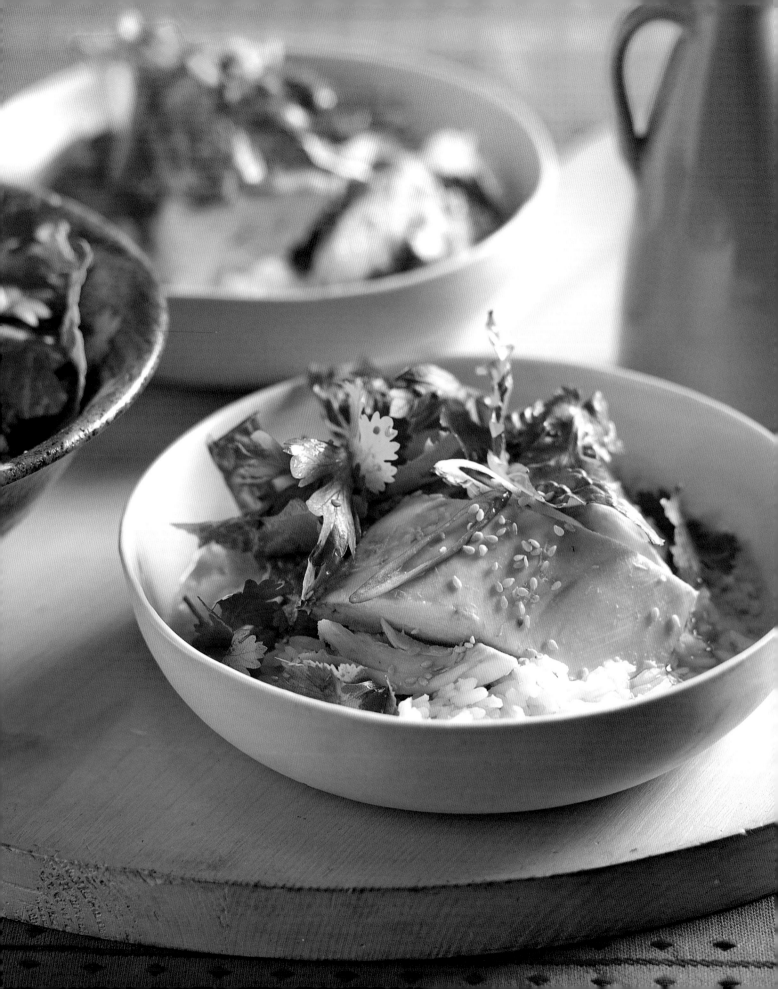

Whole chicken poached in ginger with a herb salad

1.5 kg (3 lb) whole chicken
1 cup (250 ml) Chinese rice wine
4 cloves garlic, peeled
2 x 6 cm (2$\frac{1}{2}$ inch) pieces fresh ginger,
    peeled and thickly sliced
4–6 black peppercorns
2 strips orange zest
4 whole star anise
steamed brown rice, to serve
1 tablespoon sesame seeds, toasted, to serve

Herb salad

1 baby cos (romaine) lettuce, halved,
    cut into wedges
1 cup (30 g) fresh coriander (cilantro) leaves
1 cup (30 g) fresh basil, Thai basil or flat-leaf
    (Italian) parsley
2 spring onions (scallions), finely sliced
1 tablespoon salt-reduced soy sauce
1 tablespoon sesame oil

PREPARATION 25 minutes, plus cooling
COOKING 2 hours SERVES 6

EACH SERVING PROVIDES 1204 kJ, 287 kcal, 26 g protein,
14 g fat (3 g saturated fat), 6 g carbohydrate (3 g sugars),
2 g fibre, 252 mg sodium

This is a simple and fragrant dish with the anti-oxidant benefits of ginger and fresh herbs, as well as the antibacterial power of chicken soup.

1 Wash chicken under cold running water, including cavity. Remove neck and trim off any excess fat. Put chicken in a large deep saucepan, add rice wine and enough cold water to cover the chicken by about 5 cm (2 inches). (You will need about 4 cups/1 litre water.) Add garlic, ginger, peppercorns, orange zest and star anise.

2 Slowly bring water to a simmer over medium heat. Reduce heat to low and simmer 1$\frac{1}{2}$–2 hours, or until chicken is very tender and pulling away from the bone. Leave chicken in broth until cool enough to handle. Remove chicken from pan, discard skin and bones, and store chicken meat in refrigerator until needed. Strain broth and set aside.

3 To make the herb salad, put lettuce in a serving bowl. Scatter over coriander, basil or parsley and spring onions. Combine soy sauce and sesame oil in a small bowl. Drizzle over salad just before serving.

4 Serve chicken pieces and steamed rice in serving bowls, with some of the reserved cooking broth spooned over. Sprinkle each with sesame seeds and accompany with herb salad.

COOK'S TIP You can replace Chinese rice wine with dry sherry or white wine. The flavour won't be quite the same, but the chicken and the broth will still taste delicious.

The cooking liquid makes a wonderful chicken soup. Skim off the fat from the top of the broth, then strain. Reheat the broth until boiling, add $\frac{1}{2}$ cup (15 g) coriander leaves and 2 sliced spring onions, stir for 30 seconds then serve.

Chicken lemon braise with Jerusalem artichokes

8 skinless chicken thigh cutlets, bone in
(about 1.5 kg/3 lb in total), trimmed of fat
olive oil cooking spray
freshly ground black pepper
1 tablespoon extra virgin olive oil
1 red onion, halved and sliced
2 cloves garlic, chopped
1 small lemon, halved and very thinly sliced
1 pinch saffron threads
3 cups (750 ml) homemade or salt-reduced
chicken stock
1 bay leaf
4 Jerusalem artichokes (about 400 g/14 oz),
scrubbed, cut into chunks
½ cup (10 g) flat-leaf (Italian) parsley,
roughly chopped, to serve

PREPARATION 20 minutes,
COOKING 50 minutes SERVES 4

EACH SERVING PROVIDES 1787 kJ, 427 kcal, 42 g protein,
22 g fat (6 g saturated fat), 15 g carbohydrate (6 g sugars),
4 g fibre, 668 mg sodium

Lemon, garlic and saffron – rich in anti-oxidants – combine here with Jerusalem artichokes, which are high in fibre and act as a probiotic, promoting the presence of beneficial bacteria in the gut.

1 Lightly spray both sides of chicken cutlets with cooking spray and season with pepper. Heat a large, deep frying pan over medium heat and cook chicken in batches 3–4 minutes, until lightly browned. Transfer to a plate and set aside. Repeat to cook remaining batches of chicken.

2 Heat oil in pan over medium heat. Add onion and garlic and cook, stirring frequently, until softened, about 2–3 minutes. Add lemon slices and cook a further 1 minute, until lightly browned and softened. Push onion, garlic and lemon to one side of pan. Add saffron threads and warm 5 seconds. Crush with a teaspoon, then add a little hot water to dissolve saffron.

3 Add stock and bay leaf and stir to mix well. Bring to a boil, then reduce heat to medium–low. Return chicken thighs to pan with Jerusalem artichokes and simmer, partially covered, 25–30 minutes, or until chicken is cooked and artichokes are tender. Remove lid, increase heat and cook vigorously 3–5 minutes, or until liquid has reduced and thickened slightly. Sprinkle with parsley and serve.

COOK'S TIP Serve with mashed potato and steamed green beans.

Jerusalem artichokes are an autumn and winter vegetable. These tubers look a little like a big ginger root with bumps and little lumps. They have a waxy texture and a sweet nutty taste. They are great to roast (skin on or off) and make delicious soup or purée, or they can be used in casseroles or braises. They are easier to peel if you first trim off any big bumps. They brown quickly once peeled, so put them in water with a little vinegar or lemon juice to stop discolouration. You could replace them with small potatoes in this recipe.

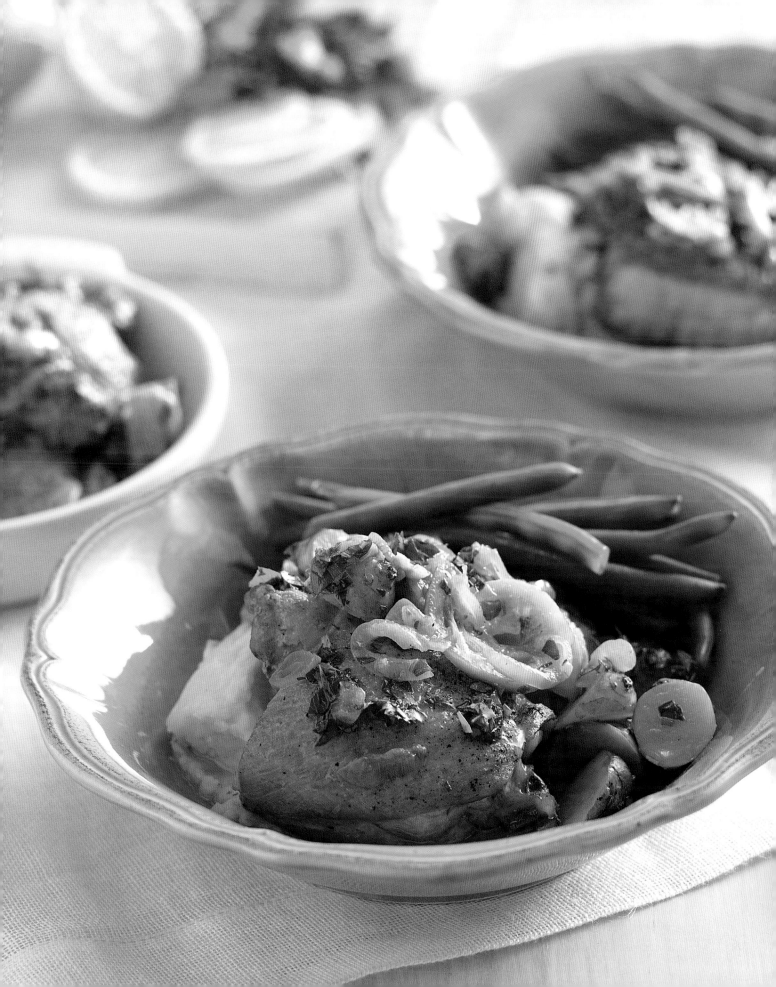

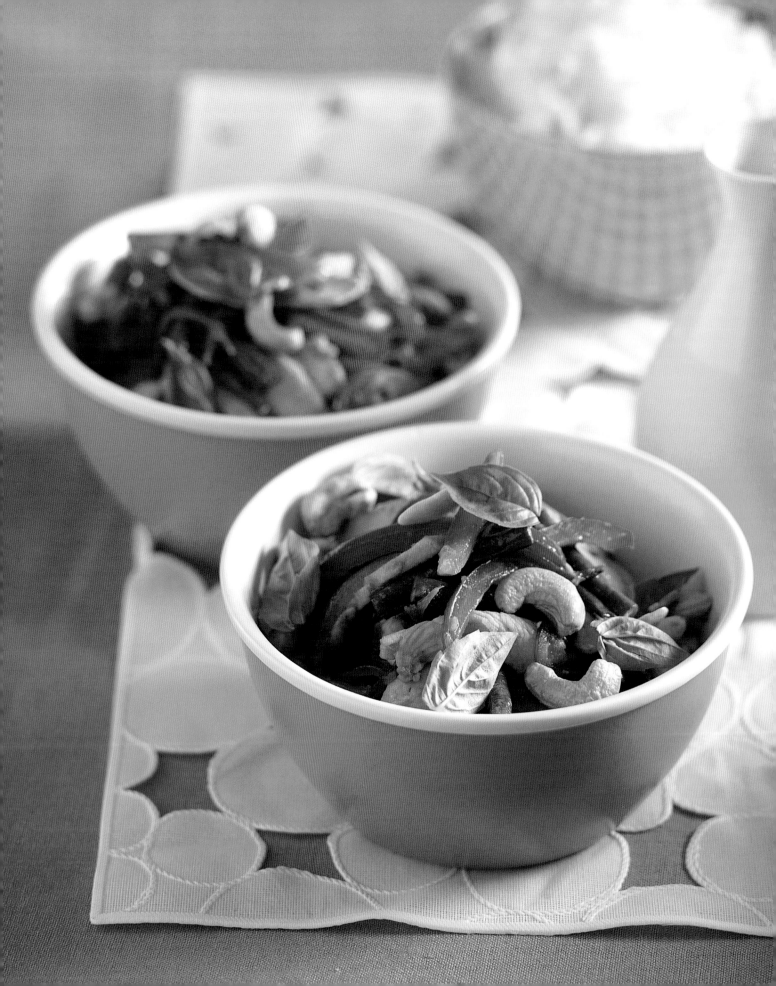

Stir-fried chicken with beans, turmeric and basil

7 chicken tenderloins (tenders) or 2 large
  boneless, skinless chicken breasts
  (about 500 g/1 lb in total), trimmed
  of sinew, cut into thin strips
2 tablespoons light olive oil
3 teaspoons grated fresh ginger
3 cm (1¼ inch) piece fresh turmeric, grated,
  or 1 teaspoon dried ground turmeric
1 small red onion, halved, cut into
  very fine wedges
1 bunch snake (yard-long) beans or
  350 g (12 oz) green beans, trimmed,
  cut into 4 cm (1½ inch) lengths
juice of 1 lime
1 tablespoon fish sauce or salt-reduced
  soy sauce
½ cup (15 g) small fresh basil leaves
½ cup (80 g) cashew nuts, toasted

PREPARATION 15 minutes,
COOKING 15 minutes SERVES 4

EACH SERVING PROVIDES 1629 kJ, 389 kcal, 33 g protein,
25 g fat (5 g saturated fat), 8 g carbohydrate (3 g sugars),
4 g fibre, 538 mg sodium

Colourful turmeric has powerful anti-oxidant and anti-inflammatory properties. It has been used in traditional medicine for thousands of years to soothe sore joints and calm the digestive system.

1 Place chicken strips in a bowl with 1 tablespoon oil and mix well.

2 Heat a wok or large frying pan over high heat until hot. Add half the chicken and stir-fry 3–4 minutes, until well browned and just cooked through. Transfer to a plate and keep warm. Reheat wok and cook remaining chicken, then set aside on the plate.

3 Reheat wok and add remaining oil. Add ginger, turmeric and onion, and stir-fry 1–2 minutes. Add beans and stir-fry 2–3 minutes, or until tender. Return chicken to wok and toss to warm through. Add lime juice, fish sauce or soy sauce, and basil leaves and stir to mix through. Reserve a few basil leaves and scatter on top before serving. Sprinkle with cashew nuts and serve immediately.

COOK'S TIP Serve this stir-fry with rice noodles or steamed rice.

Fresh turmeric's flavour is subtle, earthy and slightly bitter, but it's much more flavoursome than dried turmeric. Like the dried version, it gives a wonderful yellow hue to dishes such as curries, stir-fries and vegetable soups. Wear disposable plastic gloves to peel and grate it, as it will stain your hands. To store, wrap fresh unpeeled turmeric in foil or damp paper towel, then put in a ziplock plastic bag and keep in the refrigerator for up to 3 weeks.

Duck and lentils

2 tablespoons olive oil
1 onion (about 125 g/4 oz), finely diced
2 cloves garlic, finely diced
1 large carrot, finely diced
1 large celery stalk, finely diced
1 cup (200 g) French-style green (puy) lentils
2 cups (500 ml) homemade or salt-reduced
    chicken or vegetable stock or water
4 boneless duck breasts, with skin
    (about 150 g/5 oz each)
salt and freshly ground black pepper
olive oil, for frying
2 tablespoons chopped fresh flat-leaf
    (Italian) parsley, to garnish

PREPARATION 10 minutes, plus 5 minutes resting
COOKING 1 hour SERVES 4

EACH SERVING PROVIDES 2971 kJ, 710 kcal, 24 g protein,
65 g fat (18 g saturated fat), 8 g carbohydrate (3 g sugars),
4 g fibre, 205 mg sodium

> Lentils are legumes (pulses), and an anti-ageing dietary necessity. They add valuable protein and fibre to any dish. At the same time, they are low in fat and do not contain cholesterol-producing agents.

1 Preheat oven to 150°C (300°F/Gas 2). Heat oil in a large flameproof casserole dish. Add onions and garlic and cook over low heat 5 minutes, or until softened. Add carrot and celery and simmer until soft and starting to colour, about 10 minutes.

2 Add lentils and stock and stir well. Bring to a boil, then cover and put in oven to cook 45 minutes, until lentils are cooked through but still retain their shape.

3 Meanwhile, trim excess fat off duck breasts. Rinse duck under cold water and pat dry. Prick skin of each breast all over with point of a sharp knife, then rub well with a pinch each of salt and pepper. Leave to stand 30 minutes at room temperature.

4 Increase oven temperature to 200°C (400°F/Gas 6). Rub a little oil over a large heavy-based non-stick frying pan and heat over high heat until very hot. Add duck breasts, skin side down, sliding each a little with a 'swishing' action as they touch the hot surface to help prevent sticking. Firmly press the back of each duck breast with a metal spatula so entire skin surface is flat against pan and cook 5 minutes to crisp the skin. As the fat is rendered from the skin, pour it off into a heatproof bowl (use a spatula to hold duck in place while you pour fat out of pan), then wipe outside of pan carefully to avoid burning. Turn duck over and cook a further 1 minute.

5 Transfer duck breasts to a baking tray (sheet) and cook in oven 8 minutes, until cooked through but retaining a little pinkness. Rest in a warm place 5 minutes, then slice each breast into 4–5 slices, reserving any juices.

6 Remove lentils from oven and stir in reserved duck juices. Divide lentils among four serving plates, top each with a duck breast and sprinkle with parsley.

COOK'S TIP Duck has a reputation for being fatty, but it is high in beneficial monounsaturated fatty acids, and here the fat is reduced by the cooking method. Or remove the duck skin before cooking, if you prefer.

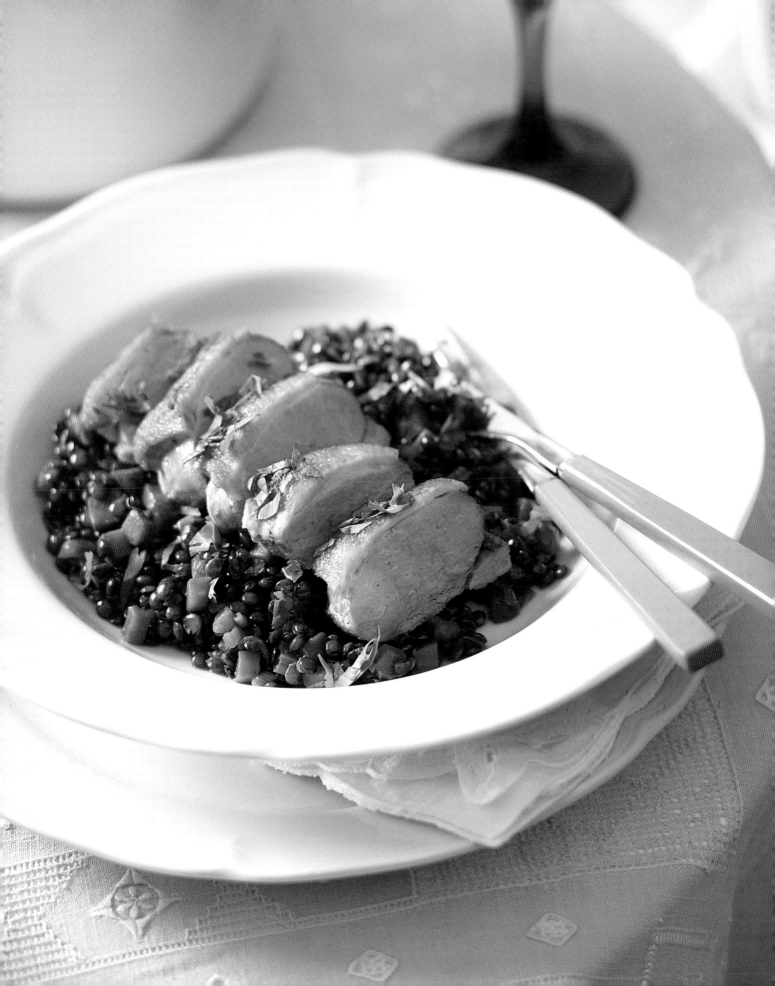

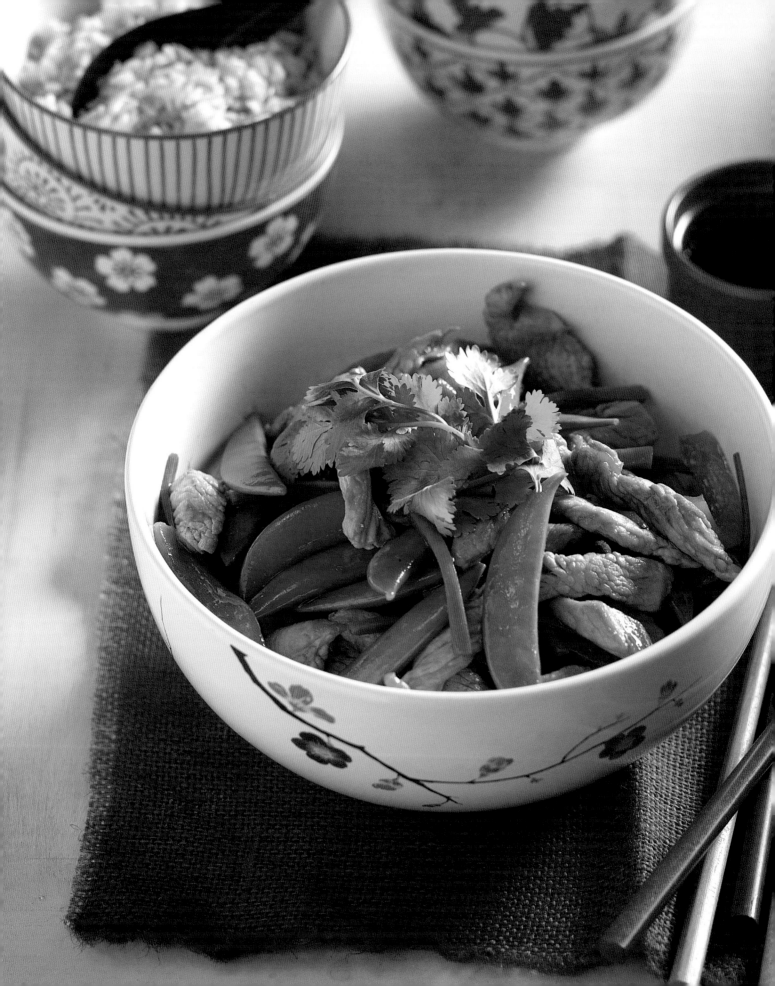

Turkey and vegetable stir-fry

500 g (1 lb) turkey breast steaks or turkey
    tenderloins (tenders), trimmed of sinew,
    cut into thin strips
2 tablespoons light olive oil
1 tablespoon salt-reduced soy sauce
1 tablespoon oyster sauce
2 teaspoons sesame oil
2 teaspoons cornflour (cornstarch)
175 g (6 oz) sugarsnap peas,
    topped and tailed
125 g (4 oz) baby corn, halved lengthwise
1 carrot, cut into thin matchsticks
2 cloves garlic, crushed
coriander (cilantro), to garnish

PREPARATION 15 minutes
COOKING 15 minutes SERVES 4

EACH SERVING PROVIDES 1216 kJ, 290 kcal, 30 g protein,
17 g fat (3 g saturated fat), 7 g carbohydrate (3 g sugars),
2 g fibre, 423 mg sodium

> Turkey is one of the best dietary sources
> of tryptophan, an amino acid (protein
> building-block) that is known to promote a
> good night's sleep, so turkey is a great basis
> for an evening meal. In this high-fibre stir-fry,
> turkey is combined with the benefits of
> anti-oxidants from the corn, sugarsnap peas,
> carrots and garlic.

1 Place turkey strips in a bowl with 1 tablespoon light olive oil and mix well. Put soy sauce, oyster sauce, sesame oil, cornflour and ¾ cup (175 ml) water in a separate bowl and stir to combine. Set aside.

2 Heat a wok or large frying pan until hot. Add half the turkey and stir-fry 3–4 minutes, until well browned and just cooked through. Transfer to a plate and set aside. Reheat wok and cook remaining turkey, then set aside on the plate.

3 Reheat wok and add remaining light olive oil. Add sugarsnap peas and corn and stir-fry 1–2 minutes. Add carrots and garlic and stir-fry 1–2 minutes, or until vegetables are just tender. Return turkey to wok, add reserved sauce mixture and stir-fry until sauce bubbles and turkey is hot. Garnish with coriander and serve immediately.

COOK'S TIP Serve this stir-fry with steamed rice.

When stir-frying, always heat the wok until it is hot before adding any oil or ingredients, and then heat it again between cooking batches of meat or vegetables.

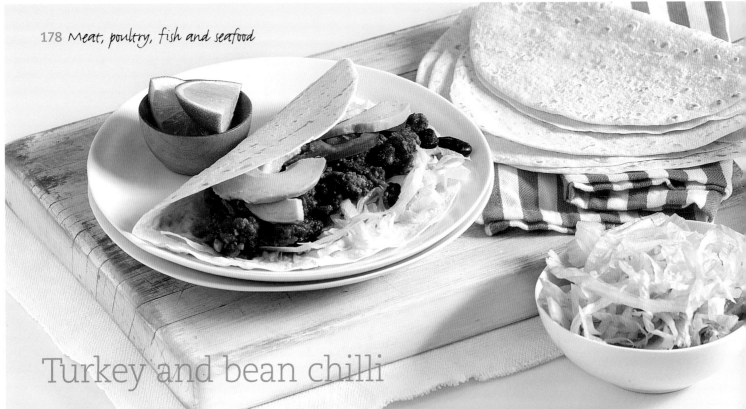

Turkey and bean chilli

500 g (1 lb) turkey mince
2 tablespoons olive oil
1 large red onion, finely diced
2 cloves garlic, finely chopped
3 teaspoons ground cumin
3 teaspoons sweet paprika
1–2 teaspoons mild chilli powder, to taste
800 g (28 oz) can chopped tomatoes
400 g (14 oz) can red kidney beans,
    rinsed and drained
warm tortillas, shredded lettuce and sliced
    tomato and avocado, to serve

PREPARATION 10 minutes

COOKING 35 minutes SERVES 4 (makes 8 tortillas)

EACH SERVING PROVIDES 2093 kJ, 487 kcal, 54 g protein,
19 g fat (4 g saturated fat), 26 g carbohydrate (12 g sugars),
8 g fibre, 456 mg sodium

The combination of kidney beans and
minced turkey makes this a high-protein,
high-fibre meal. Wild meats such as minced
venison, kangaroo or buffalo make a great
anti-inflammatory alternative to the turkey.

1 Put turkey mince in a medium bowl, drizzle over
1 tablespoon oil and mix well. Heat a large deep
non-stick frying pan over medium–high heat until
hot. Add half the turkey and cook about 2 minutes,
stirring with a wooden spoon to break up any lumps.
Cook, stirring, about a further 2 minutes, until any
liquid has evaporated and turkey is lightly browned.
Transfer to a plate and set aside. Reheat pan and cook
remaining turkey, then set aside on the plate.

2 Reduce heat to medium and reheat pan. Heat
remaining oil, then add onion and cook 2 minutes,
or until softened. Add garlic, cumin, paprika and
chilli powder and cook, stirring, 1 minute.

3 Add tomatoes and reserved turkey to pan and
mix well. Reduce heat to medium–low and simmer,
partially covered, 15 minutes. Add kidney beans and
cook uncovered a further 5 minutes, or until most of
the liquid has evaporated.

4 Serve turkey and bean mixture on plates with
tortillas, lettuce, tomato and avocado alongside.

COOK'S TIP Sweet paprika has a wonderful full-
bodied flavour, with no bitterness or heat. You could
add hot paprika (made from ground hot chillies)
instead if you prefer a little heat.

Roasted sweet potato and turkey with cranberry glaze

4 turkey drumsticks (about 300 g/10 oz each)
4 tablespoons cranberry juice
2 tablespoons hoisin sauce
2 tablespoons olive oil
1 large orange sweet potato (kumara)
    (750 g/1½ lb), peeled, cut into
    large chunks
½ cup (160 g) cranberry jelly or
    redcurrant jelly

PREPARATION 15 minutes
COOKING 30 minutes SERVES 4

EACH SERVING PROVIDES 3045 kJ, 728 kcal, 62 g protein,
30 g fat (8 g saturated fat), 47 g carbohydrate
(31 g sugars), 4 g fibre, 369 mg sodium

> Cranberries are one of the fruits with the highest anti-oxidant activity, and they also have unique antibacterial properties. Here they are combined with sweet potato, rich in anti-oxidants, and lean turkey for a low-fat, high-protein meal.

1 Preheat oven to 180°C (350°F/Gas 4). Put turkey drumsticks in a large roasting pan (baking dish). Combine 2 tablespoons cranberry juice, hoisin sauce and 1 tablespoon oil in a small bowl. Brush over turkey.

2 Toss sweet potato in remaining oil, then put in roasting pan around turkey. If the pan is not large enough, put sweet potato on a separate baking tray (sheet). Put turkey and sweet potato in oven and bake 30 minutes, or until turkey is cooked through and sweet potato is golden brown and tender.

3 Warm cranberry or redcurrant jelly and remaining cranberry juice in a saucepan over medium heat.

4 Put turkey and sweet potato on serving plates, drizzle with a little cranberry glaze and serve.

COOK'S TIP Serve with steamed green beans and broccoli. You can use chicken drumsticks instead of turkey (2 drumsticks per serve). Remove the skin before brushing the chicken drumsticks with glaze.

Cover the roasting pan with foil if the turkey is browning too quickly. Baste the turkey with cranberry juice while cooking to help keep the meat moist.

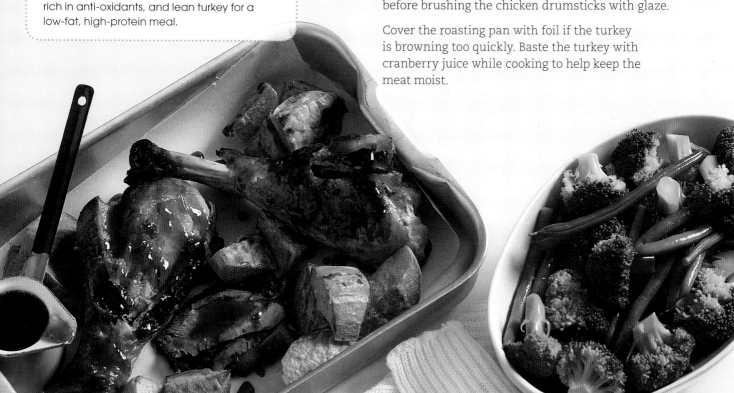

Pork with apple and blueberry relish

1 tablespoon balsamic vinegar
1 tablespoon dijon mustard
4 thick lean pork loin cutlets or chops
    (about 200 g/7 oz each), patted dry
    with paper towel
freshly ground black pepper
extra virgin olive oil cooking spray

Apple and blueberry relish

2 green apples, such as granny smith,
    peeled, cored and diced
1 small onion, finely diced
1/3 cup (80 ml) balsamic vinegar
1/4 cup (45 g) soft brown sugar
2 cloves
125 g (4 oz) fresh blueberries

PREPARATION 20 minutes, plus 30 minutes cooling
COOKING 10 minutes SERVES 4

EACH SERVING PROVIDES 1676 kJ, 400 kcal, 42 g protein,
12 g fat (4 g saturated fat), 31 g carbohydrate (30 g sugars),
2 g fibre, 250 mg sodium

> The combination of apples, blueberries
> and onions in this relish provides
> complementary anti-oxidant powers. Apples
> and onions are rich in quercetin, a flavonoid
> that appears to have promising effects on
> inflammation and some cancers. Blueberries
> contain colourful anthocyanins, which protect
> the heart and nervous system.

1 Combine balsamic vinegar and mustard in a small bowl. Brush over both sides of pork cutlets or chops and season with pepper. Leave to marinate while preparing the relish.

2 To make the apple and blueberry relish, put apples, onion, balsamic vinegar, sugar and cloves in a medium saucepan over medium heat and stir to combine. Bring to a boil, stirring to dissolve sugar. Reduce heat to low and simmer until apples and onion are just tender, about 4 minutes. Add blueberries, stir and simmer a further 3–4 minutes, or until blueberries have softened. Remove from heat. Discard cloves and leave relish to cool, about 30 minutes.

3 Lightly spray both sides of pork cutlets or chops with cooking spray. Preheat a non-stick chargrill pan to high or heat a non-stick frying pan over high heat. Add pork, reduce heat to medium and cook about 3–4 minutes, depending on thickness, until small beads of moisture appear on top of each cutlet; do not turn before then. Cook other side until done to your liking (1–2 minutes for rare, 2–3 minutes for medium and 3–4 minutes for well done). Remove from heat and rest 3–4 minutes.

4 Serve pork cutlets with a spoonful of apple and blueberry relish on the side.

COOK'S TIP Serve pork and relish accompanied by steamed green vegetables, such as broccolini, young green beans or asparagus spears. This dish also goes well with a side of quinoa. Mix together 2/3 cup cooked quinoa, 2 chopped spring onions, 1/4 cup chopped parsley and 2 teaspoons finely grated lemon rind.

Resting the pork for a few minutes before serving allows the juices driven to the centre of the meat during cooking a chance to redistribute throughout the meat. The pork will be juicier and tender, and very little juice runs out onto the plate when you cut the pork. Instead, it remains in the meat.

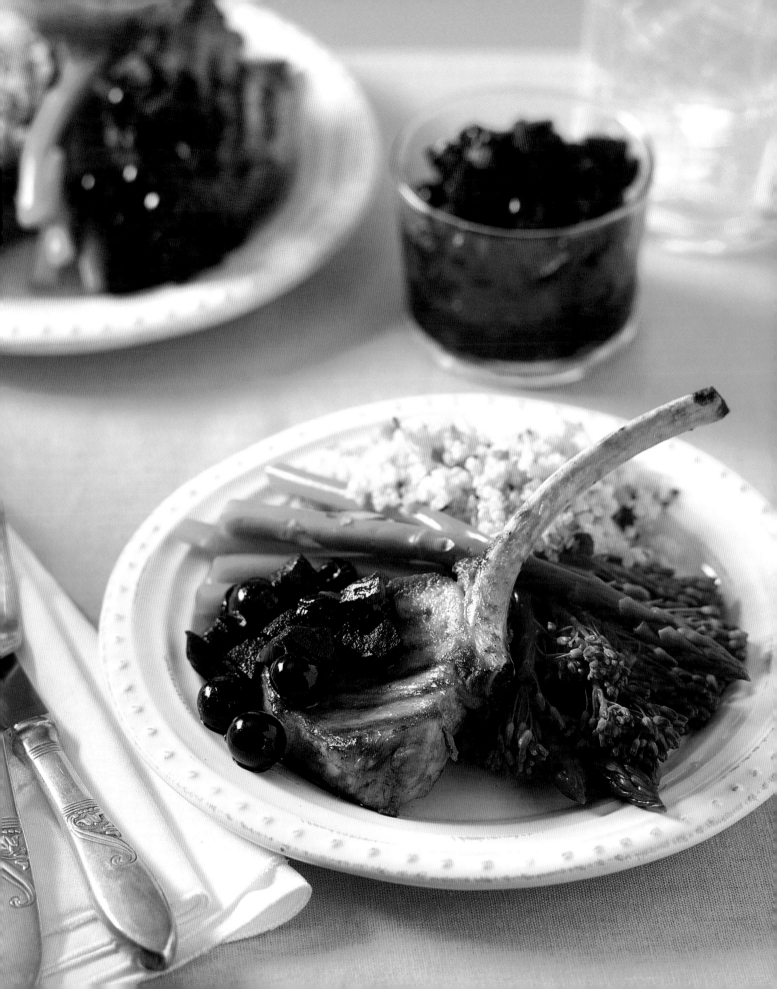

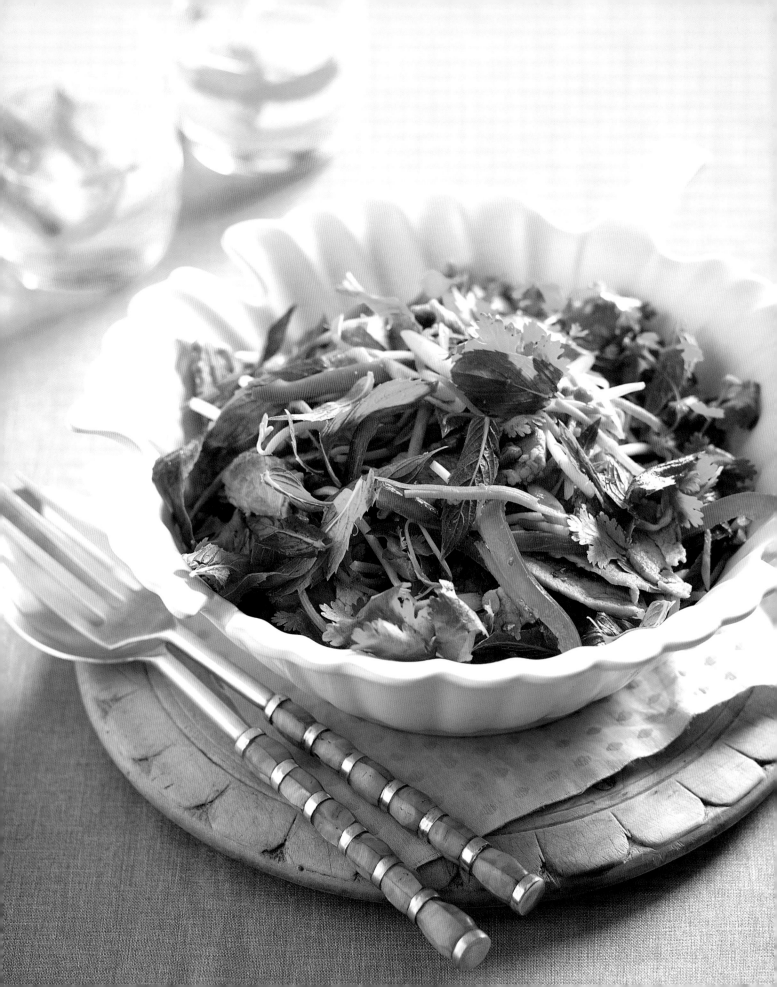

Shredded pork with Thai lime dressing

500 g (1 lb) pork fillet, finely sliced
3 teaspoons light olive oil
1 large carrot, finely shredded
6 cm (2½ inch) piece fresh ginger, peeled
    and finely shredded
2 spring onions (scallions), finely shredded
1 red capsicum (bell pepper), finely sliced
1 cup (90 g) bean sprouts, trimmed
1 tablespoon salt-reduced soy sauce
1 tablespoon fish sauce
1 tablespoon sesame oil
grated zest and juice of 2 limes
1 small red chilli, halved, seeds removed,
    finely chopped
1 cup (30 g) fresh coriander (cilantro) leaves
1 cup (30 g) small fresh mint or basil
1 bunch (125 g/4 oz) rocket (arugula), trimmed

PREPARATION 15 minutes
COOKING 10 minutes SERVES 4

EACH SERVING PROVIDES 1087 kJ, 260 kcal, 30 g protein,
11 g fat (2 g saturated fat), 9 g carbohydrate (4 g sugars),
4 g fibre, 735 mg sodium

This combination of stir-fried shredded pork with a dressing of lime juice and chilli, tossed with fresh salad vegetables and herbs, makes for a fabulously healthy meal.

1 Put pork and 2 teaspoons light olive oil in a bowl and stir to coat well.

2 Heat a large heavy-based frying pan or wok over high heat. Add remaining light olive oil and heat 10 seconds. Add carrot and ginger and cook, stirring, 30 seconds, or until just wilted. Put in a large bowl.

3 Reheat pan until hot. Stir-fry pork in three batches, 2–3 minutes for each batch, or until just cooked. Transfer each batch to a plate and reheat pan before cooking the next batch.

4 Add spring onions, capsicum and bean sprouts to carrot and ginger in the large bowl. Put soy sauce, fish sauce, sesame oil, lime zest and juice and chilli in a small bowl and mix to combine well. Pour over salad, then add pork and toss to mix through. Add coriander, basil or mint, and rocket, toss gently and serve immediately.

COOK'S TIP Add the herbs and rocket and toss through just before serving, so that the flavours are zingy and the textures remain fresh.

For a variation, omit the carrot and spring onions and stir-fry the ginger with the pork. Add two thinly sliced pears with the herbs at the end of step 4.

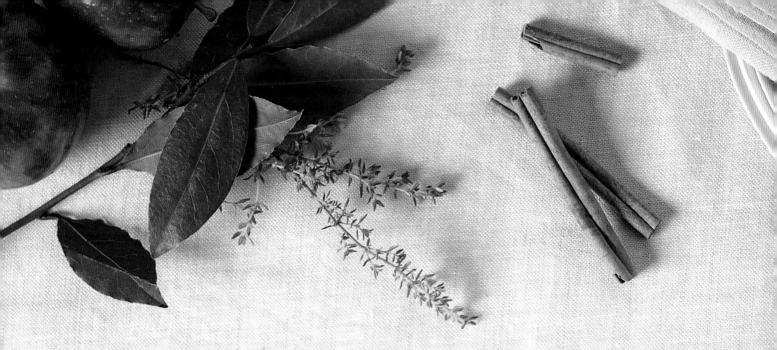

Pork with cinnamon apples

750 g (1½ lb) pork scotch (pork neck)
2 bay leaves
4 sprigs fresh thyme
olive oil, for brushing
freshly ground black pepper
4 apples, skin left on, quartered and cored
2 cinnamon sticks, broken in half
3 cups (750 ml) non-alcoholic apple cider
   or apple juice
1 French shallot (eschalot),
   very finely chopped
2 teaspoons cornflour (cornstarch)

PREPARATION 10 minutes, plus 15 minutes resting
COOKING 45 minutes SERVES 4

EACH SERVING PROVIDES 1600 kJ, 382 kcal, 40 g protein,
6 g fat (2 g saturated fat), 40 g carbohydrate (37 g sugars),
3 g fibre, 113 mg sodium

Not only is the cinnamon high in anti-oxidants but the flavonoids in apples also have powerful anti-oxidant and anti-inflammatory properties.

1 Preheat oven to 200°C (400°F/Gas 6). Tie pork in three or four places with kitchen string to help keep its shape. Slip bay leaves and thyme under the string. Lightly brush pork with oil and season with pepper.

2 Put pork in a roasting pan (baking dish) and bake 20 minutes. Remove from oven and put apple halves and cinnamon sticks around pork, then pour in 1 cup (250 ml) apple cider or juice. Return to oven and cook a further 25 minutes.

3 Transfer pork and apples to a large plate. Cover loosely with foil and leave to rest in a warm place 15 minutes.

4 Meanwhile, wrap two or three ice cubes in paper towel and skim over surface of pan juices in pan to remove fat. Put pan on stovetop and heat pan juices over medium–high heat until bubbling. Add shallot and cook, stirring, about 30 seconds. Pour in remaining cider or juice and bring to a boil, then reduce heat to medium and simmer 2–3 minutes, or until liquid has reduced by about half. Mix cornflour with a little water in a small bowl. Add to pan and cook, stirring constantly, 1–2 minutes, until mixture thickens slightly.

5 Slice pork thinly. Serve on warmed dinner plates with some roasted apple and a spoonful of pan juices.

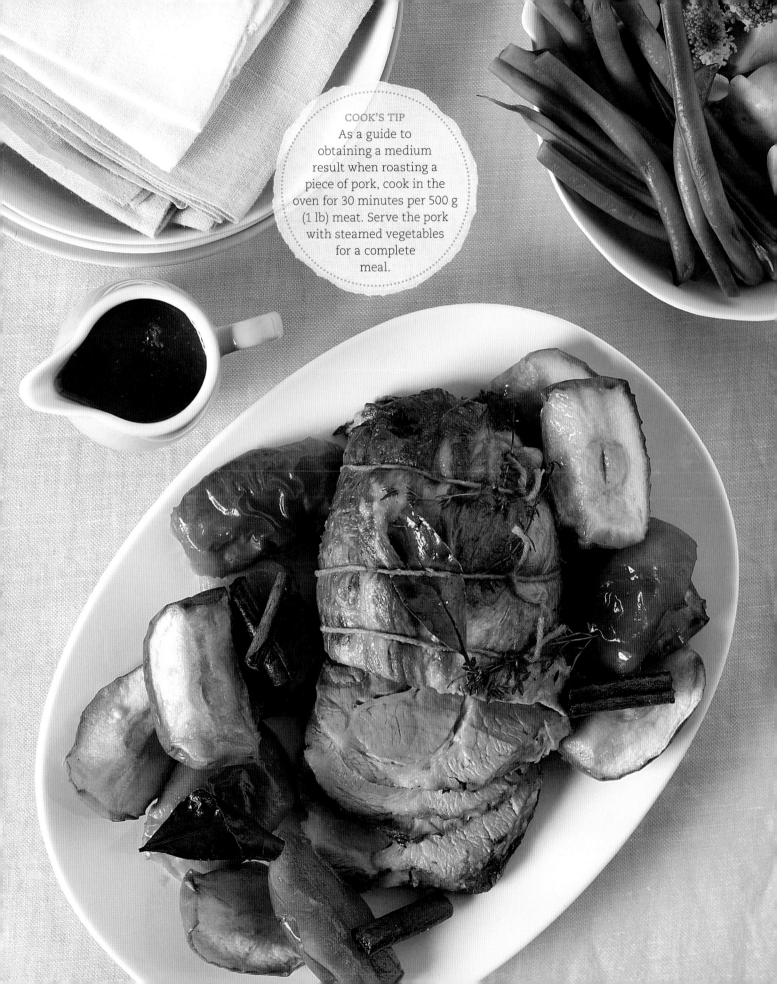

COOK'S TIP
As a guide to obtaining a medium result when roasting a piece of pork, cook in the oven for 30 minutes per 500 g (1 lb) meat. Serve the pork with steamed vegetables for a complete meal.

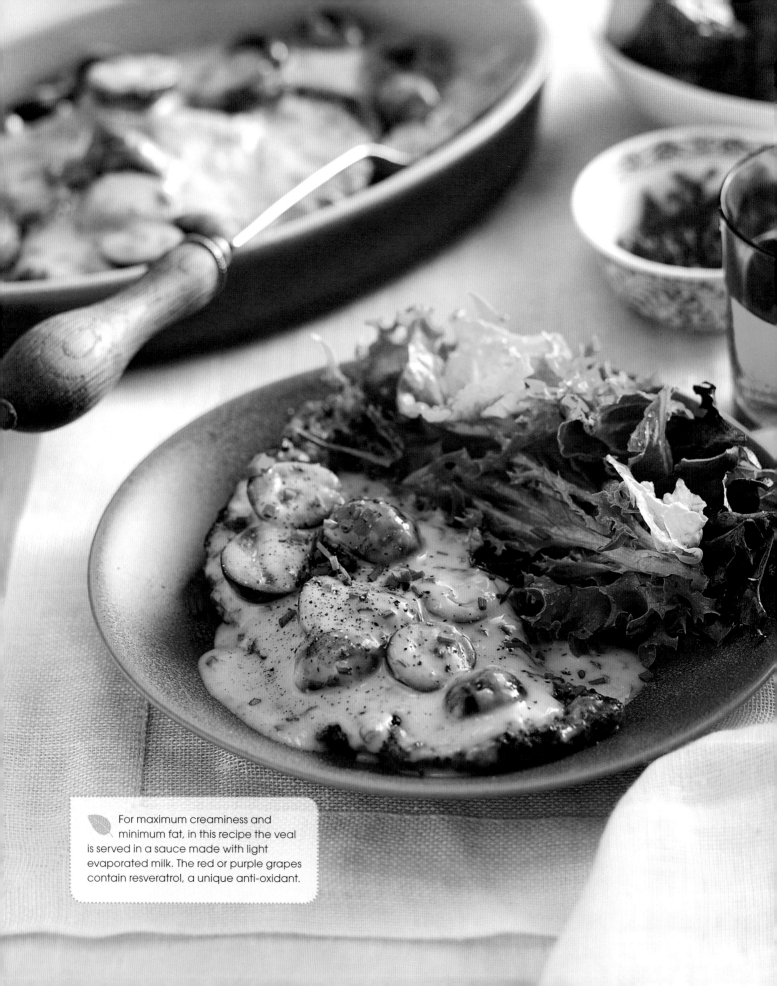

For maximum creaminess and minimum fat, in this recipe the veal is served in a sauce made with light evaporated milk. The red or purple grapes contain resveratrol, a unique anti-oxidant.

Veal with grapes 'Véronique'

2 tablespoons plain (all-purpose) flour
4 veal leg steaks (about 125 g/4 oz each)
2 tablespoons olive oil
1 clove garlic, crushed
375 ml (10 fl oz) can light evaporated milk
1 tablespoon cornflour (cornstarch)
1/3 cup (80 ml) homemade or salt-reduced
    chicken stock
1 cup (180 g) purple or red grapes, halved
1 tablespoon snipped fresh chives
freshly ground black pepper

PREPARATION 10 minutes
COOKING 20 minutes SERVES 4

EACH SERVING PROVIDES 1448 kJ, 346 kcal, 40 g protein,
13 g fat (3 g saturated fat), 18 g carbohydrate (12 g sugars),
1 g fibre, 169 mg sodium

1 Put flour on a plate. Dip the veal steaks in the flour to coat on both sides, shaking off the excess.

2 Heat oil in a large frying pan over medium–high heat. Add 2 steaks and cook 2 minutes on each side, or until golden and just cooked through. Transfer to a warmed plate and keep warm. Cook remaining veal steaks, transfer to the plate and set aside.

3 Reduce heat to medium and return pan to heat. Add garlic and cook, stirring constantly, 10 seconds, until just starting to colour. Combine evaporated milk, cornflour and stock in a small bowl, then add to pan and stir. Reduce heat to low and simmer, stirring occasionally, 3–4 minutes, or until the mixture has thickened slightly.

4 Add grapes and stir to mix through. Return veal steaks to pan and turn to coat in sauce. Cook 1–2 minutes, or until steaks and grapes are heated through. Add chives and season with pepper. Serve steaks on warmed plates and with a spoonful of grape sauce.

COOK'S TIP Serve with baked potatoes and a green salad.

Grapes make a tasty base for many salads – both fruit and savoury. For example, toss 1/2 cup (90 g) red grapes, 2 red apples, cored and chopped, and 1/4 cup (25 g) walnut halves in a dressing of extra virgin olive oil, lemon juice and 1 teaspoon wholegrain mustard. Add 2 grilled (broiled) boneless, skinless chicken breasts, shredded, and toss, then pile on top of mixed salad leaves and serve.

Crumbed veal schnitzels with purple cabbage coleslaw

4 uncrumbed veal schnitzel fillets or veal
    escalopes (about 100 g/3½ oz each)
1 cup (150 g) plain (all-purpose) flour
1 egg, lightly beaten
⅓ cup (80 ml) low-fat milk
1 cup (85 g) dry wholegrain breadcrumbs
3 teaspoons lemon pepper or
    herb and garlic seasoning
extra virgin olive oil cooking spray
1 lemon, quartered, to serve

Coleslaw

¼ purple (red) cabbage (about 350 g/12 oz),
    finely shredded
1 carrot, grated
2 celery stalks, sliced diagonally
1 apple, cored, finely sliced
¼ cup (60 g) low-fat mayonnaise
½ cup (125 g) low-fat thick Greek-style yogurt
juice of 1 lemon

PREPARATION 20 minutes, plus 10 minutes chilling
COOKING 20 minutes SERVES 4

EACH SERVING PROVIDES 2171 kJ, 519 kcal, 39 g protein,
10 g fat (3 g saturated fat), 62 g carbohydrate (18 g sugars),
8 g fibre, 404 mg sodium

This low-fat version of traditional wiener schnitzel is served with a high anti-oxidant coleslaw of carrot and purple cabbage, with a dressing of mayonnaise and yogurt to add calcium and reduce the fat content even further.

1 Put each piece of veal between two sheets of baking (parchment) paper or plastic wrap and pound with a meat mallet or rolling pin until about 5 mm (¼ inch) thick.

2 Preheat oven to 200°C (400°F/Gas 6). Put flour on a large plate. Combine egg and milk in a bowl. Mix together breadcrumbs and lemon pepper or herb and garlic seasoning on a large plate.

3 Coat each veal schnitzel in flour, shaking off any excess. Dip veal in egg and milk mixture. Then press veal into seasoned breadcrumbs to coat thoroughly, shaking off any excess. Put crumbed veal on a tray in a single layer and refrigerate about 10 minutes.

4 Line a large baking tray (sheet) with foil. Put a wire rack on the tray and spray rack with a little cooking spray. Put veal on the rack and generously spray with cooking spray. Bake 8–10 minutes on one side. Turn veal and generously spray the other side with cooking spray, then cook a further 8–10 minutes, or until crumbs are golden and crispy.

5 Meanwhile, make the coleslaw. Combine cabbage, carrot, celery and apple in a large serving bowl. Put mayonnaise, yogurt and lemon juice in a small bowl and stir to combine. Add to vegetables and toss thoroughly to mix through. Serve veal schnitzels accompanied by the coleslaw and lemon wedges.

COOK'S TIP To shred cabbage finely, first remove the thick white core from the centre. Cut the whole cabbage in half, lay the half flat side down on the board and cut a V in the centre. Turn the cabbage half over and ease the core out. Then shred the cabbage finely with a sharp, long-bladed knife.

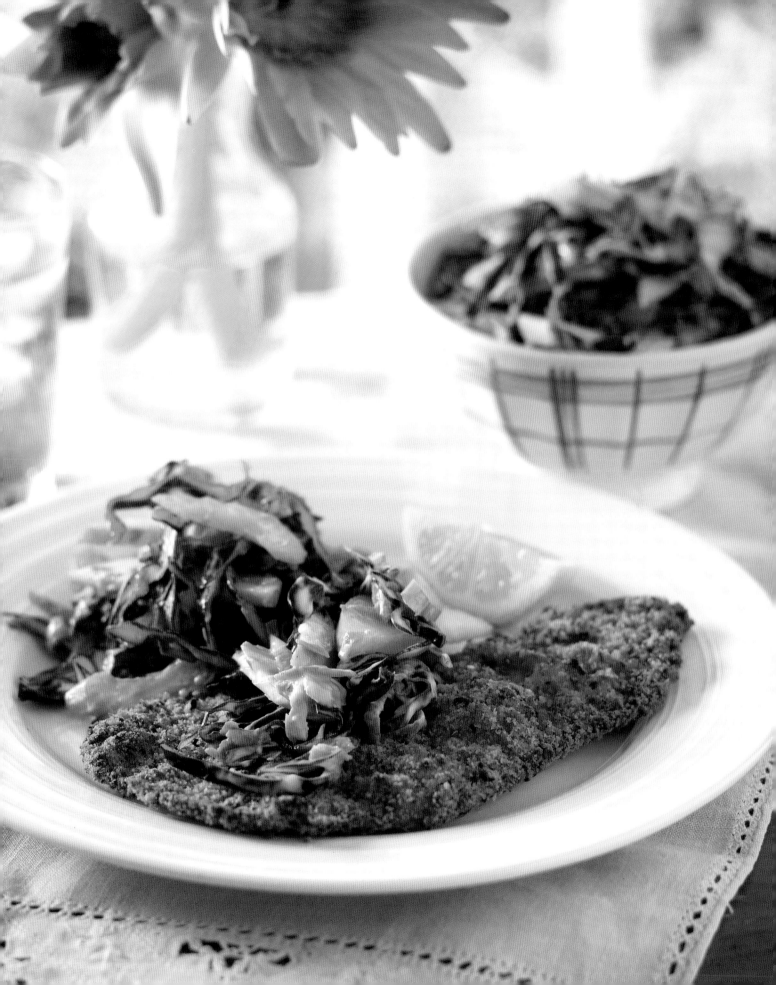

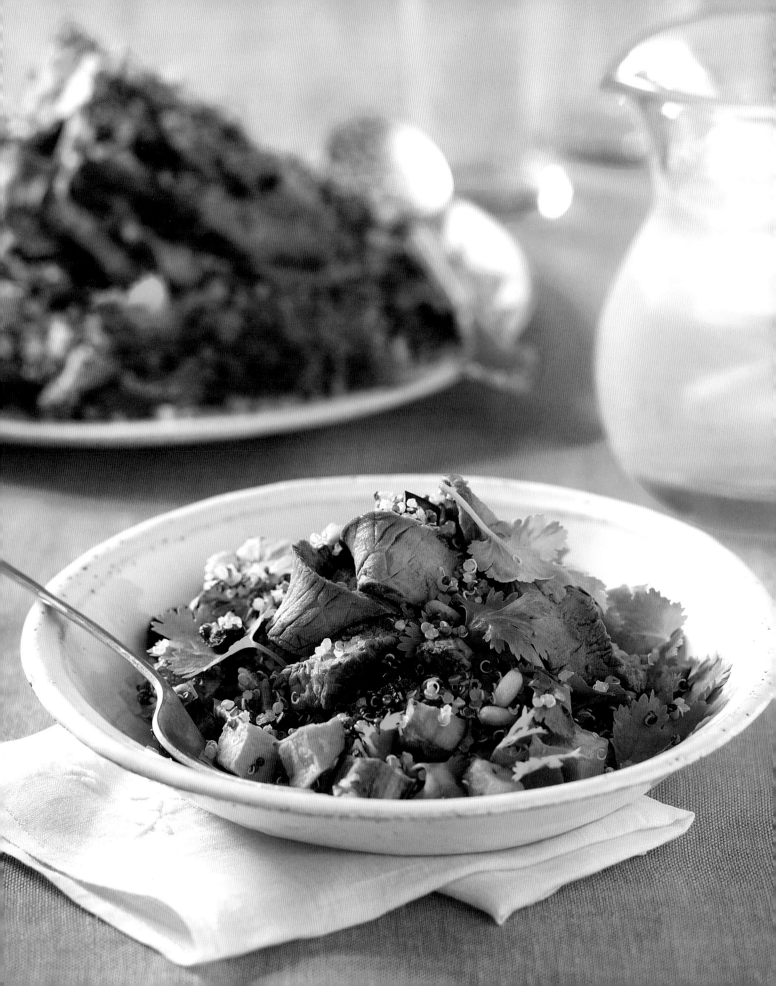

Roasted eggplant, sweet potato and quinoa with beef

½ cup (100 g) red quinoa, rinsed and drained
½ cup (100 g) white quinoa, rinsed and
   drained
2 small eggplants (aubergine), chopped
1 small orange sweet potato (kumara),
   chopped
extra virgin olive oil cooking spray
2 teaspoons ground cumin
2 teaspoons ground cardamom
300 g (10 oz) thick-cut sirloin or
   rump (round) steak
½ cup (60 g) dried cranberries,
   roughly chopped
⅓ cup (50 g) pine nuts, toasted
½ cup (15 g) fresh coriander (cilantro) leaves

PREPARATION 15 minutes, plus 5 minutes standing
COOKING 25 minutes SERVES 4

EACH SERVING PROVIDES 2125 kJ, 508 kcal, 27 g protein,
18 g fat (3 g saturated fat), 62 g carbohydrate (11 g sugars),
13 g fibre, 56 mg sodium

> Iron-rich lean beef is featured here in a salad that is high in a variety of anti-oxidants, due to its combination of quinoa, cranberries, pine nuts and spices. Using kangaroo or another lean meat provides the same good amounts of iron and protein, with a better balance of healthy fats.

1 Preheat oven to 200°C (400°F/Gas 6). Put quinoa in a heavy-based saucepan with 2 cups (500 ml) water. Bring to a boil, then cover with a lid, reduce heat to low and cook 12–15 minutes, until water has evaporated. Turn off heat and leave to stand while still covered, 10 minutes.

2 Meanwhile, line a baking tray with baking paper (baking sheet with parchment paper). Spread eggplants and sweet potato in a single layer on tray. Spray with cooking spray and sprinkle over cumin and cardamom. Roast 10–15 minutes, or until golden brown and cooked through.

3 Heat a chargrill pan or barbecue plate to high. Lightly spray steak with cooking spray. Put on pan or barbecue and cook until small beads of moisture appear on top of steak. Turn and cook other side 2–3 minutes. To test if it is cooked to your liking, prod the centre of the steak with tongs – rare will feel soft; medium will feel firm; and well done will feel very firm. Remove steak from heat, cover loosely with foil and leave to rest in a warm place 5 minutes.

4 Put quinoa in a bowl and fluff with a fork. Add eggplants, sweet potato, cranberries, pine nuts and coriander and toss to combine. Slice steak very thinly. Divide quinoa and vegetable mixture among four serving plates, top with slices of steak and serve.

COOK'S TIP This recipe will also work well with kangaroo or another lean wild meat such as venison. Make sure you leave it fairly rare as lean meats become tough if grilled too long.

Instead of quinoa, this recipe also works with brown rice, wholegrain couscous or burghul (bulgur).

Wine-braised beef

1 kg (2 lb) roasting beef or beef chuck,
trimmed of fat, cut into 3 cm
(1¼ inch) cubes
freshly ground black pepper
2 tablespoons extra virgin olive oil
1 large onion, halved and thinly sliced
2 cloves garlic, finely chopped
2 tablespoons sweet paprika
1 tablespoon caraway seeds
1 tablespoon plain (all-purpose) flour
700 g (25 oz) bottle tomato passata
(puréed tomatoes)
1 cup (250 ml) red wine
5 sprigs fresh thyme or 1 teaspoon dried
thyme or marjoram
2 large red capsicums (bell peppers),
cut into chunks
½ cup (125 g) low-fat thick Greek-style yogurt
2 teaspoons cornflour (cornstarch)
1 tablespoon snipped fresh chives, to garnish

PREPARATION 20 minutes
COOKING 2 hours SERVES 4

EACH SERVING PROVIDES 2441 kJ, 583 kcal, 63 g protein,
21 g fat (6 g saturated fat), 26 g carbohydrate (14 g sugars),
7 g fibre, 79 mg sodium

Beef cooked with paprika and red
wine and finished with yogurt gives a
rich-tasting, low-fat stroganoff-style casserole.
The paprika and wine make this dish very
high in anti-oxidants.

1 Preheat oven to 180°C (350°F/Gas 4). Season beef
with pepper. Heat 1 tablespoon oil in a large frying
pan over medium heat. Add half the beef and cook,
stirring frequently, 4–5 minutes, until lightly
browned. Transfer to a plate. Cook remaining beef,
transfer to the plate and set aside.

2 Heat remaining oil in a large flameproof casserole
dish over medium–low heat. Add onion and garlic
and cook 2 minutes, or until onion has softened,
stirring occasionally. Add paprika and caraway seeds
and cook, stirring, 30 seconds. Add flour and cook,
stirring constantly, 1 minute.

3 Stir in passata, red wine and thyme or marjoram.
Bring to a boil, then reduce heat to low. Return
browned beef and any juices to pan, add capsicums
and stir to mix.

4 Cover casserole dish and cook in oven about
1½ hours, or until beef is tender. Stir occasionally
during cooking time and add a little water if needed,
so that beef is just covered with liquid.

5 Mix together yogurt and cornflour in a small
bowl. Add 2 spoonfuls of hot liquid from casserole
and mix until smooth. Pour into casserole and stir
to mix through. Return to oven and cook a further
5–10 minutes to thicken slightly. Sprinkle the beef
with chives and serve.

COOK'S TIP Serve this rich stew with mashed or
baked potato and steamed vegetables.

Beef chuck is an inexpensive cut that becomes
meltingly tender with long, slow cooking. It is
important that the casserole simmers but does not
boil to ensure the beef becomes tender. Beef shin
could also be used. For a quicker option, use 1 kg
(2 lb) boneless, skinless chicken thighs; cook for
about 40 minutes.

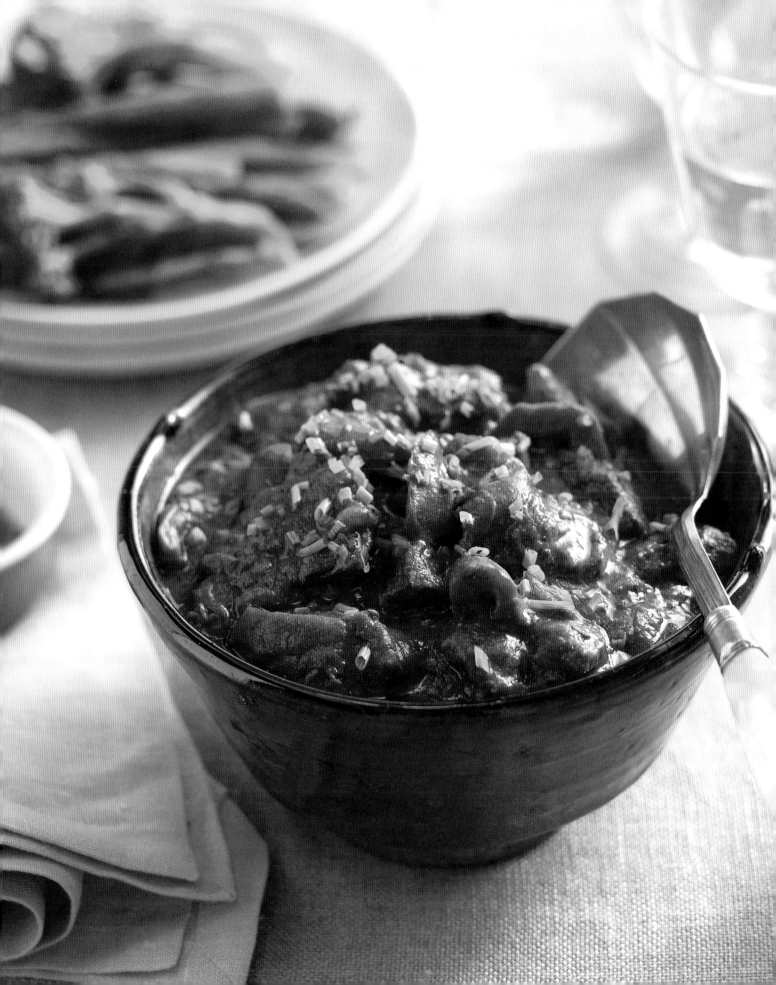

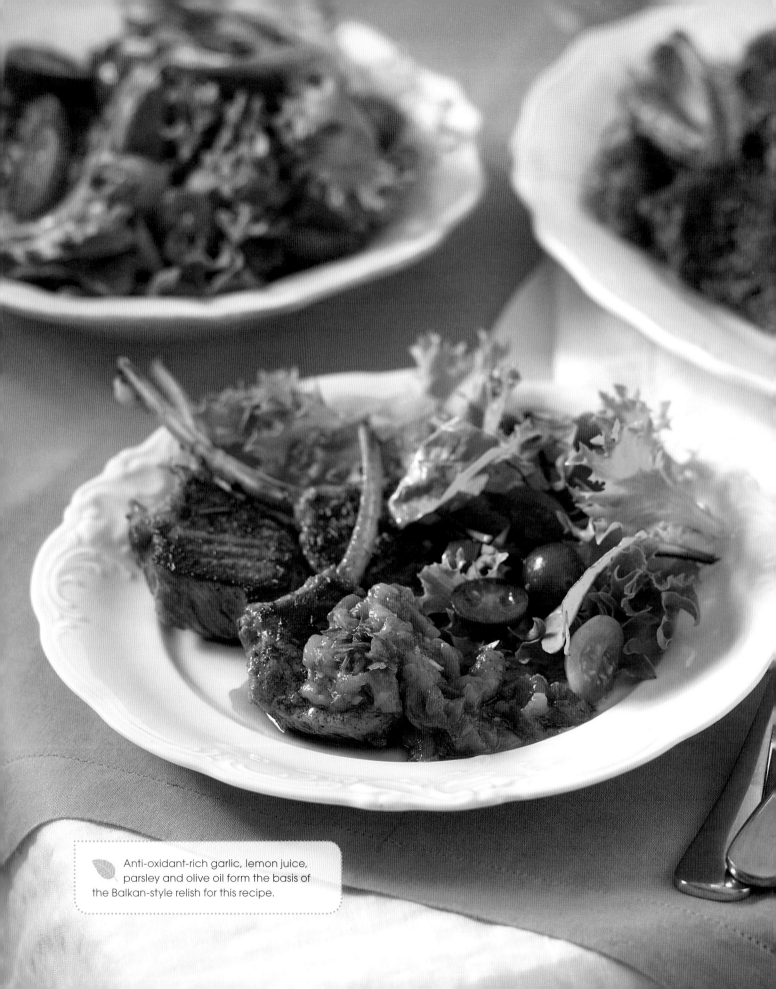

Anti-oxidant-rich garlic, lemon juice, parsley and olive oil form the basis of the Balkan-style relish for this recipe.

Lamb cutlets with eggplant and capsicum relish

1 tablespoon chopped fresh rosemary
grated zest of 1 small lemon
1 tablespoon extra virgin olive oil
12 lamb cutlets, French trimmed
freshly ground black pepper
mixed salad leaves, to serve

Eggplant and capsicum relish

2 eggplant (aubergine)
2 large red capsicums (bell peppers)
1 large red chilli (optional)
2 cloves garlic, chopped
1/3 cup (7 g) fresh flat-leaf (Italian) parsley
1/4 cup (60 ml) extra virgin olive oil
grated zest and juice of 1 lemon

PREPARATION 15 minutes
COOKING 50 minutes SERVES 4

EACH SERVING PROVIDES 1710 kJ, 409 kcal, 29 g protein,
31 g fat (8 g saturated fat), 7 g carbohydrate (6 g sugars),
5 g fibre, 93 mg sodium

1 To make the eggplant and capsicum relish, preheat oven to 180°C (350°F/Gas 4). Prick eggplant two or three times with a fork. Put eggplant, capsicums and chilli, if using, directly on an oven rack and put a baking tray (sheet) on the oven rack below them. Cook 35–40 minutes, turning two or three times, until skins are charred and browned. Remove capsicums and chilli before eggplant if they cook more quickly. Leave to cool.

2 Cut capsicums and chilli in half, remove seeds and membrane, and put in a large bowl. Cut eggplant in half and spoon flesh into the bowl. Add garlic, parsley, oil and lemon zest and juice. Mash roughly until evenly mixed and starting to look creamy.

3 Preheat barbecue plate or chargrill pan to hot. Combine rosemary, lemon zest and oil in a small bowl. Brush each lamb cutlet with the mixture, then season with pepper.

4 Put cutlets on barbecue or chargrill and cook until small beads of moisture appear on top of cutlets; do not turn before then. Cook other side until done to your liking (1–2 minutes for rare, 2–3 minutes for medium and 3–4 minutes for well done). Remove from heat and rest 3 minutes.

5 Divide lamb cutlets among four serving plates and serve with a dollop of eggplant and capsicum relish and some salad leaves on the side.

....

COOK'S TIP The leftover relish can be stored in an airtight container in the refrigerator for up to 3 days. You could use it as a bruschetta topping or dolloped on hot pasta.

Red wine lamb shanks

8 lamb shanks (about 250 g/8 oz each),
    French trimmed (see page 197)
freshly ground black pepper
2 tablespoons extra virgin olive oil
1 large onion, diced
2 small carrots, diced
2 celery stalks, diced
1 tablespoon plain (all-purpose) flour
2 cups (500 ml) homemade or
    salt-reduced beef stock
1 cup (250 ml) red wine
410 g (15 oz) can chopped tomatoes
1 bay leaf
2 sprigs fresh rosemary
5 sprigs fresh thyme
chopped parsley, to serve

PREPARATION 20 minutes
COOKING 1 hour 45 minutes SERVES 4

EACH SERVING PROVIDES 2191 kJ, 523 kcal, 55 g protein,
24 g fat (8 g saturated fat), 11 g carbohydrate (7 g sugars),
3 g fibre, 851 mg sodium.

1 Preheat oven to 180°C (350°F/Gas 4). Season lamb shanks with pepper. Heat 1 tablespoon oil in a large frying pan over medium heat. Add lamb shanks and cook until well browned on all sides, 3–6 minutes. Remove from heat and set aside.

2 Heat remaining olive oil in a large flameproof casserole dish over medium–low heat. Add onion, carrot and celery, and cook, stirring occasionally, 2–3 minutes, or until onion and celery are soft. Add flour and cook, stirring constantly, 1 minute.

3 Stir in stock, red wine, tomatoes, bay leaf, rosemary and thyme and bring to a boil. Reduce heat to low and add lamb shanks. Cover casserole dish with lid and cook in oven 1½ hours, or until lamb shanks are very tender. Stir occasionally during cooking time and add a little water if needed to keep lamb shanks just covered with liquid. Top with parsely and serve immediately.

This is a hearty dish, rich in anti-oxidants. To remove some of the fat, refrigerate overnight, then scrape or lift off the fat that has set on the top of the dish. Reheat until thoroughly hot.

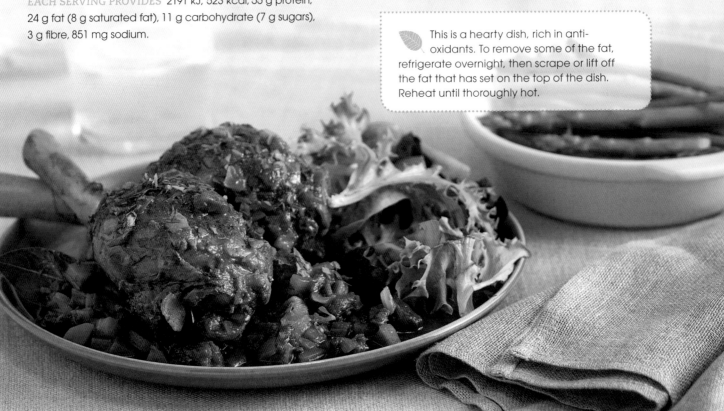

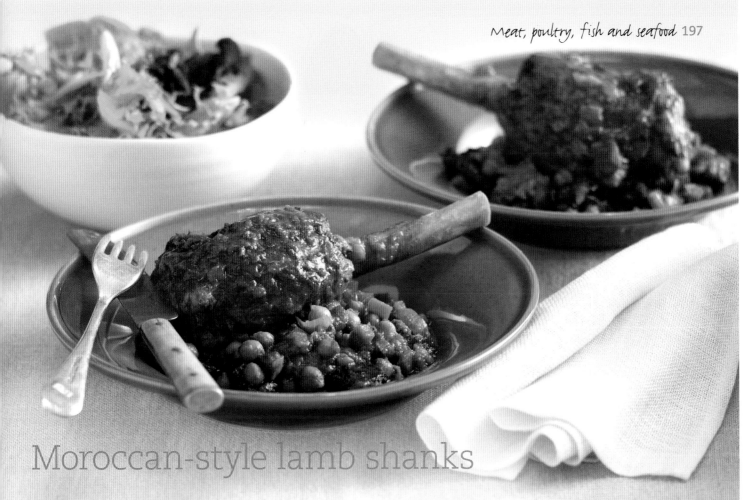

Moroccan-style lamb shanks

4 lamb shanks (about 1 kg/2 lb),
    French trimmed
1 apple, peeled, cored and diced
1 onion, finely chopped
410 g (15 oz) can chopped tomatoes
1 carrot, finely diced
400 g (14 oz) can chickpeas,
    rinsed and drained
8 kalamata olives
8 pitted prunes
2 tablespoons chopped preserved lemon
1 cinnamon stick
1/4 teaspoon ground ginger
1/4 teaspoon ground cumin
1/4 teaspoon ground turmeric

PREPARATION 10 minutes
COOKING 4 hours SERVES 4

EACH SERVING PROVIDES 2005 kJ, 479 kcal, 57 g protein,
15 g fat (5 g saturated fat), 25 g carbohydrate (13 g sugars),
7 g fibre, 963 mg sodium

1 Preheat oven to 150°C (300°F/Gas 2).

2 Put lamb shanks, apple, onion, tomatoes, carrot, chickpeas, olives, prunes, preserved lemon, cinnamon, ginger, cumin and turmeric in a large casserole dish with a tight-fitting lid, or a tagine. Stir to mix well, then cover with lid.

3 Bake 4 hours, then serve hot.

COOK'S TIP To French trim lamb shanks, cut the meat and fat away from the end of the shank to expose the bone.

Tagines are usually high in fibre as they feature legumes and dried fruits such as prunes or figs; these ingredients also lower the glycaemic index of this dish. The herbs and spices provide a range of different anti-oxidants.

Diced lamb with chickpeas and figs

1 lamb shoulder (about 1 kg/2 lb)
    or 1 kg (2 lb) lean lamb leg steaks,
    cut into 3 cm (1¼ inch) cubes
freshly ground black pepper
2 tablespoons extra virgin olive oil
1 large onion, chopped
2 cloves garlic, chopped
2 teaspoons ground coriander
2 teaspoons ground cumin
1 teaspoon ground ginger
1 tablespoon plain (all-purpose) flour
3 cups (750 ml) homemade or
    salt-reduced beef stock
3 tomatoes, chopped
2 strips orange zest
1 cinnamon stick, broken
½ cup (95 g) chopped dried figs
300 g (10 oz) can chickpeas, rinsed and
    drained, or 1 cup (160 g) cooked
    chickpeas
¼ cup (7 g) chopped fresh parsley or
    coriander (cilantro) leaves

PREPARATION 20 minutes

COOKING 1 hour 45 minutes SERVES 4

EACH SERVING PROVIDES 2389 kJ, 571 kcal, 60 g protein,
25 g fat (8 g saturated fat), 27 g carbohydrate (18 g sugars),
8 g fibre, 1109 mg sodium

This fragrant tagine-style dish features lamb and the high fibre content of chickpeas and figs. It is cooked in a spicy sauce rich in anti-oxidants.

1 Preheat oven to 180°C (350°F/Gas 4). Season lamb with pepper. Heat 1 tablespoon oil in a large frying pan over medium heat. Add half the lamb and cook, stirring frequently, 4–5 minutes, or until browned. Transfer to a plate. Cook remaining lamb, transfer to the plate and set aside.

2 Heat remaining oil in a large flameproof casserole dish over medium–low heat. Add onion and garlic and cook, stirring occasionally, 2 minutes, or until onion is soft. Add coriander, cumin and ginger, and cook, stirring, 1 minute. Add flour and cook, stirring constantly, 1 minute.

3 Stir in stock and tomatoes, add orange zest and cinnamon, and bring to a boil. Reduce heat to low. Add lamb and stir to combine. Cover casserole dish and cook in oven 60 minutes.

4 Add figs and chickpeas, cover and cook a further 30 minutes, or until lamb is tender. Stir occasionally during cooking time, and add a little water if needed to keep the lamb just covered.

5 Stir in parsley or coriander and serve.

COOK'S TIP This stew goes well with a side serve of wholegrain couscous. The recipe also works well with kangaroo or another lean wild meat, cut in narrow strips.

Taking time to brown the lamb well in step 1 will result in a richly flavoured dish. Don't overcrowd the pan when you brown the meat, so that the meat colours to a deep golden brown rather than stewing.

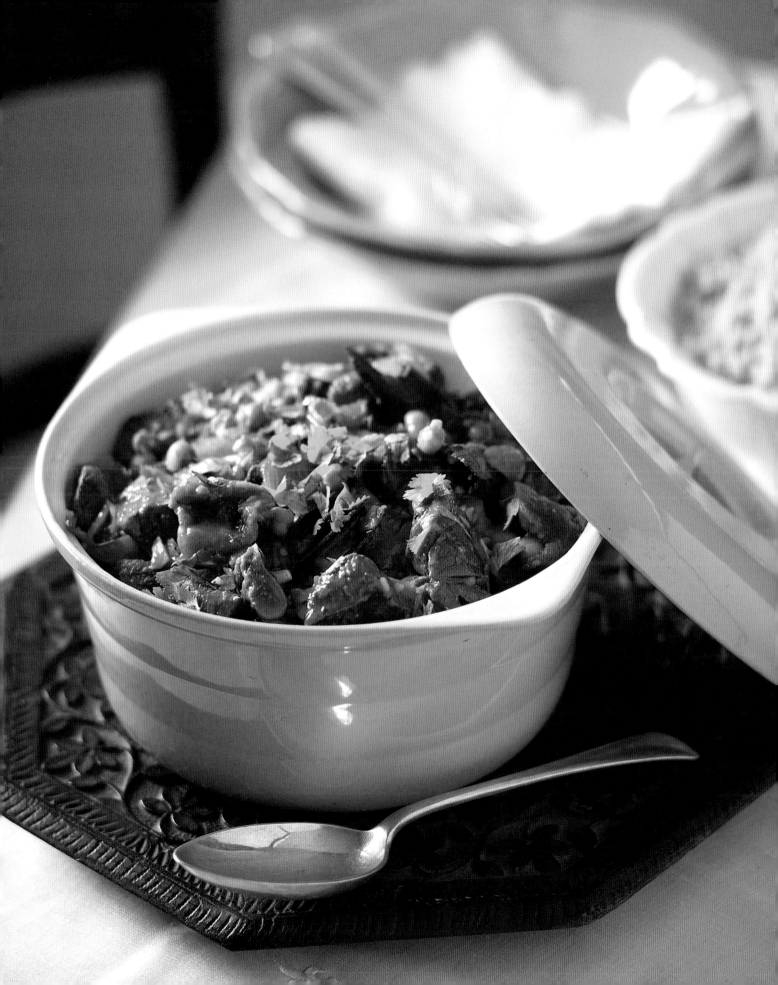

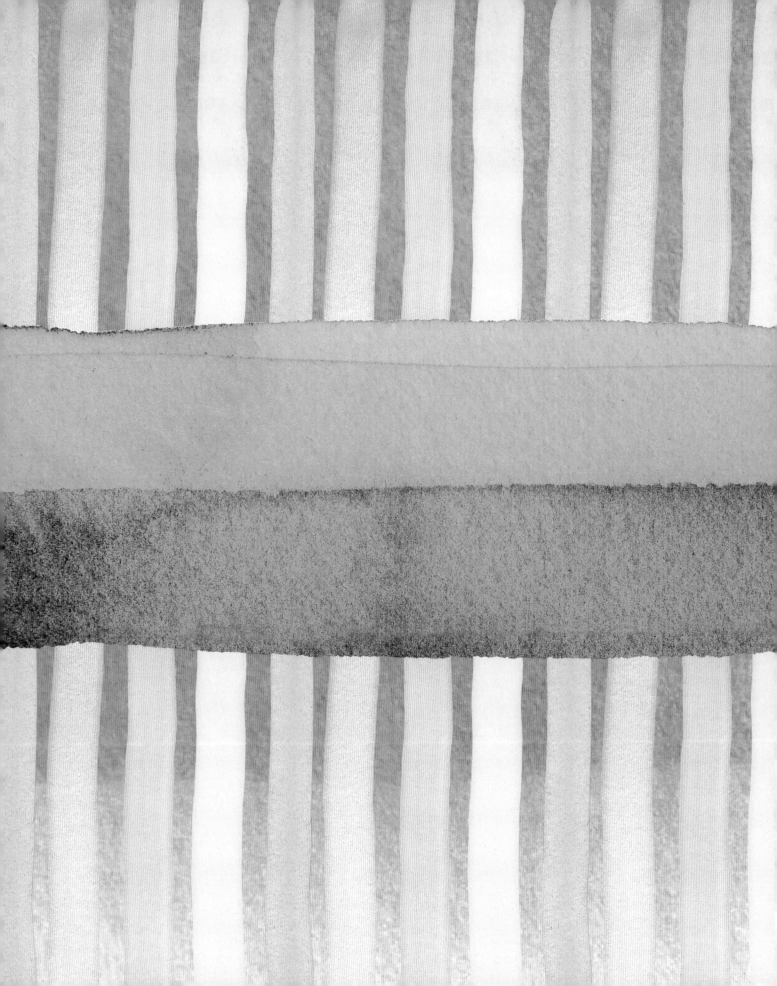

Desserts
and baking

Relax! Hidden anti-ageing nutrients mean these treats are healthy, too.

Mixed grape salad with ginger syrup

1 cup (250 ml) water
4 cm (1½ inch) piece fresh ginger, peeled,
    cut into thin matchsticks
3 cm (1¼ inch) strip lemon zest
2 tablespoons honey
250 g (8 oz) white seedless grapes
250 g (8 oz) red grapes, halved

PREPARATION 15 minutes, plus 30 minutes chilling
COOKING 10 minutes SERVES 4

EACH SERVING PROVIDES 536 kJ, 128 kcal, 1 g protein,
<1 g fat (<1 g saturated fat), 32 g carbohydrate
(31 g sugars), 1 g fibre, 10 mg sodium

1 Combine water, ginger, lemon zest and honey in a medium saucepan over medium heat. Stir until mixture comes to a boil. Reduce heat to low and simmer 8–10 minutes, or until slightly thickened. Remove and discard zest. Leave syrup to cool.

2 Combine white and red grapes in a serving bowl. Pour over ginger syrup. Cover with plastic wrap and refrigerate 30 minutes before serving.

COOK'S TIP You could replace the honey with agave syrup.

Grapes have a unique anti-oxidant, resveratrol, which is sometimes referred to as an anti-ageing substance.

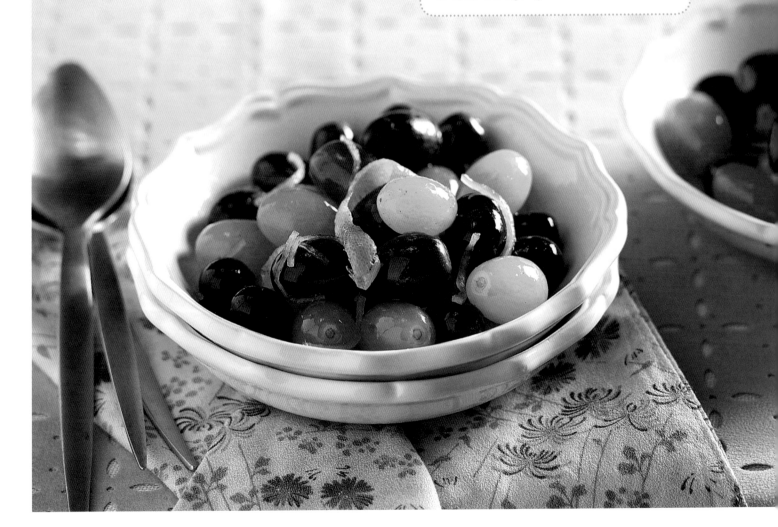

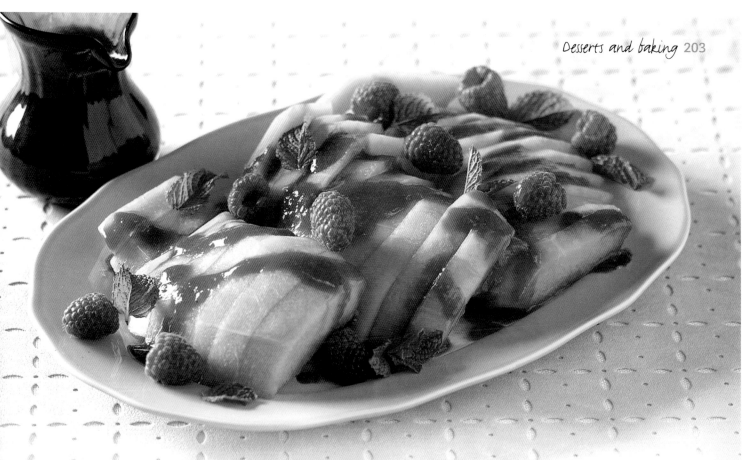

Melon with raspberry sauce

350 g (12 oz) fresh or frozen raspberries
1 teaspoon lemon juice
2 tablespoons honey
1 large ripe rockmelon (cantaloupe)
fresh mint leaves, to garnish

PREPARATION 20 minutes
SERVES 4

EACH SERVING PROVIDES 511 kJ, 122 kcal, 2 g protein,
<1 g fat (0 g saturated fat), 27 g carbohydrate
(26 g sugars), 7 g fibre, 24 mg sodium

Whether you call it rockmelon, cantaloupe, muskmelon, netted melon or spanspek, this member of the melon family is an excellent source of the anti-oxidant beta-carotene.

1 Reserve a few raspberries to garnish. Purée remaining raspberries in a food processor or blender until smooth. Press purée through a medium mesh strainer into a bowl.

2 Add lemon juice and honey and stir to mix well. Set aside.

3 Cut melon into quarters and remove seeds and fibres. Peel the quarters. Using a sharp knife, slice each quarter lengthwise without cutting completely through. Open out each quarter into a fan shape.

4 Divide raspberry purée among four serving plates. Place a melon fan on each plate and decorate with mint leaves and reserved raspberries.

COOK'S TIP Look for melons with a yellowish cast to the rind and a pleasant aroma, and that yield slightly to light pressure. After buying, keep 2–4 days at room temperature to allow for completion of ripening. Once cut, keep the melon in the refrigerator.

Watermelon granita

½ small seedless watermelon (about 1.5 kg/ 3 lb), rind removed, roughly chopped
2 tablespoons lime juice
2 teaspoons finely grated lime zest
1 tablespoon honey or agave syrup

PREPARATION 10 minutes, plus overnight freezing
SERVES 6

EACH SERVING PROVIDES 107 kJ, 25 kcal, <1 g protein, <1 g fat (0 g saturated fat), 7 g carbohydrate (6 g sugars), <1 g fibre, 1 mg sodium

This refreshing pink granita is a great way to store and use leftover watermelon while retaining all the nutrients of the fresh fruit.

1 Put watermelon, lime juice, zest (reserving a little for garnish) and honey or agave syrup in a food processor or blender and process until smooth. Pour into a 4 cup (1 litre) plastic container. Cover and freeze for 3 hours or until almost set.

2 Remove granita from freezer. Using a fork, scrape granita from bottom and sides of container, mixing frozen and unfrozen mixture. Cover and freeze overnight or until set.

3 Using a fork, scrape granita into shards and spoon into serving glasses. Serve sprinkled with grated lime zest, if desired.

COOK'S TIP This recipe can also be made with mango, banana, berries or other types of melon. You will need approximately 500 g (1 lb) of peeled, seeded fruit.

Agave syrup, also known as agave nectar, is made from the juice of a spiky desert plant. The juice is concentrated to make a sweet, mild-flavoured syrup that is often used as a vegan alternative to honey. It has become more popular recently after research found it has a very low glycaemic index, releasing its energy gradually to keep your blood glucose stable and stave off hunger for longer.

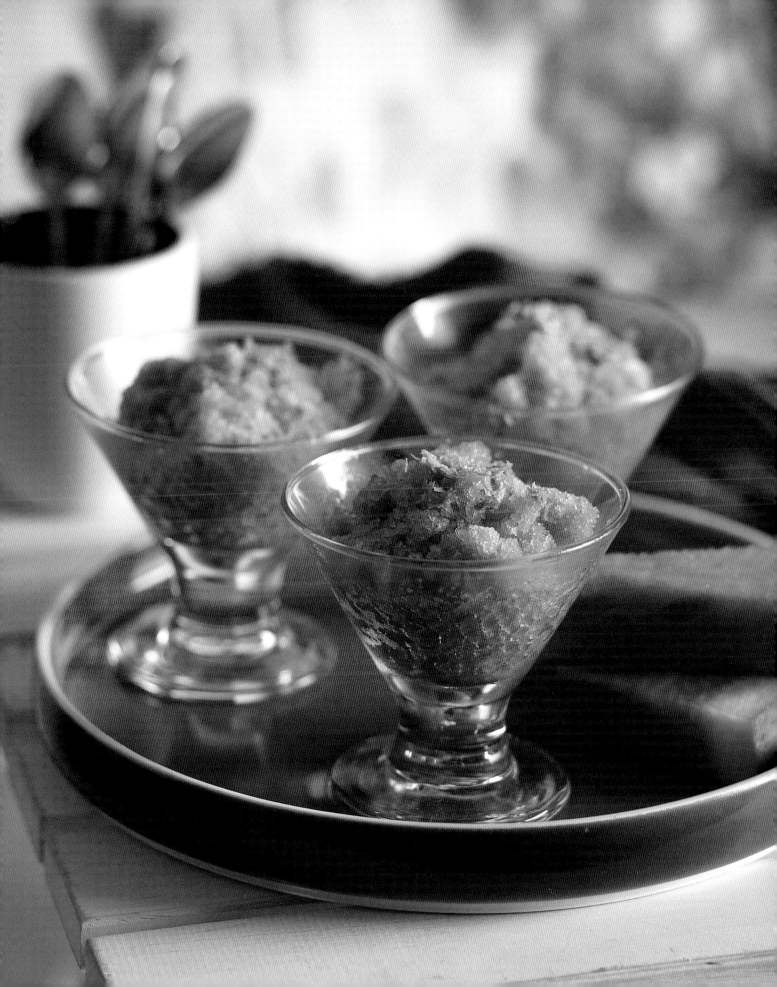

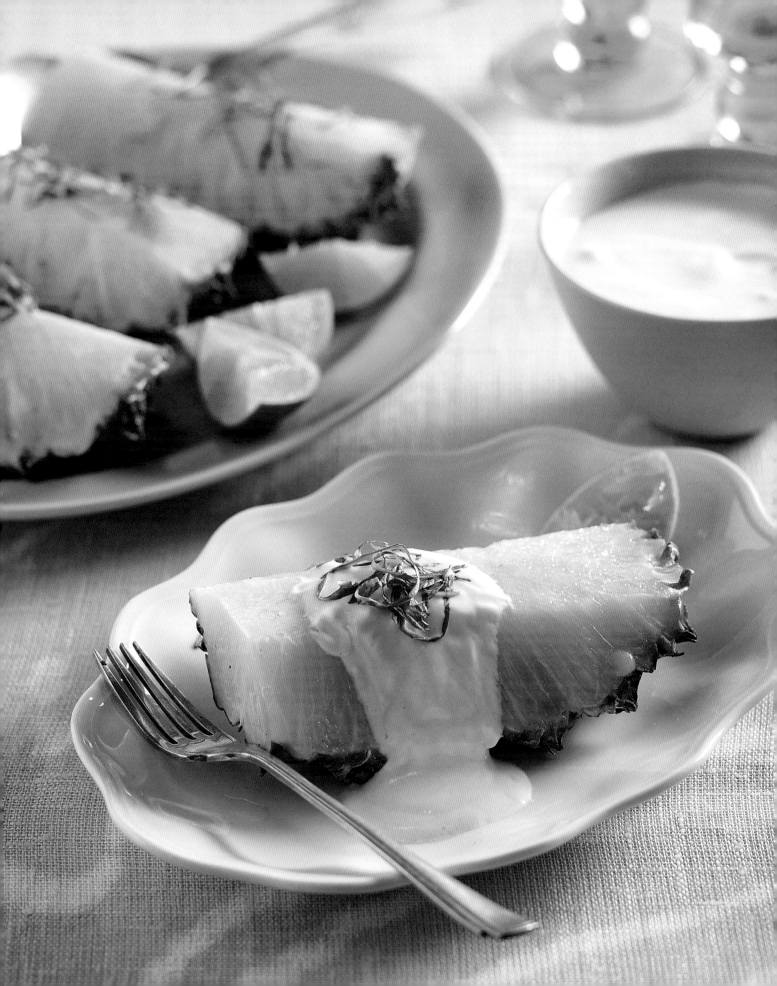

Baked pineapple with ginger yogurt

1 pineapple (about 1.25 kg/2½ lb)
1 cup (250 g) low-fat thick Greek-style yogurt
2 teaspoons honey
½ teaspoon ground ginger
lime wedges, to serve
2 teaspoons grated lime zest, to garnish

PREPARATION 10 minutes, plus 10 minutes cooling
COOKING 1 hour 45 minutes SERVES 4

EACH SERVING PROVIDES 836 kJ, 200 kcal, 8 g protein,
2 g fat (1 g saturated fat), 36 g carbohydrate
(33 g sugars), 6 g fibre, 100 mg sodium

> This dessert is high in fibre and low in fat.
> Pineapples contain bromelain, an enzyme
> that has anti-inflammatory effects. Very high
> doses of bromelain, in supplement form, are
> often used as part of arthritis treatment. Fresh
> pineapple does not contain such large amounts,
> but the bromelain is more concentrated in the
> core and stem of the pineapple, so you will
> obtain more anti-inflammatory benefits if you
> eat the middle of the pineapple.

1 Preheat oven to 180°C (350°F/Gas 4). Put whole pineapple on a large baking tray (sheet). Bake in oven, turning every 20 minutes, 1¾ hours, or until pineapple feels soft when squeezed gently. Leave to cool 10 minutes.

2 Meanwhile, combine yogurt, honey and ginger in a small bowl.

3 With a sharp knife, remove top from cooled pineapple and quarter lengthwise. Remove core from each quarter, if desired.

4 Put each quarter, skin side down, on a serving plate. Top with a dollop of ginger yogurt and a sprinkle of lime zest. Serve with lime wedges on the side.

COOK'S TIP For another cooked pineapple dessert, remove skin from 1 small pineapple and cut in half lengthwise. Cook halves under a hot grill (broiler) 5 minutes, then turn and sprinkle with a little soft brown sugar and ground ginger and cook about 5 minutes, until the sugar is caramelised.

Date and orange salad

½ cup (125 ml) water
1 pinch saffron threads
3 cardamom pods, bruised
3 cm (1¼ inch) strip lemon zest
1 tablespoon honey
1 teaspoon rosewater
3 large oranges, peeled, thickly sliced
8 fresh dates, pitted, quartered
2 tablespoons pistachios, toasted, chopped
2 tablespoons slivered almonds, toasted

PREPARATION 15 minutes, plus 1 hour chilling
COOKING 10 minutes SERVES 4

EACH SERVING PROVIDES 774 kJ, 185 kcal, 4 g protein,
5 g fat (<1 g saturated fat), 32 g carbohydrate
(30 g sugars), 6 g fibre, 9 mg sodium

Dates are high in fibre, anti-oxidants and valuable minerals, and here they are combined with other ingredients rich in anti-oxidants, such as oranges, spices and nuts.

1 Combine water, saffron threads, cardamom, lemon zest and honey in a medium saucepan over medium heat. Stir until mixture comes to a boil. Reduce heat to low and simmer 4–5 minutes, or until slightly thickened. Remove zest and discard. Stir in rosewater and leave to cool.

2 Combine oranges and dates in a serving bowl. Pour over rosewater syrup, then cover and refrigerate 1 hour.

3 Sprinkle salad with pistachios and almonds and serve.

COOK'S TIP You could serve this Middle Eastern–influenced dessert with a spoonful of low-fat thick Greek-style yogurt.

Bruise cardamom pods by putting them on a chopping board and gently pressing down with the flat side of a knife blade until the pods flatten and open slightly at one end. This helps release the flavour of the cardamom.

Rosewater is used in Middle Eastern and Greek cooking and is available from Middle Eastern and specialty food stores.

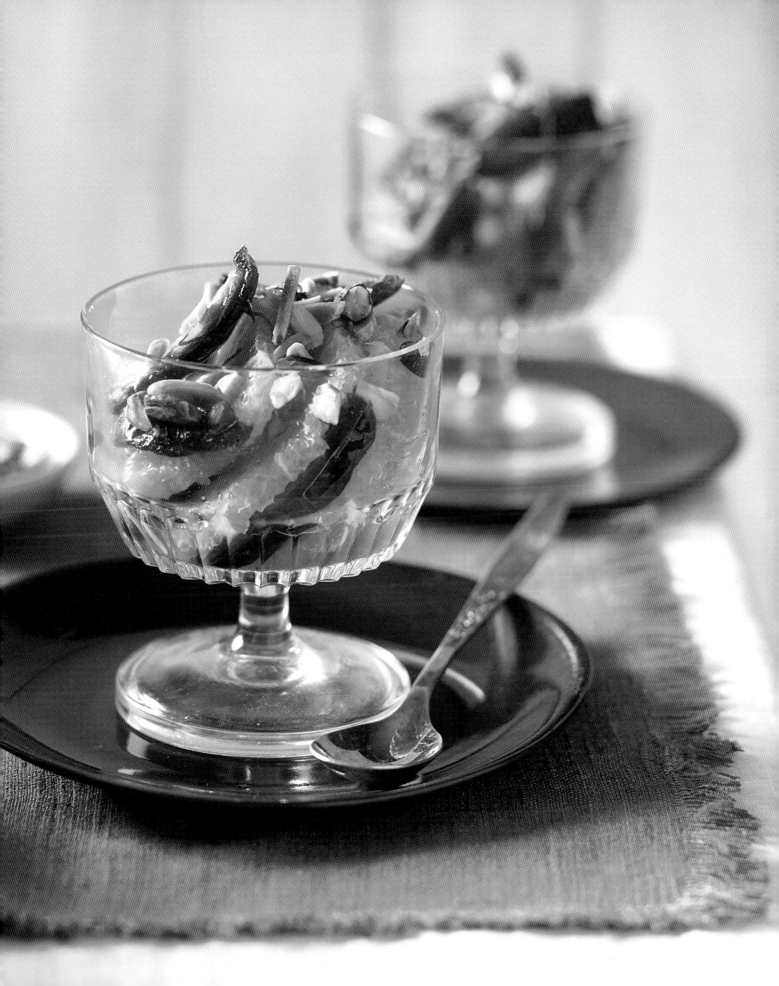

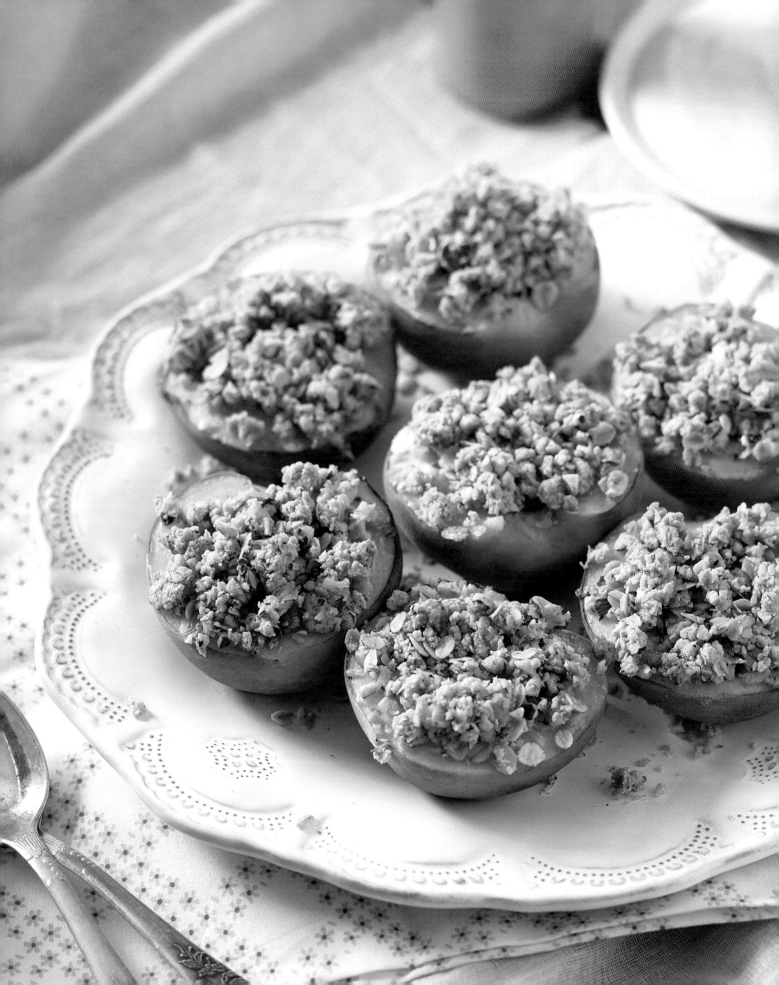

Peach crumbles with cinnamon yogurt

¼ cup (40 g) wholemeal (whole-wheat)
   self-raising flour
1 tablespoon soft brown sugar
2 tablespoons (40 g) olive oil spread
¼ cup (25 g) rolled (porridge) oats
¼ cup (35 g) hazelnuts, finely chopped
4 peaches (about 600 g/1¼ lb), halved,
   stones removed
¾ cup (185 g) low-fat thick Greek-style yogurt
1 teaspoon honey
½ teaspoon ground cinnamon

PREPARATION 15 minutes
COOKING 15 minutes SERVES 4

EACH SERVING PROVIDES 1126 kJ, 269 kcal, 8 g protein,
13 g fat (3 g saturated fat), 30 g carbohydrate
(18 g sugars), 5 g fibre, 109 mg sodium

1 Preheat oven to 180°C (350°F/Gas 4). Line a baking tray with baking paper (or a baking sheet with parchment paper). Combine flour and sugar in a medium bowl. With your fingertips, rub spread into flour and sugar until mixture resembles coarse breadcrumbs. Stir in oats and hazelnuts.

2 Put peach halves, cut side up, on the prepared baking tray. Press crumble onto each peach. Bake 12–15 minutes, or until peaches are tender and crumble is golden.

3 Meanwhile, combine yogurt, honey and cinnamon in a small bowl.

4 Put two peach halves in each dessert bowl and serve with a generous dollop of cinnamon yogurt.

COOK'S TIP Apricots, plums or nectarines can be used instead of peaches.

Peaches are rich in anti-oxidants, as is cinnamon, which is added to yogurt for a high-calcium garnish. The crumble in this recipe has a low glycaemic index thanks to the hazelnuts and the wholegrain content of the flour and oats.

Low-fat berry mousse

300 g (10 oz) fresh or frozen mixed berries,
 such as blackberries, blueberries and
 raspberries, plus extra fresh berries,
 to serve (optional)
1 tablespoon powdered gelatin
¼ cup (60 ml) hot water
375 ml (13 fl oz) can light evaporated milk,
 chilled
2 tablespoons caster (superfine) sugar
1 tablespoon lemon juice
½ cup (125 g) low-fat natural (plain) yogurt

PREPARATION 15 minutes, plus chilling
SERVES 8

EACH SERVING PROVIDES 285 kJ, 68 kcal, 4 g protein,
<1 g fat (<1 g saturated fat), 11 g carbohydrate
(10 g sugars), 2 g fibre, 38 mg sodium

> This mousse is a low-fat alternative
> to the usual cream-based mousses,
> thanks to its use of high-protein light
> evaporated milk. It is also a good source
> of anti-oxidants from the berries.

1 Put berries in a food processor or blender and
blend until smooth. Push berry purée through a
mesh strainer into a bowl. Discard seeds.

2 Combine gelatin and hot water in a small bowl and
stir until gelatin dissolves. Leave to cool.

3 Put chilled evaporated milk, sugar and lemon juice
in a medium bowl and beat with an electric mixer
3–4 minutes, or until light and fluffy. Beat in gelatin
mixture, yogurt and strained berry purée.

4 Spoon mousse into eight dessert glasses.
Refrigerate 30 minutes – 1 hour, or until set.
Serve decorated with extra berries, if desired.

COOK'S TIP This recipe can be made with raspberries,
blackberries or any other berry or combination of
berries. If using frozen mixed berries, thaw them
thoroughly before puréeing.

Chilling the evaporated milk helps it become light
and fluffy when whipped.

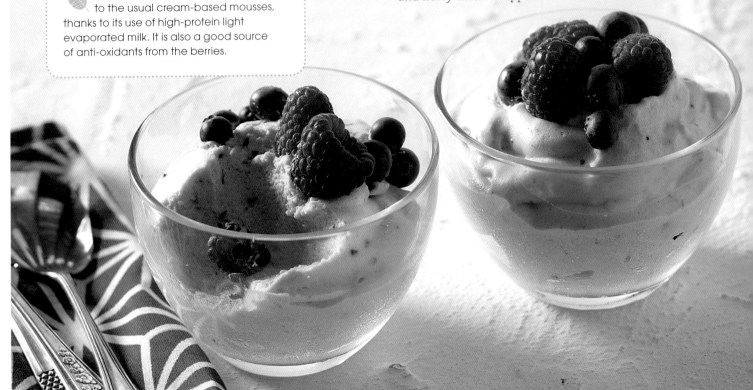

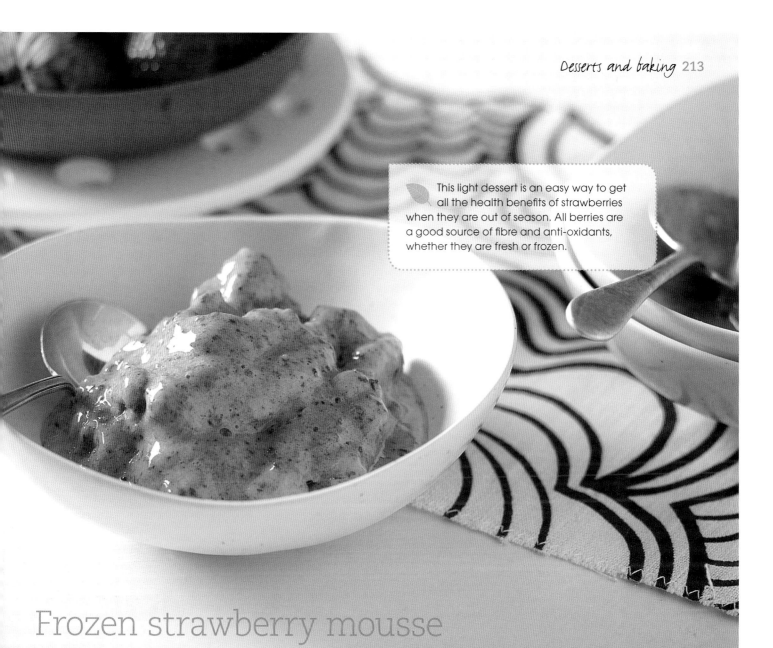

This light dessert is an easy way to get all the health benefits of strawberries when they are out of season. All berries are a good source of fibre and anti-oxidants, whether they are fresh or frozen.

Frozen strawberry mousse

1 cup (250 ml) light evaporated milk, chilled
2 tablespoons icing (confectioners') sugar
1 teaspoon grated orange zest
2 cups (300 g) frozen strawberries

PREPARATION 5 minutes
SERVES 4

EACH SERVING PROVIDES 250 kJ, 60 kcal, 3 g protein, <1 g fat (<1 g saturated fat), 11 g carbohydrate (11 g sugars), 2 g fibre, 30 mg sodium

1 Combine evaporated milk, icing sugar and orange zest in a measuring cup.

2 Put strawberries in a food processor or blender and pulse just until shaved. With the motor running, gradually add evaporated milk mixture and process just until the ingredients are combined.

3 Divide mousse among four dessert bowls and serve immediately.

COOK'S TIP You could use frozen mixed berries instead of strawberries.

Baked Greek yogurt

2 cups (500 g) low-fat thick Greek-style yogurt
reduced-fat canola spread, for greasing
1 tablespoon caster (superfine) sugar
2 eggs, separated
1 teaspoon finely grated lemon zest
2 tablespoons honey, plus extra honey,
    to serve (optional)
4 fresh figs, halved, or 2 fresh figs, sliced

PREPARATION 15 minutes, plus 2 hours draining
COOKING 15 minutes SERVES 4

EACH SERVING PROVIDES 1073 kJ, 256 kcal, 15 g protein,
8 g fat (4 g saturated fat), 30 g carbohydrate
(24 g sugars), 1 g fibre, 234 mg sodium

This light yet satisfying dessert is high in protein and calcium, and low in fat. To reduce the fat content even further, you can omit the egg yolks and make this recipe with eggwhites only.

1 Put yogurt in a medium mesh strainer set over a bowl. Cover and refrigerate overnight or at least 2 hours to drain.

2 Preheat oven to 200°C (400°F/Gas 6). Grease four ¾ cup (180 ml) ovenproof dishes with spread, then evenly coat the insides with caster sugar.

3 Whisk egg yolks, lemon zest and honey in a medium bowl until smooth. Discard any liquid from the strained yogurt. Add strained yogurt to egg yolk mixture and mix to combine well.

4 Put eggwhites in a clean medium bowl and beat with an electric mixer until stiff. Fold into yogurt mixture.

5 Pour yogurt mixture into prepared dishes. Bake 10–15 minutes, or until puffy and golden brown.

6 Top each baked yogurt with fig halves or slices, drizzle over a little more honey, if desired, and serve.

COOK'S TIP Straining the yogurt separates some of the curds from the whey, making it thicker and less likely to separate during baking. For draining to be most effective, make sure the strainer sits high enough above the base of the bowl so that the yogurt does not touch the drained liquid in the bowl.

For a change of flavour, replace the lemon zest with lime or orange zest, or the strained pulp of 1 passionfruit.

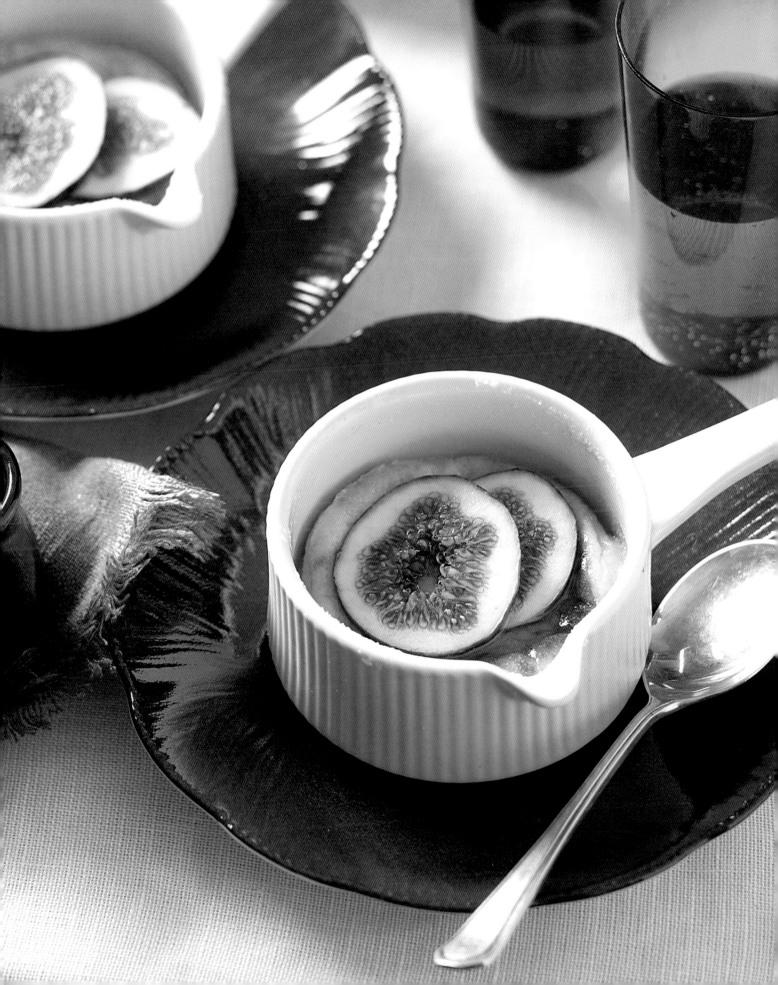

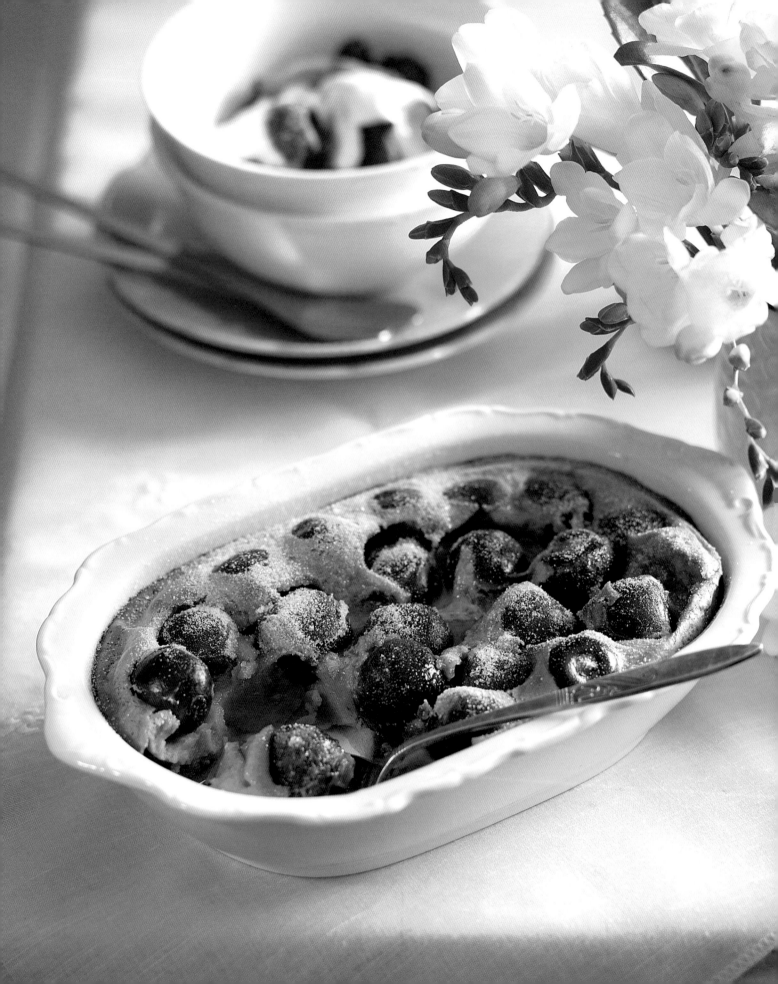

Cherry clafoutis

2 eggs
1/3 cup (50 g) plain (all-purpose) flour
1/2 teaspoon ground cinnamon
3/4 cup (180 ml) light evaporated milk
2 tablespoons honey or agave syrup
1 teaspoon vanilla extract
reduced-fat canola spread, for greasing
200 g (7 oz) fresh, canned or frozen pitted
    black cherries, thawed
2 teaspoons caster (superfine) sugar

PREPARATION 15 minutes, plus 5 minutes standing
COOKING 25 minutes SERVES 4

EACH SERVING PROVIDES 755 kJ, 180 kcal, 8 g protein,
5 g fat (1 g saturated fat), 27 g carbohydrate
(21 g sugars), 1 g fibre, 79 mg sodium

> Cherries contain a combination of anti-oxidants such as phenols, quercetin and anthocyanins at very high levels, which puts cherries in the category of 'anti-ageing superfood'. Anthocyanins, in particular, are the subject of current research into inflammatory conditions such as gout and arthritis, and cherries are thought to be protective against gout due to their high anthocyanin content.

1 Preheat oven to 200°C (400°F/Gas 6). Whisk eggs in a large bowl until smooth, then gradually beat in flour and cinnamon. While beating continuously, add evaporated milk, honey or agave syrup, and vanilla extract. Continue beating until smooth.

2 Lightly grease a shallow 3 cup (750 ml) ovenproof dish with spread, and set the dish on a baking tray (sheet). Spread cherries in a single layer over base of prepared dish. Pour batter over cherries.

3 Bake 20–30 minutes, or until cooked and well risen, and a skewer inserted in the centre comes out clean. Sprinkle with sugar and leave to stand 5 minutes. Serve warm.

COOK'S TIP You will need about 280 g (10 oz) unpitted fresh cherries for this recipe. Fresh or canned pitted plums, peaches or apricots can replace the cherries.

If using a deeper ovenproof dish, place it in a large roasting pan (baking dish), pour boiling water into the pan to come one-third of the way up the side of the dish, then bake until just set.

Remove the clafoutis from the oven as soon as it is set all the way through, as overcooking can cause the texture to become rubbery.

Baked custard with prunes

150 g (5 oz) pitted prunes, halved
1 cinnamon stick
1 star anise
2 whole cloves
1/3 cup (80 ml) water
reduced-fat canola spread, for greasing
4 eggs
1 tablespoon plain (all-purpose) flour
1 tablespoon honey
1 teaspoon vanilla extract
2 1/2 cups (625 ml) low-fat milk, warmed
ground cinnamon, for dusting

PREPARATION 15 minutes, plus 15 minutes standing
COOKING 55 minutes SERVES 4

EACH SERVING PROVIDES 1120 kJ, 267 kcal, 15 g protein,
7 g fat (2 g saturated fat), 36 g carbohydrate
(28 g sugars), 3 g fibre, 165 mg sodium

Egg custard baked with prunes that
have been stewed with cinnamon, star
anise and cloves – all rich in anti-oxidants –
creates a high-protein dessert that is a good
complement to a light main meal.

1 Put prunes, cinnamon, star anise, cloves and water in a medium saucepan over medium heat and bring to a boil. Reduce heat to low and simmer, uncovered, 5–7 minutes, or until water has evaporated. Remove from heat and leave to stand 10 minutes. Remove spices and discard.

2 Preheat oven to 160°C (320°F/Gas 2–3). Grease four 1 1/2 cup (375 ml) ovenproof dishes with spread. Divide prunes among the dishes.

3 Whisk eggs, flour, honey and vanilla extract in a medium bowl until well combined. Gradually whisk in warm milk, then pour over prunes in dishes.

4 Put dishes in a large roasting pan (baking dish) and carefully add enough boiling water to the pan to come halfway up sides of dishes. Bake 40–45 minutes, or until just set. Remove custards from pan, dust with ground cinnamon and leave to stand 5 minutes before serving.

COOK'S TIP If you tie the spices in a piece of muslin (cheesecloth), it will be easier to remove them from the prune mixture at the end of step 1.

Once the custards are cooked, they must be removed from the water bath immediately so that they don't continue cooking.

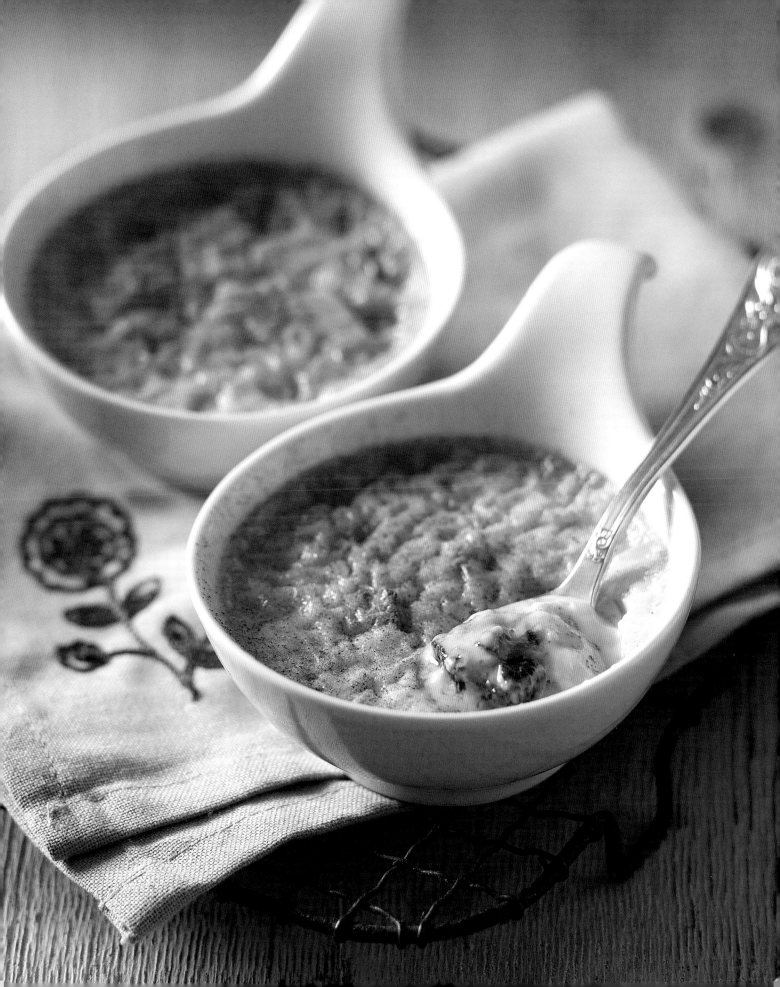

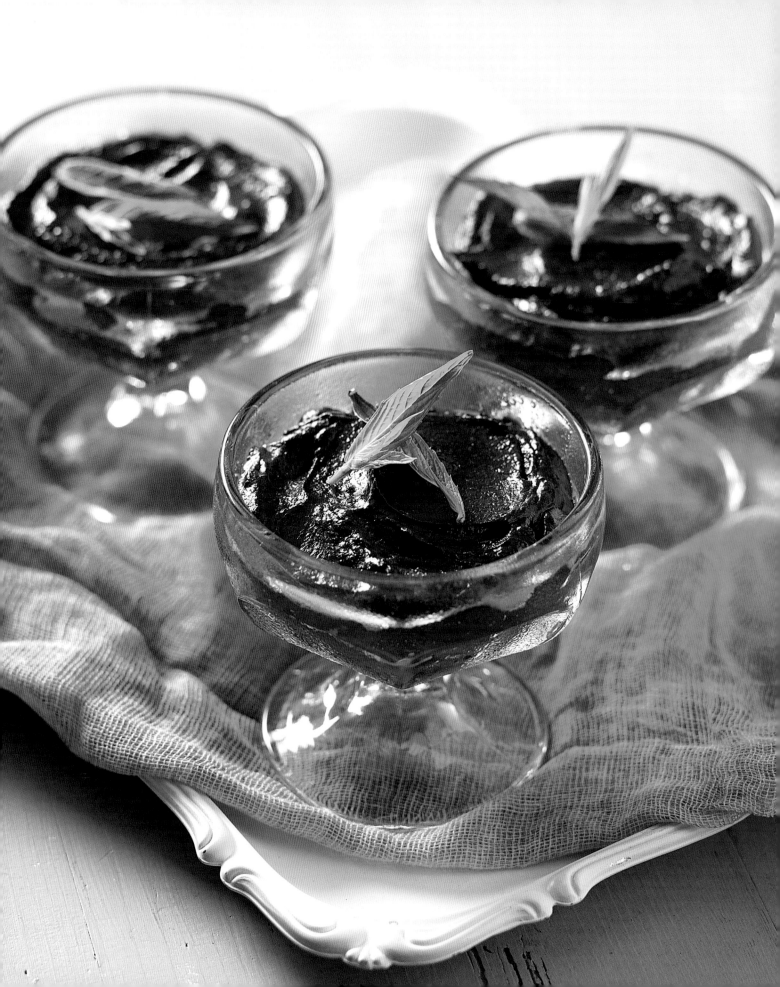

Surprise chocolate mousse

¾ cup (135 g) pitted dates
1 large ripe avocado, roughly chopped
1 tablespoon maple syrup
⅓ cup (40 g) unsweetened cocoa powder
1 teaspoon vanilla extract

PREPARATION 15 minutes, plus 10 minutes standing
and 1 hour chilling SERVES 4

EACH SERVING PROVIDES 1126 kJ, 269 kcal, 4 g protein,
15 g fat (3 g saturated fat), 30 g carbohydrate
(27 g sugars), 5 g fibre, 33 mg sodium

Avocado in a dessert sounds odd, but makes a dairy-free version of chocolate mousse that contains only good fats and very little added sugar. It tastes rich and chocolatey and yet it is packed with anti-oxidants.

1 Put dates in a medium heatproof bowl. Cover with boiling water and stand 10 minutes, or until softened. Drain, reserving soaking liquid.

2 Put dates in a food processor or blender and process until smooth. Add avocado and process until smooth. Add maple syrup, cocoa powder and vanilla extract and process until well combined, adding a little of the reserved soaking liquid (about 2 tablespoons), to form the desired consistency.

3 Spoon mousse into four ½ cup (125 ml) dessert glasses. Refrigerate 1 hour, or until chilled. Serve.

COOK'S TIP Use a good-quality unsweetened raw or regular cocoa powder to ensure that the mousse has a rich chocolate taste.

Strawberry and yogurt cupcakes

100 g (3½ oz) light olive oil spread
½ cup (115 g) caster (superfine) sugar
1 teaspoon vanilla extract
2 eggs
¾ cup (110 g) self-raising flour
½ cup (75 g) wholemeal plain flour
    (whole-wheat all-purpose flour)
⅔ cup (160 g) low-fat thick Greek-style yogurt
150 g (5 oz) strawberries, hulled,
    finely chopped
icing (confectioners') sugar, for dusting

PREPARATION 10 minutes, plus cooling
COOKING 25 minutes MAKES 9 cupcakes

EACH CUPCAKE PROVIDES 896 kJ, 214 kcal, 6 g protein,
8 g fat (2 g saturated fat), 30 g carbohydrate
(14 g sugars), 2 g fibre, 168 mg sodium

Yogurt is great as a low-fat, high-calcium component of cake batter. Here it is combined with pieces of fresh strawberry to make these delightfully fruity little cupcakes.

1 Preheat oven to 180°C (350°F/Gas 4). Line 9 holes of a deep, flat-based patty pan or standard ⅓ cup muffin tin with paper cases.

2 Put spread, caster sugar and vanilla extract in a medium bowl and beat with an electric mixer 3–4 minutes, or until pale and creamy. Add eggs, one at a time, beating well after each addition.

3 Sift together self-raising and wholemeal plain flour, then stir into creamed mixture until well combined. Add yogurt and strawberries. Stir until well combined. Spoon mixture into paper cases.

4 Bake cupcakes 20–25 minutes, or until a skewer inserted in the centre comes out clean. Cool cupcakes 5 minutes before transferring to a wire rack to cool completely.

5 Serve cupcakes dusted with a little icing sugar.

COOK'S TIP Strawberries can be replaced with 150 g (5 oz) fresh raspberries or blueberries.

You can store the cupcakes in an airtight container for up to 3 days.

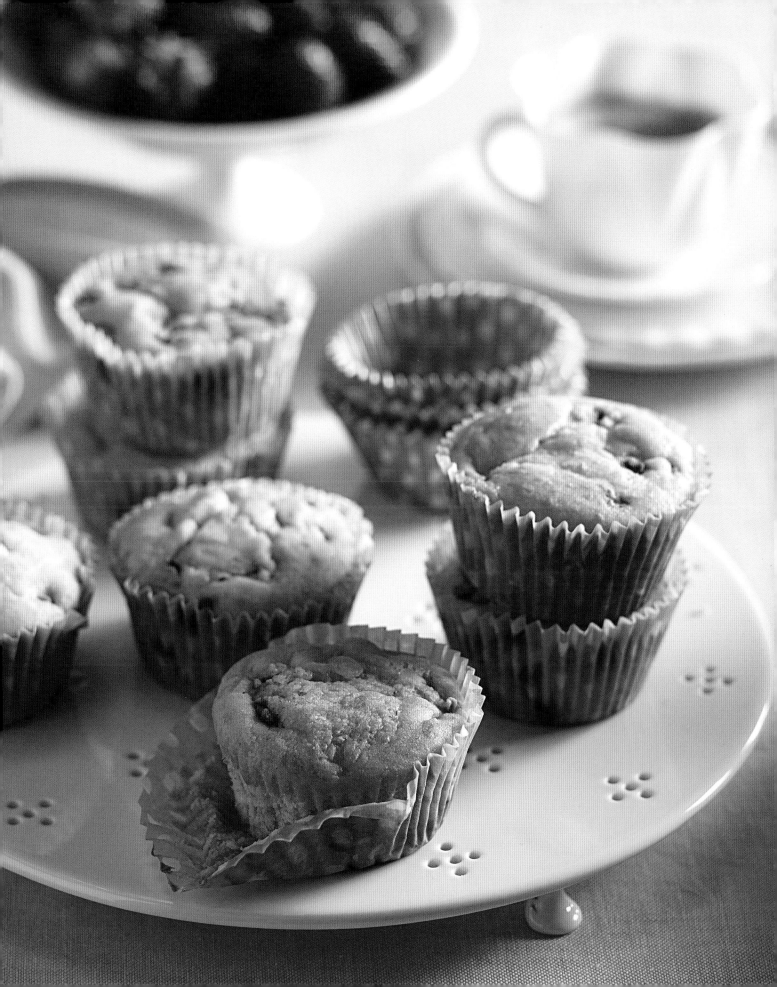

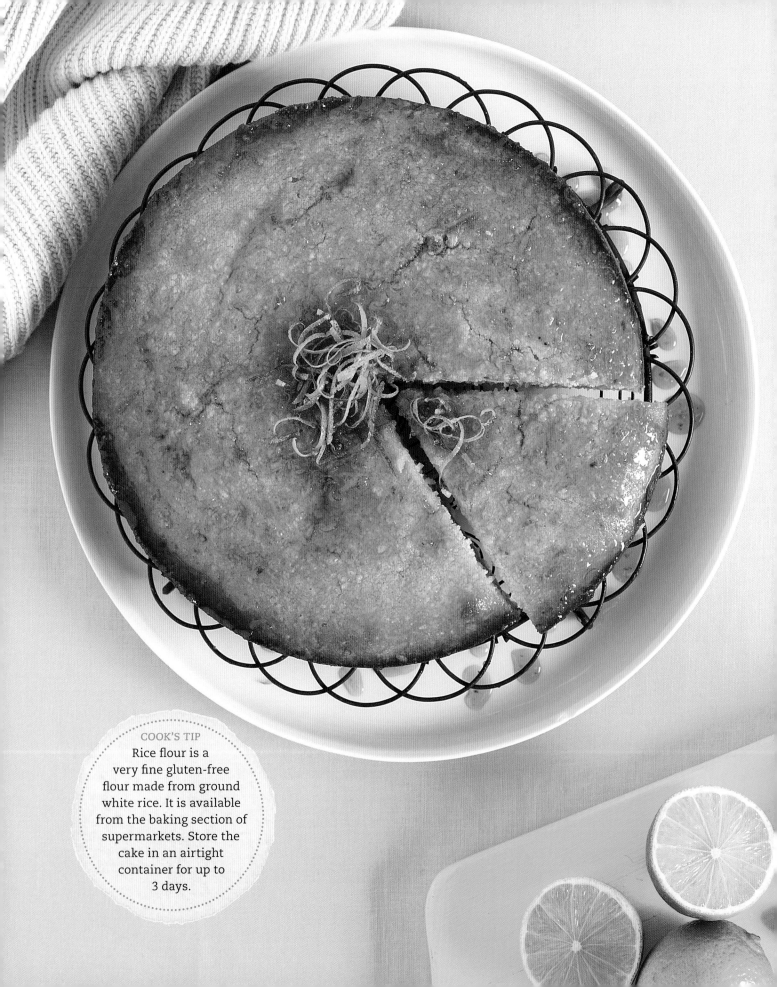

COOK'S TIP
Rice flour is a
very fine gluten-free
flour made from ground
white rice. It is available
from the baking section of
supermarkets. Store the
cake in an airtight
container for up to
3 days.

Lime and almond syrup cake

light olive oil spread, for greasing
1½ cups (240 g) raw unblanched almonds
   or 1½ cups (155 g) almond meal
   (ground almonds)
150 g (5 oz) light olive oil spread
½ cup (115 g) caster (superfine) sugar
3 teaspoons finely grated lime zest
3 eggs
½ cup (90 g) rice flour
2 tablespoons lime juice
low-fat vanilla yogurt, to serve (optional)

Lime syrup

⅓ cup (80 ml) agave syrup or honey
finely grated zest of 1 lime
¼ cup (60 ml) lime juice

PREPARATION 20 minutes, plus cooling
COOKING 50 minutes **SERVES** 12

EACH SERVING PROVIDES 1226 kJ, 293 kcal, 6 g protein,
21 g fat (4 g saturated fat), 24 g carbohydrate
(18 g sugars), 2 g fibre, 64 mg sodium

1 Preheat oven to 180°C (350°F/Gas 4). Grease a
20 cm (8 inch) round spring-form cake tin. Line base
and side with baking (parchment) paper. If using raw
unblanched almonds, put in a food processor or
blender and process until finely ground. Set aside.

2 Put spread, sugar and 2 teaspoons zest in a
medium bowl and beat with an electric mixer
3–4 minutes, or until pale and creamy. Add eggs,
one at a time, beating well after each addition.

3 Stir in finely ground unblanched almonds or
almond meal, rice flour and lime juice until
combined. Spoon mixture into prepared tin and
smooth the surface.

4 Bake 45–50 minutes, or until a skewer inserted in
the centre comes out clean. Cool 5 minutes before
removing cake from tin.

5 Meanwhile, make the lime syrup. Combine agave
syrup or honey, lime zest and lime juice in a small
saucepan over high heat. Bring to a boil, then reduce
heat to low and simmer 2–3 minutes, or until slightly
thickened. Pour hot syrup over warm cake. Garnish
with remaining lime zest.

6 Serve cake warm or cold with a dollop of yogurt,
if desired.

> This cake uses almond meal from whole
> almonds as a base, increasing the fibre
> and anti-oxidant content. Lime zest gives the
> cake a gorgeous lime fragrance and the
> cake is finished with a syrup made from lime
> juice giving it the benefits of both the citrus
> peel and the juice.

Steamed fruit pudding

3 cups (550 g) mixed dried fruit
1 cup (160 g) chopped dates
½ cup (95 g) chopped dried figs
¾ cup (180 ml) orange juice
¾ cup (165 g) firmly packed soft brown sugar
125 g (4 oz) olive oil spread, plus extra,
   for greasing
1 teaspoon bicarbonate of soda
   (baking soda)
2 eggs, lightly beaten
¾ cup (110 g) self-raising flour
½ cup (75 g) plain (all-purpose) flour
½ cup (55 g) almond meal (ground
   almonds)
2 teaspoons curry powder, toasted
1 teaspoon ground turmeric, toasted
1 teaspoon mixed (pumpkin pie) spice
2 tablespoons brandy
low-fat custard or low-fat ice cream, to serve
   (optional)

PREPARATION 20 minutes, plus 30 minutes cooling and
10 minutes standing COOKING 4 hours SERVES 12

EACH SERVING PROVIDES 1533 kJ, 366 kcal, 5 g protein,
10 g fat (2 g saturated fat), 64 g carbohydrate
(52 g sugars), 5 g fibre, 272 mg sodium

> This Christmas-type plum pudding is rich in fibre, minerals and anti-oxidants thanks to its dried fruit content and the additional spices, which include, surprisingly, curry powder and turmeric. These spices are not identifiable when you eat the finished dessert but add to the richness of its overall flavour.

1 Combine mixed dried fruit, dates, figs, orange juice, sugar and spread in a large saucepan over medium heat. Stir until sugar dissolves, then bring to a boil. Reduce heat and simmer, uncovered, 5 minutes. Stir in bicarbonate of soda. Transfer mixture to a large bowl and leave to cool 30 minutes.

2 Stir in eggs, self-raising and plain flours, almond meal, curry powder, turmeric, mixed spice and brandy until well combined.

3 Grease an 8 cup (2 litre) pudding steamer. Spoon mixture into steamer. Cut a circle of baking (parchment) paper about 10 cm (4 inches) wider in diameter than the top of the steamer. Fold a 4 cm (1½ inch) wide pleat in the centre of the circle. Lay this over pudding batter, then secure steamer lid.

4 Put pudding steamer in a large saucepan. Pour in enough boiling water to come halfway up the side of steamer. Cover saucepan with a tight-fitting lid and bring to a boil over high heat. Reduce heat to low and simmer 4 hours, or until a skewer inserted in the centre of the pudding comes out clean. Replenish water as necessary to maintain the water level.

5 Leave pudding to stand in steamer 10 minutes, then turn out onto a serving plate. Serve with custard or ice cream, if desired.

COOK'S TIP Pleat the baking paper on top of the pudding batter so that it expands as the pudding rises during cooking.

To toast curry powder and turmeric, put in a small saucepan over low heat and cook, stirring, until fragrant. Remove from heat immediately and transfer to a bowl to cool.

You can store this Christmas pudding in an airtight container in the refrigerator for up to 6 weeks or freeze it for up to 8 months. To reheat, stand at room temperature 6 hours, then cover with plastic wrap and microwave on Medium 10–12 minutes.

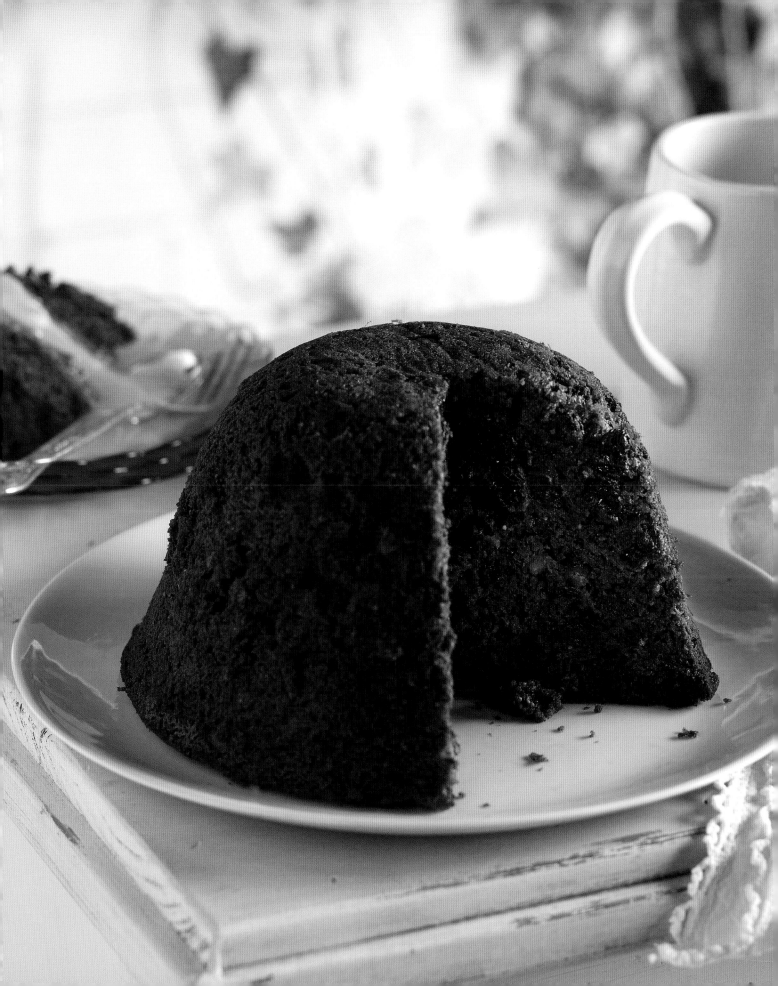

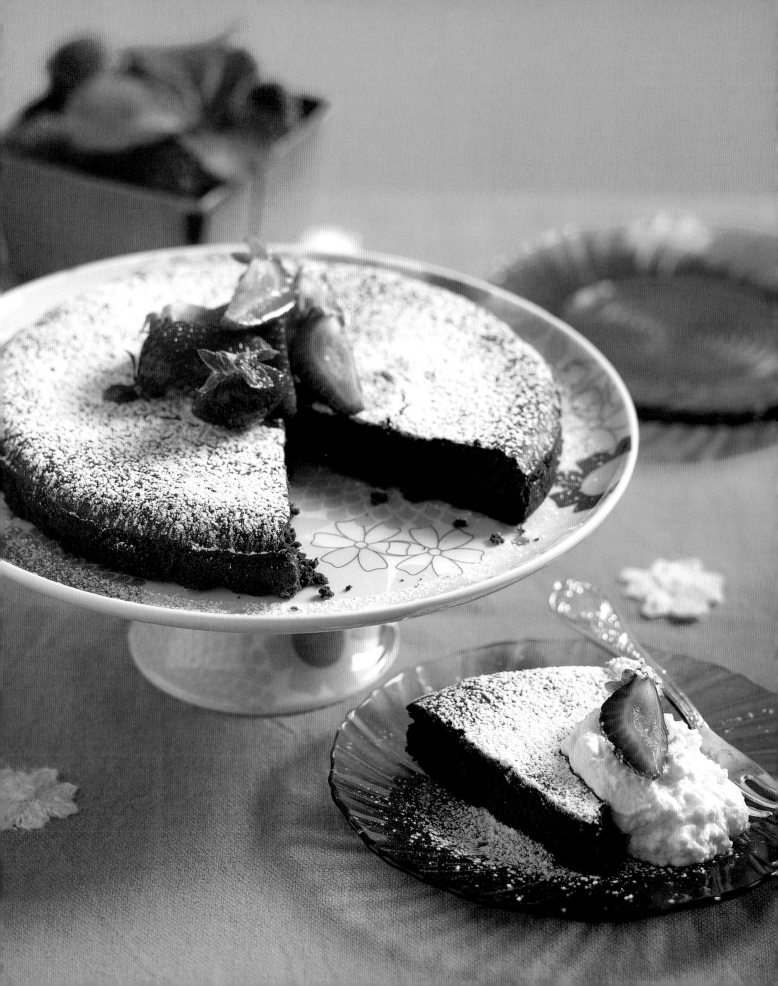

Secret ingredient chocolate cake

canola oil cooking spray, for greasing
125 g (4 oz) dark (bittersweet) chocolate
    (70% cacao), broken into pieces
400 g (14 oz) can red kidney beans or black
    beans, rinsed and drained
2 large eggs, lightly beaten
½ cup (110 g) sugar
¼ teaspoon baking powder
2 teaspoons vanilla extract
icing (confectioners') sugar, for dusting
500 g (1 lb) fresh strawberries or raspberries,
    sliced
reduced-fat ricotta, to serve (optional)

PREPARATION 20 minutes, plus cooling
COOKING 45 minutes SERVES 8

EACH SERVING PROVIDES 958 kJ, 229 kcal, 6 g protein,
10 g fat (4 g saturated fat), 28 g carbohydrate
(24 g sugars), 5 g fibre, 155 mg sodium

> This cake has the intense chocolate flavour and fudge-like texture of a rich flourless chocolate cake, but it contains a fraction of the saturated fat. You cannot taste the red kidney beans or black beans, but the fibre and protein from them helps to balance the carbohydrate and lower the glycaemic index of the cake.

1 Preheat oven to 180°C (350°F/Gas 4). Coat a 20 cm (8 inch) round cake tin with cooking spray. Line base with baking (parchment) paper.

2 Melt chocolate in a plastic or glass bowl in the microwave on High, about 1–2 minutes. Alternatively, melt chocolate in a heatproof bowl over a small saucepan of simmering water, stirring occasionally.

3 Put beans in a food processor or blender and process to a purée. Add eggs, sugar, baking powder and vanilla extract. Process until smooth and creamy, stopping several times to scrape down sides of bowl. Add melted chocolate and pulse several times until thoroughly blended. Scrape batter into prepared cake tin.

4 Bake 35–45 minutes, until the top springs back when touched lightly. (The cake will look cracked.) Cool in the tin on a wire rack 5 minutes, then loosen edges, invert cake onto rack and peel off baking paper. Leave to cool.

5 Dust cake with icing sugar. Serve slightly warm, or at room temperature for the fudgiest texture, accompanied by strawberries or raspberries. Serve with ricotta on the side, if desired.

COOK'S TIP For a special presentation, place a paper doily over the cake before dusting with the icing sugar. You can also create your own stencil using strips of baking (parchment) paper.

Greek walnut cake

light olive oil spread, for greasing
2 cups (200 g) walnut halves, plus extra
 walnut halves (about 12), for decorating
100 g (3½ oz) light olive oil spread
⅔ cup (145 g) caster (superfine) sugar
3 eggs, separated
1 cup (150 g) self-raising flour
¾ cup (185 g) low-fat thick Greek-style
 yogurt, plus extra, to serve (optional)
12 small walnuts (40 g), halved

Syrup

⅓ cup (80 ml) water
⅓ cup (115 g) honey
5 cm (2 inch) strip lemon zest
1 cinnamon stick
3 whole cloves

PREPARATION 25 minutes, plus cooling
COOKING 55 minutes SERVES 12

EACH SERVING PROVIDES 1306 kJ, 312 kcal, 6 g protein,
18 g fat (3 g saturated fat), 31 g carbohydrate
(22 g sugars), 2 g fibre, 160 mg sodium

This cake uses walnut meal from whole walnuts as a base, increasing the amount of fibre, anti-oxidants and omega-3 oils that it provides, along with yogurt, which increases the calcium content. A syrup with the anti-oxidant properties of lemon zest, cinnamon, cloves and honey is poured over at the end.

1 Preheat oven to 180°C (350°F/Gas 4). Grease a 20 cm (8 inch) round springform cake tin. Line base and side with baking (parchment) paper. Put 2 cups walnuts in a food processor or blender and process until finely ground.

2 Put spread and sugar in a medium bowl and beat with an electric mixer 3–4 minutes, or until pale and creamy. Add egg yolks, one at a time, beating well after each addition. Stir in flour, finely ground walnuts and ¾ cup yogurt until combined.

3 Put eggwhites in a small bowl that is thoroughly clean and dry, and beat with the electric mixer until soft peaks form. Gently fold half the eggwhites into walnut mixture, then repeat with remaining eggwhites. Spoon mixture into prepared tin and smooth the surface. Press extra walnut halves into top of mixture for a decorative effect.

4 Bake 50–55 minutes, or until a skewer inserted in the centre comes out clean. Cool 5 minutes before removing cake from tin.

5 Meanwhile, make the syrup. Combine water, honey, lemon zest, cinnamon and cloves in a small saucepan. Bring to a boil over high heat. Reduce heat to low and simmer 5–6 minutes, or until slightly thickened. Discard zest and spices, then pour hot syrup over warm cake.

6 Serve slices of cake warm or cold with a dollop of yogurt, if desired.

COOK'S TIP The processed walnuts will resemble fine fresh breadcrumbs. You will need about 1¼ cups walnut meal (ground walnuts) for this recipe.

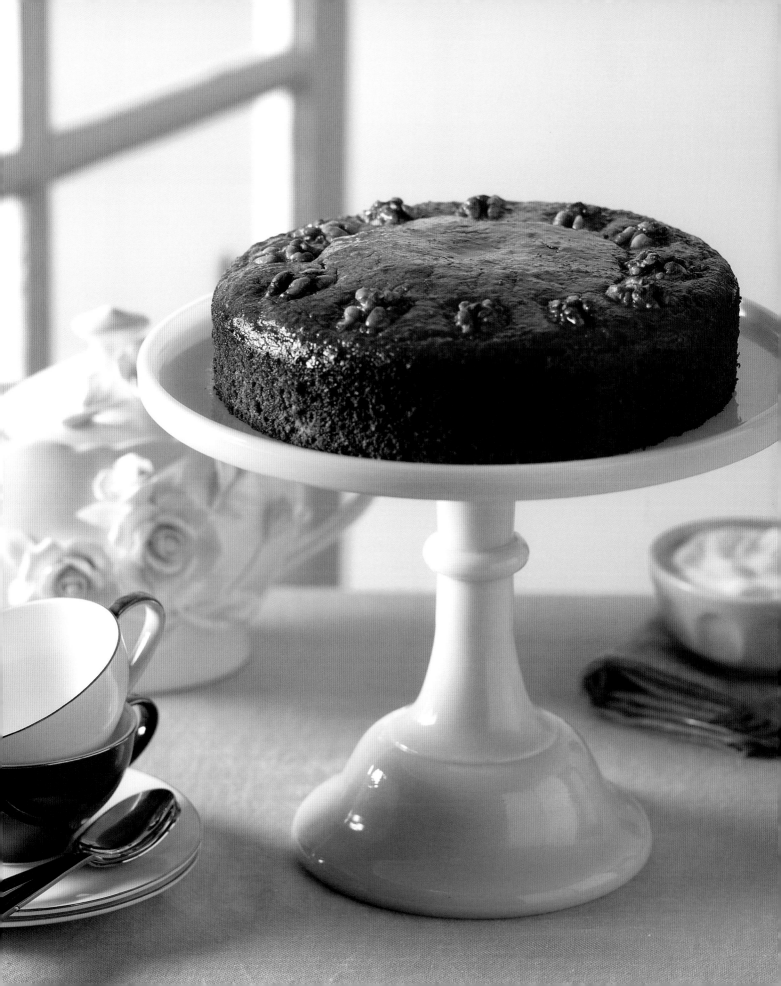

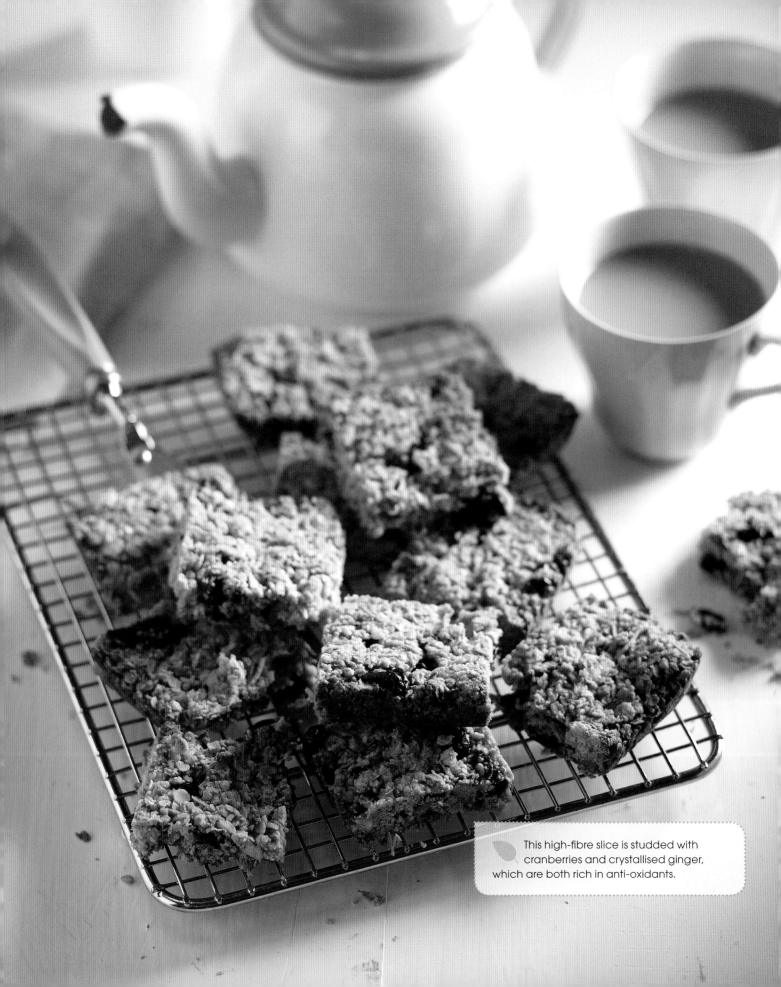

This high-fibre slice is studded with cranberries and crystallised ginger, which are both rich in anti-oxidants.

Ginger and cranberry oat slice

olive oil spread, for greasing
1 cup (125 g) rolled (porridge) oats
²/₃ cup (100 g) wholemeal (whole-wheat)
　　self-raising flour
½ cup (60 g) dried cranberries
⅓ cup (20 g) shredded coconut
2 tablespoons finely chopped crystallised
　　ginger
¼ cup (35 g) chopped pistachios
100 g (3½ oz) olive oil spread
¼ cup (45 g) firmly packed soft brown sugar
2 tablespoons honey

PREPARATION 15 minutes, plus cooling
COOKING 35 minutes MAKES 15 pieces

EACH PIECE PROVIDES 610 kJ, 146 kcal, 2 g protein,
7 g fat (2 g saturated fat), 20 g carbohydrate
(8 g sugars), 3 g fibre, 72 mg sodium

1 Preheat oven to 180°C (350°F/Gas 4). Grease an
18 cm x 28 cm (7 x 11 inch) baking tin. Line base and
sides with baking (parchment) paper, extending it
2.5 cm (1 inch) from edges of tin.

2 Combine oats, flour, cranberries, coconut, ginger
and pistachios in a large bowl. Put spread, sugar and
honey in a small saucepan and stir over low heat
until melted and smooth. Add to oat mixture and stir
to combine.

3 Press mixture into prepared tin and smooth the
surface. Bake 25–30 minutes, or until golden and just
firm to touch. Leave to cool in tin.

4 Cut slice into 15 pieces and serve.

COOK'S TIP Store the slice in an airtight container for
up to 7 days.

Crystallised ginger can be replaced with glacé
(candied) ginger if you prefer.

Orange cake

olive oil spread, for greasing
3 eggs
1 cup (230 g) caster (superfine) sugar
finely grated zest of 1 orange
1¼ cups (185 g) self-raising flour
1 cup (150 g) wholemeal plain flour
    (whole-wheat all-purpose flour)
½ cup (125 ml) olive oil
¼ cup (60 ml) orange juice
¼ cup (60 ml) buttermilk
icing (confectioners') sugar, for dusting

PREPARATION 20 minutes, plus cooling
COOKING 50 minutes SERVES 12

EACH SERVING PROVIDES 1173 kJ, 280 kcal, 5 g protein,
11 g fat (2 g saturated fat), 40 g carbohydrate
(21 g sugars), 2 g fibre, 127 mg sodium

In this light cake, olive oil – rich
in anti-oxidants – is used as a
fruity-flavoured alternative to butter.

1 Preheat oven to 180°C (350°F/Gas 4). Grease a
20 cm (8 inch) square cake tin. Line base and sides
with baking (parchment) paper.

2 Put eggs, caster sugar and orange zest in a
medium bowl and beat with an electric mixer
5–6 minutes, or until thick and creamy and sugar
is dissolved. Transfer mixture to a large bowl.

3 Sift together self-raising and wholemeal plain
flours. Beat together oil, orange juice and buttermilk
in a small bowl. Stir half the dry ingredients and half
the oil mixture into the creamed eggs and sugar until
combined. Repeat with remaining dry ingredients
and remaining oil mixture, stirring until thoroughly
combined. Pour into prepared tin.

4 Bake 50 minutes, or until a skewer inserted in the
centre comes out clean. Cool 10 minutes before
turning out onto a wire rack to cool completely.

5 Serve cake dusted with a little icing sugar. Top
with orange slices, if desired.

COOK'S TIP Store the cake in an airtight container
for up to 4 days.

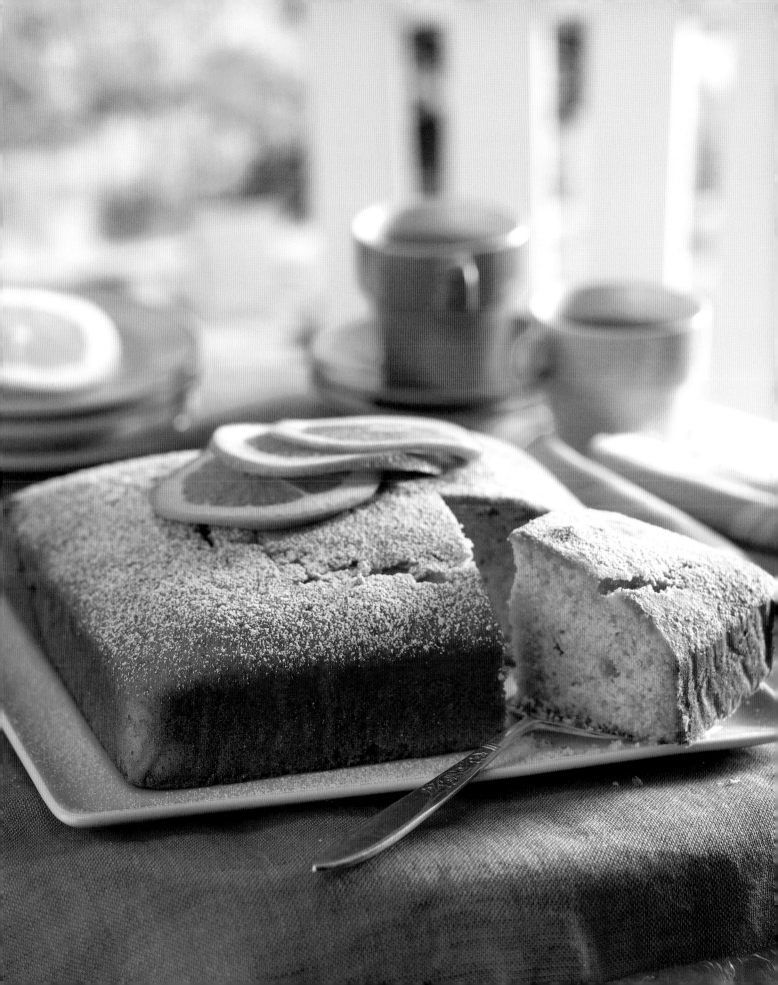

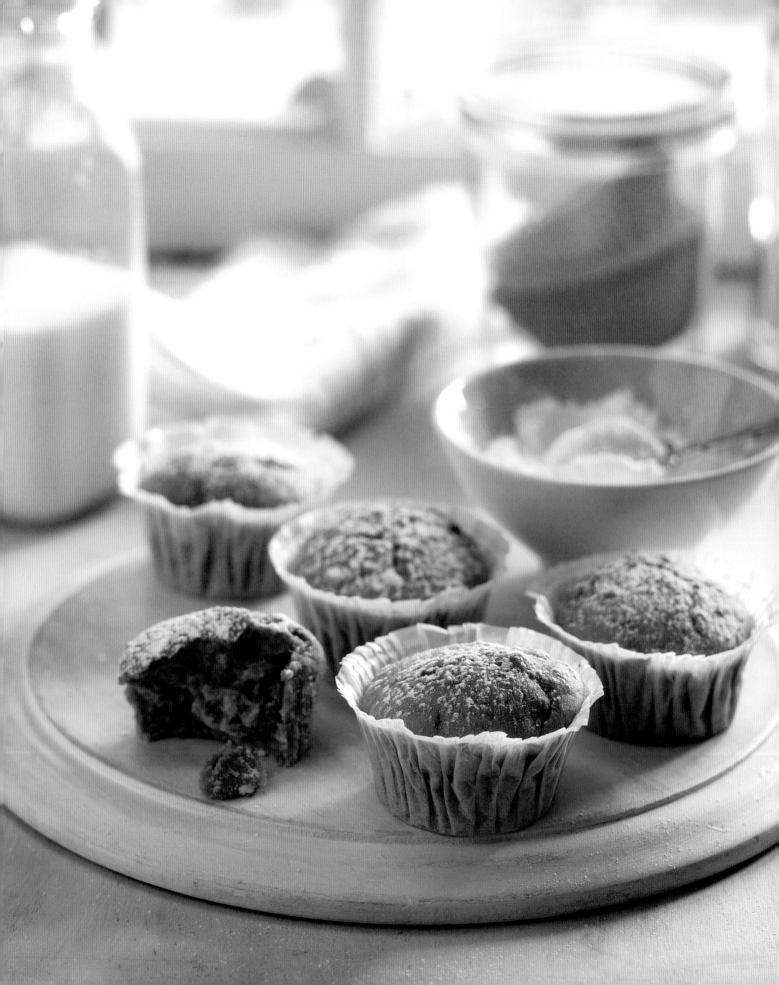

Sweet potato cupcakes

125 g (4 oz) light olive oil spread
1/3 cup (80 g) firmly packed soft brown sugar
1 tablespoon golden syrup or honey
2 eggs
3/4 cup (110 g) white self-raising flour
1/2 cup (75 g) wholemeal (whole-wheat)
    self-raising flour
1 cup (250 g) mashed orange sweet potato
    (kumara)
1 teaspoon mixed (pumpkin pie) spice
1/4 cup (60 ml) low-fat milk
icing (confectioners') sugar, for dusting

PREPARATION 18 minutes, plus cooling
COOKING 20 minutes MAKES 9 cupcakes

EACH CUPCAKE PROVIDES 915 kJ, 219 kcal, 5 g protein,
9 g fat (2 g saturated fat), 30 g carbohydrate
(14 g sugars), 2 g fibre, 218 mg sodium

Sweet potatoes are high in anti-oxidants and here form the basis for a soft, mildly sweet cupcake that has a low glycaemic index. This is thanks to the wholemeal flour and sweet potato, both of which release their energy more slowly than highly processed white flour.

1 Preheat oven to 180°C (350°F/Gas 4). Line 9 holes of a deep, flat-based patty pan or standard 1/3-cup muffin tin with paper cases.

2 Put spread, brown sugar and golden syrup or honey in a medium bowl and beat with an electric mixer 3–4 minutes, or until pale and creamy. Add eggs, one at a time, beating well after each addition.

3 Sift together white self-raising and wholemeal self-raising flour, then stir into creamed mixture with sweet potato and mixed spice. Add milk and stir until well combined. Spoon mixture into paper cases.

4 Bake 15–20 minutes, or until a skewer inserted in the centre comes out clean. Cool cupcakes 5 minutes before transferring to a wire rack to cool completely.

5 Serve cupcakes dusted with a little icing sugar.

COOK'S TIP You will need 400 g (14 oz) orange sweet potato to make 1 cup mashed sweet potato for this recipe. Peel and roughly chop the sweet potato, then cook in a saucepan of boiling water 8–10 minutes, or until tender. Drain well before mashing.

Ginger and Brazil nut biscuits

75 g (2½ oz) light olive oil spread, plus extra,
    for greasing
¼ cup (55 g) firmly packed soft brown sugar
2 tablespoons golden syrup or honey
1¼ cups (185 g) plain (all-purpose) flour
½ teaspoon bicarbonate of soda
    (baking soda)
2 teaspoons ground ginger
½ teaspoon ground cinnamon
¼ cup (35 g) chopped Brazil nuts,
    plus 16 small Brazil nuts, for decorating
1 tablespoon chopped crystallised ginger

PREPARATION 15 minutes, plus cooling
COOKING 20 minutes MAKES 16 biscuits

EACH BISCUIT PROVIDES 429 kJ, 102 kcal, 2 g protein,
4 g fat (1 g saturated fat), 15 g carbohydrate
(6 g sugars), <1 g fibre, 57 mg sodium

1 Preheat oven to 180°C (350°F/Gas 4). Grease and line two baking trays with baking paper (baking sheets with parchment paper).

2 Put spread, sugar and golden syrup or honey in a medium saucepan and stir over low heat until melted and smooth. Remove from heat.

3 Sift together flour, bicarbonate of soda, ground ginger and cinnamon. Stir into melted mixture. Stir in chopped Brazil nuts and crystallised ginger until well combined. Leave to cool 10 minutes.

4 Roll level tablespoons of mixture into balls. Space balls about 3 cm (1¼ inch) apart on prepared trays. With your hand, press balls to flatten slightly, then press 1 Brazil nut into the top of each biscuit. Bake 12–15 minutes, or until golden. Leave to cool on trays.

COOK'S TIP You will need about 200 g (7 oz) Brazil nuts for this recipe.

These crunchy biscuits have the anti-oxidant benefits of both ground ginger and chunks of crystallised ginger, and selenium-rich Brazil nut pieces for extra crunch.

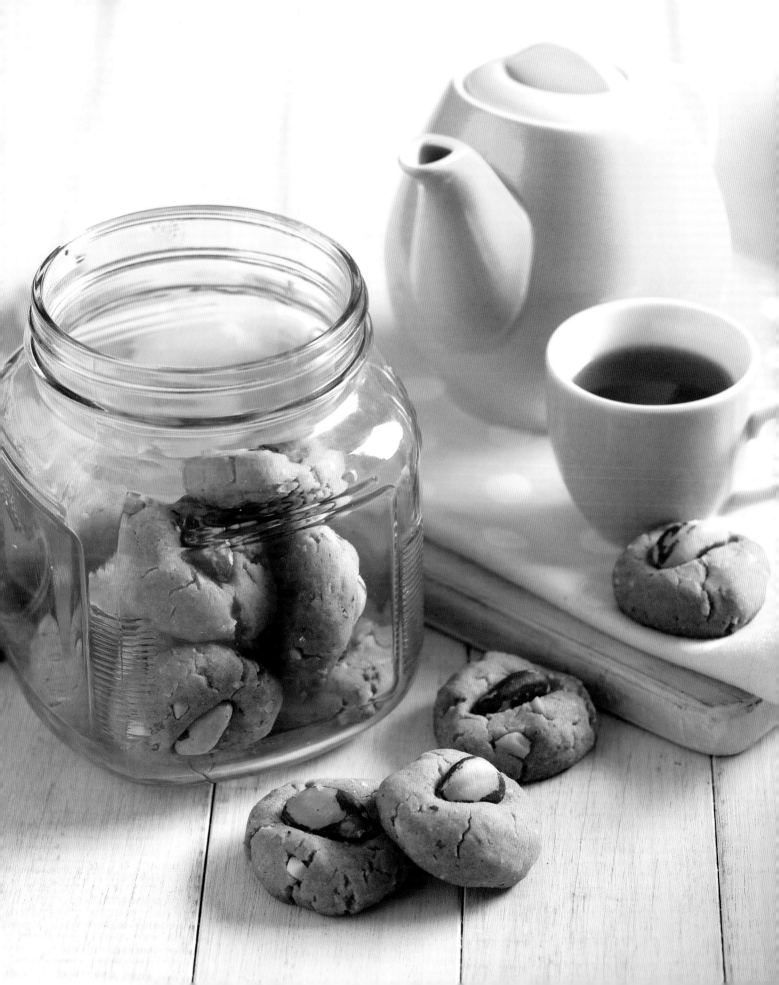

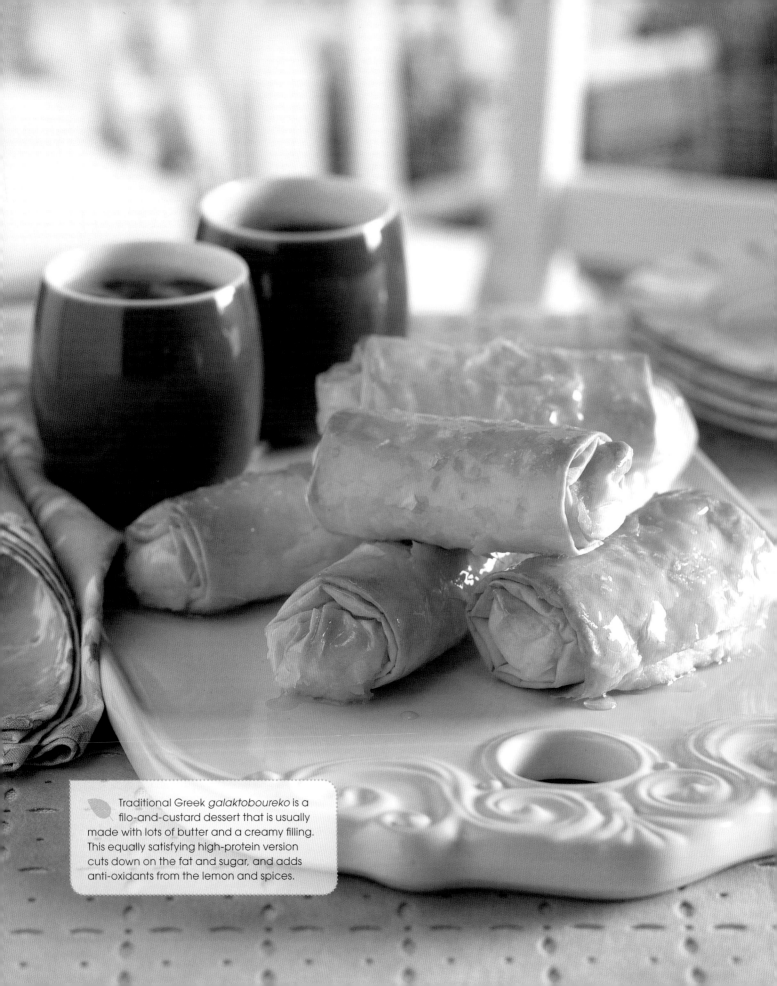

Traditional Greek *galaktoboureko* is a filo-and-custard dessert that is usually made with lots of butter and a creamy filling. This equally satisfying high-protein version cuts down on the fat and sugar, and adds anti-oxidants from the lemon and spices.

Filo custard fingers with lemon and spice syrup

1 cup (250 ml) low-fat milk
2 eggs
1½ tablespoons cornflour (cornstarch)
1 tablespoon plain (all-purpose) flour
2 tablespoons caster (superfine) sugar
½ teaspoon vanilla extract
2 whole cloves
olive oil cooking spray
6 sheets filo pastry

Lemon and spice syrup

⅓ cup (115 g) honey
grated zest of 1 lemon
¼ cup (60 ml) lemon juice
1 cinnamon stick
3 cardamom pods, bruised

PREPARATION 30 minutes, plus 1 hour chilling
and 1 hour cooling
COOKING 20 minutes SERVES 6

EACH SERVING PROVIDES 806 kJ, 192 kcal, 6 g protein,
3 g fat (1 g saturated fat), 36 g carbohydrate
(25 g sugars), <1 g fibre, 150 mg sodium

1 Put ¼ cup (60 ml) milk, eggs, cornflour, flour, sugar and vanilla extract in a medium heatproof bowl and whisk until well combined.

2 Put cloves and remaining milk in a medium saucepan over medium heat. Stir until mixture comes to a boil, then remove from heat and discard cloves. Gradually pour onto the egg mixture, whisking continuously. Return to saucepan, reduce heat to low and cook, stirring, 2–3 minutes, or until custard boils and thickens. Transfer custard to a bowl and cover with plastic wrap. Refrigerate 1 hour, or until cold.

3 Preheat oven to 200°C (400°F/Gas 6). Coat a small ovenproof dish with cooking spray.

4 Lay 1 sheet filo pastry on workbench and spray lightly with cooking spray. Repeat with a further 2 sheets pastry to make a stack of 3 sheets. Cut stack crosswise into 3 equal pieces. Put 3 tablespoons custard on a short end of each strip, leaving a 3 cm (1¼ inch) border from the edge. Roll up each pastry strip to enclose filling and form a cigar shape. Put in prepared dish. Repeat with remaining 3 sheets pastry and custard to make 6 fingers in total.

5 Bake 15 minutes, or until pastry is crisp and golden.

6 Meanwhile, make the lemon and spice syrup. Combine honey, lemon zest and juice, cinnamon and cardamom in a small saucepan. Bring to a boil over high heat. Reduce heat to low and simmer 4–5 minutes, or until thickened slightly. Discard cinnamon and cardamom, then pour hot syrup over hot pastry fingers. Leave to cool about 1 hour. Serve at room temperature.

COOK'S TIP Make sure you do not roll the pastry fingers too tightly or they will split during baking, causing the custard to ooze out.

Apple gingerbread

light olive oil spread, for greasing
2 small apples, peeled, quartered and
    cored, thinly sliced, or 150 g (5 oz)
    apple purée
1/3 cup (115 g) golden syrup or honey
1/2 cup (125 ml) cold tea or water
1/3 cup (80 g) firmly packed soft brown sugar
100 g (3 1/2 oz) light olive oil spread
3/4 cup (110 g) wholemeal plain flour
    (whole-wheat all-purpose flour)
1 cup (150 g) white plain (all-purpose) flour
1 teaspoon bicarbonate of soda
    (baking soda)
1 tablespoon ground ginger
1/2 teaspoon ground cinnamon
1/2 teaspoon ground nutmeg
1/2 cup (125 g) glacé (candied) or crystallised
    ginger, chopped
3 teaspoons raw (demerara) sugar

PREPARATION 20 minutes, plus cooling
COOKING 1 hour SERVES 12

EACH SERVING PROVIDES 791 kJ, 189 kcal, 3 g protein,
5 g fat (1 g saturated fat), 34 g carbohydrate
(19 g sugars), 2 g fibre, 161 mg sodium

This gingerbread cake is studded with chunks of ginger and has a rich deep flavour thanks to its anti-oxidant-rich tea and spice blend. Puréed apple is used to replace some of the butter that traditionally makes this cake moist – adding fibre and anti-oxidants instead of fat.

1 Preheat oven to 160°C (320°F/Gas 2–3). Grease a 20 cm (8 inch) square cake tin. Line base and sides with baking (parchment) paper.

2 If using small apples for the purée, put the apple slices and 1 tablespoon water in a medium saucepan over low heat and simmer, stirring occasionally, 10–15 minutes, or until soft and well cooked. Mash well with a fork to make a purée, or purée in a food processor or blender.

3 Meanwhile, put golden syrup or honey, tea or water, brown sugar and spread in a medium saucepan and stir over low heat until melted and smooth. Bring to a boil. Remove from heat and stir in apple purée. Cool 10 minutes.

4 Sift together wholemeal and white flours, bicarbonate of soda, ground ginger, cinnamon and nutmeg. Stir into melted mixture until well combined, then fold in chopped ginger. Spoon mixture into prepared tin and smooth the surface with a spatula. Sprinkle with raw sugar.

5 Bake 50–55 minutes, or until a skewer inserted in the centre comes out clean. Cool 10 minutes before turning out onto a wire rack to cool completely.

COOK'S TIP The uncooked gingerbread mixture is quite thick and sticky. Dip the spatula in hot water to make it easier to smooth the surface.

Replacing water with cold tea in this recipe is an easy way to boost the anti-oxidant content and enrich the cake's flavour. Try using milky cold tea instead of milk in other cake recipes.

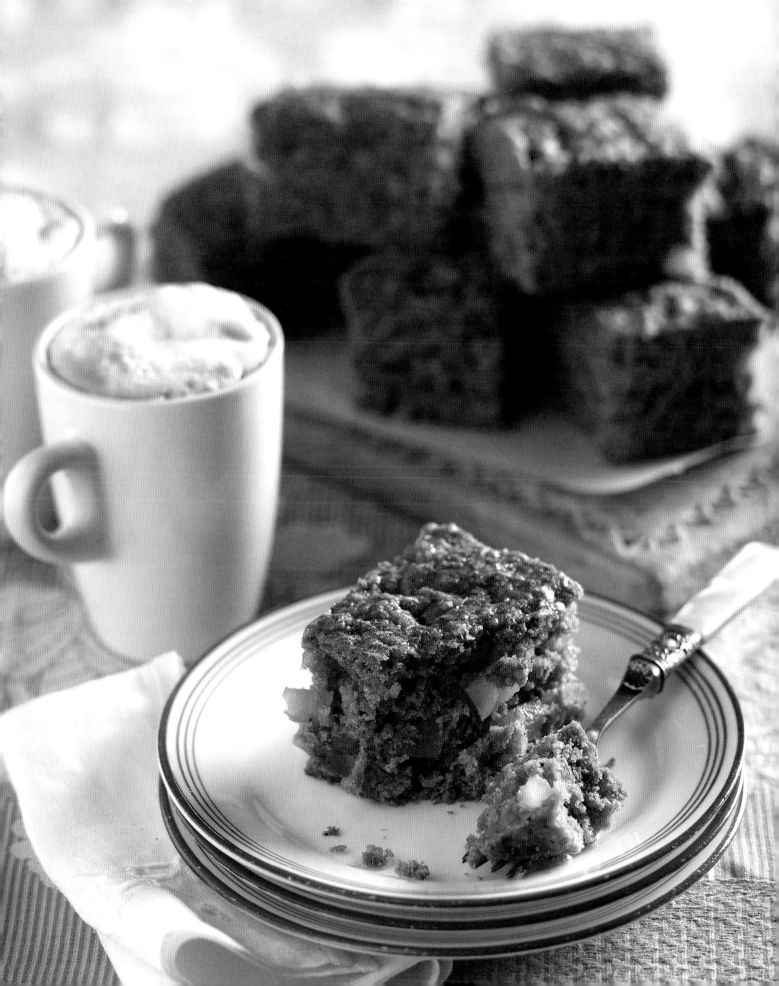

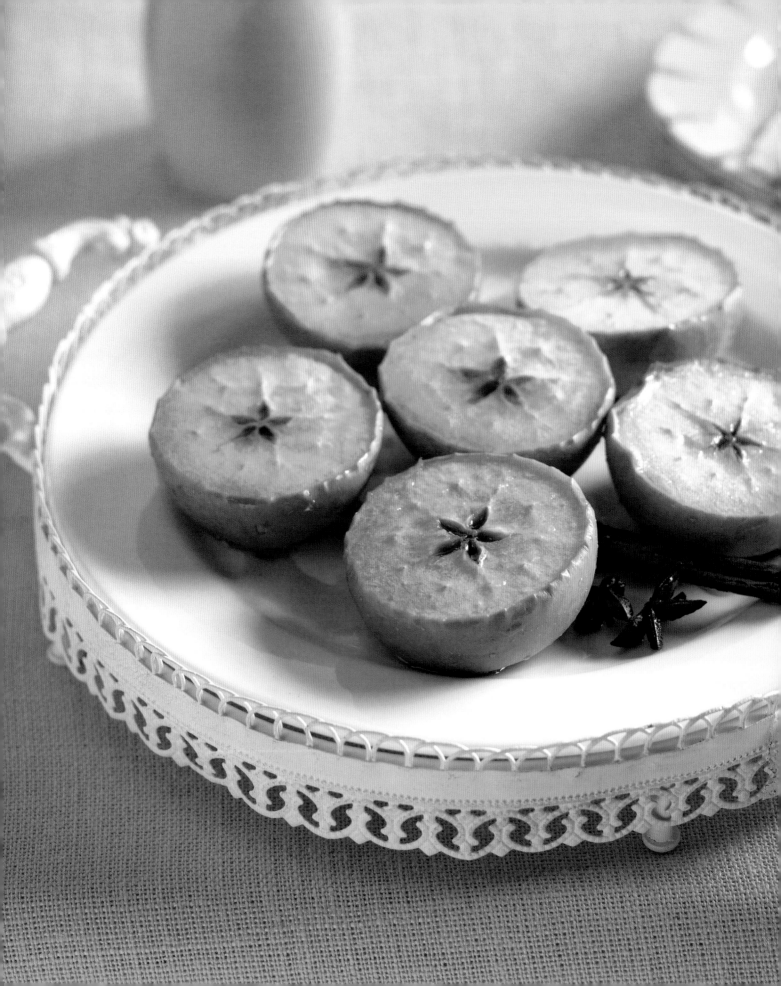

Baked apples

⅓ cup (80 ml) unsweetened apple juice
2 tablespoons maple syrup
1 cinnamon stick
1 star anise
5 cm (2 inch) strip orange zest
4 large tart yellow or green apples, such as
    golden delicious or granny smith (about
    800 g/1¾ lb in total), stalks discarded,
    halved crosswise
½ cup (125 g) low-fat vanilla yogurt, to serve

PREPARATION 15 minutes, plus 5 minutes cooling
COOKING 30 minutes SERVES 4

EACH SERVING PROVIDES 715 kJ, 171 kcal, 3 g protein,
<1 g fat (<1 g saturated fat), 39 g carbohydrate
(36 g sugars), 4 g fibre, 30 mg sodium

> Quercetin is one of the flavonoid group
> of anti-oxidants – polyphenols that
> have both anti-oxidant and anti-inflammatory
> powers. This means quercetin is beneficial in
> protecting against cardiovascular diseases
> and helping reduce the risk of stroke. Apples
> and onions appear to have the highest
> quercetin content of all foods.

1 Preheat oven to 200°C (400°F/Gas 6).

2 Combine apple juice, maple syrup, cinnamon, star anise and orange zest in a small saucepan over medium heat. Stir until mixture comes to a boil. Reduce heat to low and simmer 4–5 minutes, or until slightly thickened. Cool 5 minutes.

3 Arrange apples, cut side up, in a small ovenproof dish. Pour syrup over apples. Bake 20–25 minutes, or until apples are tender.

4 Serve apples in individual dishes, each drizzled with pan juices and a dollop of yogurt.

COOK'S TIP Maple syrup can be replaced with honey or agave syrup.

You can bake the apples in bulk beforehand and keep them in the refrigerator until ready to use.

Burghul pudding

1/3 cup (60 g) fine or medium burghul
  (bulgur), rinsed
1/4 teaspoon ground cardamom
1 1/4 cups (310 ml) low-fat milk
2/3 cup (85 g) sultanas (golden raisins)
1/4 teaspoon ground cinnamon
1 tablespoon honey or agave syrup
1 large egg
4 teaspoons grated lemon zest
1/2 teaspoon vanilla extract
4 tablespoons chopped pistachios or toasted
  slivered almonds, to garnish

PREPARATION 10 minutes, plus 20 minutes soaking
and 2 hours chilling COOKING 10 minutes SERVES 6

EACH SERVING PROVIDES 665 kJ, 159 kcal, 6 g protein,
4 g fat (<1 g saturated fat), 25 g carbohydrate
(18 g sugars), 3 g fibre, 51 mg sodium

Creamy and comforting, this Middle
Eastern-inspired dessert is a wholegrain
alternative to rice pudding. Burghul is a
cracked wheat product that retains the
nutrients of the whole wheat grain without
the long cooking times that are usually
needed with wholegrain foods.

1 Combine burghul, cardamom and 1 cup (250 ml)
water in a saucepan over medium–high heat. Bring to
a simmer. Immediately remove from heat, cover and
let stand until burghul is tender, about 20 minutes.
Drain and press out excess water, then return
burghul to pan.

2 Add milk, sultanas, cinnamon and honey or agave
syrup and bring to a simmer over medium–high heat,
stirring often. Reduce heat to medium–low and cook,
stirring, 2 minutes.

3 Whisk egg in a medium bowl. Gradually stir in
burghul mixture. Return to pan and cook over
medium–low heat, stirring constantly, 1–2 minutes,
until slightly thickened. (Do not allow the mixture
to boil. You can use an instant-read thermometer
to gauge readiness; the pudding should reach a
temperature of 70°C/158°F.)

4 Transfer mixture to a clean bowl and stir in
2 teaspoons lemon zest and vanilla extract. Allow
to cool slightly, then cover and refrigerate until
chilled, about 2 hours.

5 Divide burghul pudding among four dessert bowls
and sprinkle each with 1 tablespoon pistachios or
almonds. Top with remaining lemon zest.

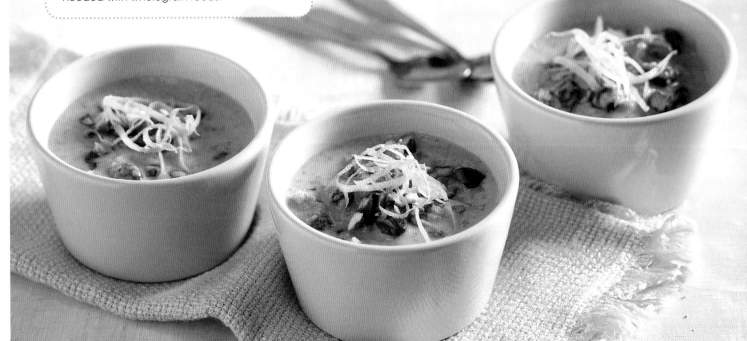

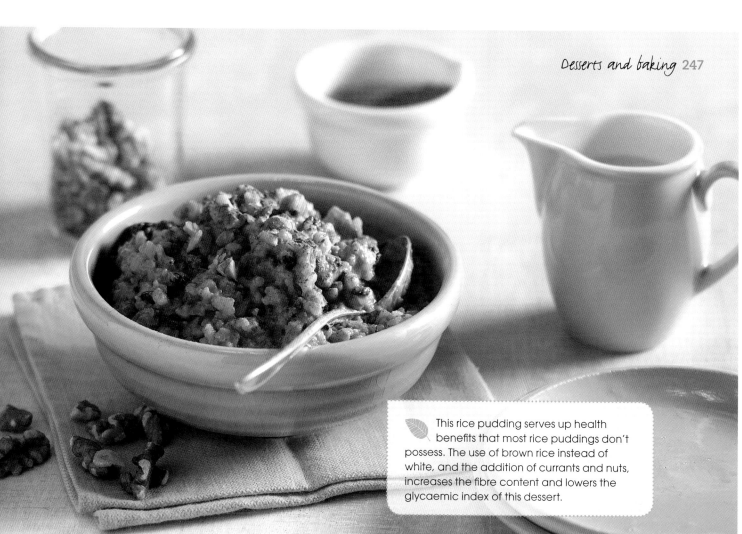

This rice pudding serves up health benefits that most rice puddings don't possess. The use of brown rice instead of white, and the addition of currants and nuts, increases the fibre content and lowers the glycaemic index of this dessert.

Brown rice pudding

3 cups (750 ml) vanilla-flavoured sweetened
    soy milk
²/₃ cup (140 g) medium-grain brown rice
½ teaspoon ground cinnamon
2 eggs, at room temperature
½ cup (75 g) currants
½ cup (60 g) chopped nuts, such as
    Brazil nuts, almonds or walnuts

PREPARATION 5 minutes, plus cooling
COOKING 1 hour 35 minutes **SERVES** 4

EACH SERVING PROVIDES 1607 kJ, 384 kcal, 15 g protein, 14 g fat (2 g saturated fat), 41 g carbohydrate (12 g sugars), 3 g fibre, 120 mg sodium

1 Put milk, rice and cinnamon in a medium saucepan over medium heat and stir to combine. Bring to a simmer, then reduce heat to low, cover and simmer 1½ hours. Remove from heat and allow to cool 5 minutes.

2 Put eggs in a bowl and beat lightly. Stir in ½ cup cooked rice mixture, stirring constantly. Gradually stir this back into rice mixture in the pan. Cook over low heat, stirring constantly, until thickened, about 5 minutes. Stir in currants and nuts.

3 Serve rice pudding warm, or refrigerate and serve cold. Sprinkle with extra nuts and cinnamon, if desired.

COOK'S TIP Soy milk can easily be substituted for cow's milk in most baked goods.

Index

Note to Readers

WEIGHTS AND MEASURES

The following metric cup and spoon measurements have been used throughout this book: 1 cup = 250 ml; 1 tablespoon = 20 ml and 1 teaspoon = 5 ml. If using the smaller imperial cup and spoon measures (where 1 cup = 235 ml and 1 tablespoon = 15 ml), some adjustments may need to be made. A small variation in the weight or volume of most ingredients is unlikely to adversely affect a recipe. The exceptions are yeast, baking powder and bicarbonate of soda (baking soda). For these ingredients adjust the recipe accordingly. All cup and spoon measures are level, unless stated otherwise.

Ingredients are generally listed by their weight or volume with cup measurements given for convenience, unless the conversion is imperfect, whereby the ingredients are listed by weight or volume only.

Sometimes conversions within a recipe are not exact but are the closest conversion that is a suitable measurement for each system. Use either the metric or the imperial measurements; do not mix the two systems.

CAN SIZES

Can sizes vary between countries and manufacturers; if the stated size is unavailable, use the nearest equivalent. Here are the metric and imperial measurements for can sizes used in this book: 225 g = 8 oz; 300 g = 10 oz; 350 g = 12 oz; 400/410 g = 14 oz = 398 ml/410 ml; 425 g = 15 oz = 540 ml; 800 g = 28 oz = 796 ml.

Alternative terms and substitutes

burghul – bulgur

butterbeans – lima beans

capsicum – bell pepper, sweet pepper

Chinese five spice – five-spice powder

coriander – cilantro

corn cob – sweetcorn

cos lettuce – romaine lettuce

eggplant – aubergine

English spinach – baby spinach; not the heavily veined, thick-leafed vegetable sold as spinach or silver beet

filo – phyllo

fish substitutes – for blue-eye, bream, ling, snapper, flathead, use any firm, white-fleshed fish such as cod or hake

fresh shiitake mushrooms – rehydrated dried shiitake mushrooms

light evaporated milk – evaporated skim milk, low-fat evaporated milk

low-fat milk – 1% milk

oregano – oreganum

passionfruit – granadilla

pepitas – pumpkin seeds

rice noodles – rice vermicelli

rockmelon – cantaloupe

salt-reduced – low-sodium

self-raising flour – self-rising flour

sunflower seeds – sunflower kernels

vanilla extract – vanilla essence

Vietnamese mint – mint or combination of cilantro and mint

wholemeal – whole-wheat

witlof – chicory, Belgian endive

zucchini – baby marrow, courgette

NUTRITIONAL ANALYSIS

Each recipe is accompanied by a nutrient profile showing kilojoules (kJ), calories (kcal), protein, fat (including saturated fat), carbohydrate (including sugars), fibre and sodium. <1 means less than 1 g. Serving suggestions, garnishes and optional ingredients are not included in the nutritional analysis. For the recipe analysis we used FoodWorks ®. In line with current nutritional recommendations, use salt-reduced stock and soy sauce wherever possible.

OVEN TEMPERATURES

These recipes have been written for a regular oven. If you have a fan-forced (convection) oven, reduce the temperature by 20°C.

If you have a broiler (grill) where the temperature cannot be adjusted by a temperature dial or knob, lower the rack down from the element as follows:
Medium – about half or two-thirds of the way down.
Medium–hot – about a third of the way down.

Anti-Ageing *diet* COOKBOOK

CONSULTANT Suzie Ferrie, Advanced Accredited
Practising Dietitian

RECIPES Jo Anne Calabria, Dixie Elliott, Cathie Lonnie,
Jan Purser, Tracy Rutherford

EDITOR Bronwyn Sweeney

DESIGNER Clare O'Loughlin

FOR VIVAT DIRECT

EDITORIAL DIRECTOR Julian Browne

MANAGING EDITOR Nina Hathway

PICTURE RESOURCE MANAGER Eleanor Ashfield

PRE-PRESS TECHNICAL MANAGER Dean Russell

PRODUCT PRODUCTION MANAGER Claudette Bramble

PRODUCTION CONTROLLER Jan Bucil

Colour origination FMG

Printed in China

*The information in this book should not be substituted for,
or used to alter, medical therapy without your doctor's advice.
For a specific health problem or dietary concern, consult your
doctor for guidance.*

ANTI-AGEING DIET COOKBOOK
Published in 2013 in the United Kingdom by Vivat Direct Limited
(t/a Reader's Digest), 157 Edgware Road, London W2 2HR
First published in 2012 by Reader's Digest (Australia) Pty Limited

This edition first published in 2013

We are committed both to the quality of our products and the
service we provide to our customers. We value your comments,
so please do contact us on 0871 351 1000 or via our website at
www.readersdigest.co.uk

If you have any comments or suggestions about the content of
our books, email us at gbeditorial@readersdigest.co.uk

Book code 400-628 UP0000-1
ISBN 978-1-78020-171-9